# Biomedical and Pharmacological Applications of Marine Collagen

# Biomedical and Pharmacological Applications of Marine Collagen

Editor

**Sik Yoon**

MDPI • Basel • Beijing • Wuhan • Barcelona • Belgrade • Manchester • Tokyo • Cluj • Tianjin

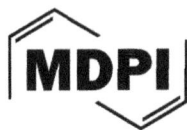

*Editor*
Sik Yoon
Department of Anatomy,
College of Medicine,
Pusan National University,
Yangsan, Republic of Korea

*Editorial Office*
MDPI
St. Alban-Anlage 66
4052 Basel, Switzerland

This is a reprint of articles from the Special Issue published online in the open access journal *Marine Drugs* (ISSN 1660-3397) (available at: https://www.mdpi.com/journal/marinedrugs/special_issues/Marine_Collagen_II).

For citation purposes, cite each article independently as indicated on the article page online and as indicated below:

LastName, A.A.; LastName, B.B.; LastName, C.C. Article Title. *Journal Name* **Year**, *Volume Number*, Page Range.

**ISBN 978-3-0365-6352-7 (Hbk)**
**ISBN 978-3-0365-6353-4 (PDF)**

© 2023 by the authors. Articles in this book are Open Access and distributed under the Creative Commons Attribution (CC BY) license, which allows users to download, copy and build upon published articles, as long as the author and publisher are properly credited, which ensures maximum dissemination and a wider impact of our publications.
The book as a whole is distributed by MDPI under the terms and conditions of the Creative Commons license CC BY-NC-ND.

# Contents

About the Editor . . . . . . . . . . . . . . . . . . . . . . . . . . . . . . . . . . . . . . . . . . . . . . . . . . vii

Preface to "Biomedical and Pharmacological Applications of Marine Collagen" . . . . . . . . . ix

**Junde Chen, Guangyu Wang and Yushuang Li**
Preparation and Characterization of Thermally Stable Collagens from the Scales of Lizardfish (*Synodus macrops*)
Reprinted from: *Mar. Drugs* **2021**, *19*, 597, doi:10.3390/md19110597 . . . . . . . . . . . . . . . . . 1

**Baolin Ge, Chunyu Hou, Bin Bao, Zhilin Pan, José Eduardo Maté Sánchez de Val, Jeevithan Elango and Wenhui Wu**
Comparison of Physicochemical and Structural Properties of Acid-Soluble and Pepsin-Soluble Collagens from Blacktip Reef Shark Skin
Reprinted from: *Mar. Drugs* **2022**, *20*, 376, doi:10.3390/md20060376 . . . . . . . . . . . . . . . . . 19

**Sijia Wu, Longhe Yang and Junde Chen**
Preparation and Characterization of Tilapia Collagen-Thermoplastic Polyurethane Composite Nanofiber Membranes
Reprinted from: *Mar. Drugs* **2022**, *20*, 437, doi:10.3390/md20070437 . . . . . . . . . . . . . . . . . 33

**Jian Li, Jun-Hui Cheng, Zhao-Jie Teng, Xia Zhang, Xiu-Lan Chen, Mei-Ling Sun, et al.**
A Novel Gelatinase from Marine *Flocculibacter collagenilyticus* SM1988: Characterization and Potential Application in Collagen Oligopeptide-Rich Hydrolysate Preparation
Reprinted from: *Mar. Drugs* **2022**, *20*, 48, doi:10.3390/md20010048 . . . . . . . . . . . . . . . . . . 53

**Sara Freitas-Ribeiro, Gabriela S. Diogo, Catarina Oliveira, Albino Martins, Tiago H. Silva, Mariana Jarnalo, et al.**
Growth Factor-Free Vascularization of Marine-Origin Collagen Sponges Using Cryopreserved Stromal Vascular Fractions from Human Adipose Tissue
Reprinted from: *Mar. Drugs* **2022**, *20*, 623, doi:10.3390/md20100623 . . . . . . . . . . . . . . . . . 71

**Anastasia Frolova, Nadezhda Aksenova, Ivan Novikov, Aitsana Maslakova, Elvira Gafarova, Yuri Efremov, et al.**
A Collagen Basketweave from the Giant Squid Mantle as a Robust Scaffold for Tissue Engineering
Reprinted from: *Mar. Drugs* **2021**, *19*, 679, doi:10.3390/md19120679 . . . . . . . . . . . . . . . . . 87

**Se-Chang Kim, Seong-Yeong Heo, Gun-Woo Oh, Myunggi Yi and Won-Kyo Jung**
A 3D-Printed Polycaprolactone/Marine Collagen Scaffold Reinforced with Carbonated Hydroxyapatite from Fish Bones for Bone Regeneration
Reprinted from: *Mar. Drugs* **2022**, *20*, 344, doi:10.3390/md20060344 . . . . . . . . . . . . . . . . . 113

**Marina Pozzolini, Eleonora Tassara, Andrea Dodero, Maila Castellano, Silvia Vicini, Sara Ferrando, et al.**
Potential Biomedical Applications of Collagen Filaments derived from the Marine Demosponges *Ircinia oros* (Schmidt, 1864) and *Sarcotragus foetidus* (Schmidt, 1862)
Reprinted from: *Mar. Drugs* **2021**, *19*, 563, doi:10.3390/md19100563 . . . . . . . . . . . . . . . . . 131

**Won Hoon Song, Hye-Yoon Kim, Ye Seon Lim, Seon Yeong Hwang, Changyong Lee, Do Young Lee, et al.**
Fish Collagen Peptides Protect against Cisplatin-Induced Cytotoxicity and Oxidative Injury by Inhibiting MAPK Signaling Pathways in Mouse Thymic Epithelial Cells
Reprinted from: *Mar. Drugs* **2022**, *20*, 232, doi:10.3390/md20040232 . . . . . . . . . . . . . . . . . 157

# About the Editor

**Sik Yoon**

Sik Yoon, M.D., Ph.D., is a professor at the Department of Anatomy and Cell Biology, Pusan National University School of Medicine, Yangsan, Korea. He has served as president of the Korean Association of Anatomists and is currently serving as the Director of the Immune Reconstitution Center of the Pusan National University Medical Research Institute. He received his M.S. and Ph.D. degrees from the Pusan National University, Korea, and studied immune cell biology at Washington University School of Medicine, USA, as a visiting scientist. He joined the Pusan National University School of Medicine in 2000. He pursues a broad range of research interests that include the nano-engineering of cells for biomedical applications, biomaterials, marine biology, the development and application of 3D cell culture technology for drug discovery and diagnostic tools, the development of therapeutic strategies to combat antitumor drug resistance and to modulate immune function, and synthetic biology for T cell regeneration.

# Preface to "Biomedical and Pharmacological Applications of Marine Collagen"

Biomimetic polymers and materials have been widely used in a variety of biomedical and pharmacological applications. Collagen-based biomaterials in particular have been extensively applied in various biomedical fields, for example, as scaffolds in tissue engineering. However, there are many challenges associated with the use of mammalian collagen, including the issues of religious constraints, allergic or autoimmune reactions, and the spread of animal diseases such as bovine spongiform encephalopathy, transmissible spongiform encephalopathy, and foot-and-mouth disease.

Over the past few decades, marine collagen has emerged as a promising biomaterial for biomedical and pharmacological applications. Marine organisms are a rich source of structurally novel and biologically active compounds, and to date, many biological components have been isolated from various marine resources. Marine collagen offers advantages over mammalian collagen due to its water solubility, easy extractability, low immunogenicity, safety, biocompatibility, biodegradability, antimicrobial activity, functionality, and low production costs. Due to its characteristics and physicobiochemical properties, it has tremendous potential for use as a scaffold biomaterial in tissue engineering and regenerative medicine, in drug delivery systems, and as a therapeutic agent.

In this book, some recent innovativeapplications of these proteins have been discussed that could potentially be applied in scientific and industrial research. This book covers recent trends in all aspects of basic and applied scientific research on marine collagen, with a particular focus on their biotechnological, biomedical and pharmacological uses.

**Sik Yoon**
*Editor*

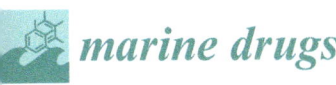 

Article

# Preparation and Characterization of Thermally Stable Collagens from the Scales of Lizardfish (*Synodus macrops*)

Junde Chen *, Guangyu Wang and Yushuang Li

Technical Innovation Center for Utilization of Marine Biological Resources, Third Institute of Oceanography, Ministry of Natural Resources, Xiamen 361005, China; 17859733637@163.com (G.W.); liyushuang@tio.org.cn (Y.L.)
* Correspondence: jdchen@tio.org.cn; Tel./Fax: +86-0592-215527

**Abstract:** Marine collagen is gaining vast interest because of its high biocompatibility and lack of religious and social restrictions compared with collagen from terrestrial sources. In this study, lizardfish (*Synodus macrops*) scales were used to isolate acid-soluble collagen (ASC) and pepsin-soluble collagen (PSC). Both ASC and PSC were identified as type I collagen with intact triple-helix structures by sodium dodecyl sulfate-polyacrylamide gel electrophoresis and spectroscopy. The ASC and PSC had high amino acids of 237 residues/1000 residues and 236 residues/1000 residues, respectively. Thus, the maximum transition temperature ($T_{max}$) of ASC (43.2 °C) was higher than that of PSC (42.5 °C). Interestingly, the $T_{max}$ of both ASC and PSC was higher than that of rat tail collagen (39.4 °C) and calf skin collagen (35.0 °C), the terrestrial collagen. Solubility tests showed that both ASC and PSC exhibited high solubility in the acidic pH ranges. ASC was less susceptible to the "salting out" effect compared with PSC. Both collagen types were nontoxic to HaCaT and MC3T3-E1 cells, and ASC was associated with a higher cell viability than PSC. These results indicated that ASC from lizardfish scales could be an alternative to terrestrial sources of collagen, with potential for biomedical applications.

**Keywords:** lizardfish scale; marine collagen; thermal stability; cell viability

## 1. Introduction

Collagen is an important structural protein of connective tissue, and it is also a principal component of the natural extracellular matrix (ECM) that plays a dominant role in providing overall tissue stiffness and integrity [1]. The main feature of collagen is its triple helical structure. In collagen type I, this structure consists of two identical polypeptide chains, α1, and one polypeptide chain, α2, with each chain containing one or more repeating amino-acid motifs (Gly–X–Y), where X is proline or hydroxyproline and Y represents any amino acid [2,3]. So far, 29 types of collagen (I–XXIX) have been identified and characterized. Among them, fibril-forming type I collagen with a high structural order and high stiffness is the most widely distributed type of collagen in connective tissue, accounting for 80–85% of collagen in the body [4,5]. Due to its excellent biocompatibility, low antigenicity, and high biodegradability, type I collagen is regarded as one of the promising biomaterials and is widely used in tissue engineering and the pharmaceutical and biomedical industry [6,7].

Collagen's preferred sources are the skin and tendons of bovine and porcine. However, as collagen of mammals has the risk of triggering an immune reaction and transferring zoonosis and transmissible spongiform encephalopathies, marine collagen has attracted interest in recent years [2,8]. Marine collagen has lower gelling and melting temperatures than mammalian collagen, but marine collagen is cheaper to extract and easier to prepare than mammalian collagen [8,9]. Marine collagen, such as that from sponges, jellyfish, squids, octopuses, cuttlefish, and fish skin, bone, and scales, comes from both marine vertebrates and invertebrates [9,10]. There is great demand for marine collagen, and this is now the main source of collagen globally. Sourour Addad et al. (2011) obtained

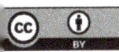

collagen from Jellyfish [11], Tziveleka et al. (2017) isolated the collagen from marine sponges *Axinella cannabina* and *Suberites carnosus* [12] and skin and Cruz-López et al. (2018) extracted collagen from gulf corvina skin and swim bladder [10]. As reported in the literature, the marine collagen market is expected to reach USD 983.84 million by 2025, with a compound annual growth rate of 7.4% [13]. Marine collagen, compared with collagen from terrestrial sources, is more easily extracted [2], has high biocompatibility [5], is without the risks of animal diseases and pathogens; has a higher absorption capacity (up to 1.5 times more efficient entry into the body), and is not associated with religious and ethical restrictions [14,15]. This provides an opportunity for fish scales. Namely, fish scales are the waste product from the fish processing industry, and they represent on average 2% of fish body weight [16]. The poor biodegradability of scales makes them difficult to be managed as waste [16]. However, scales are a safe and good source of marine type I collagen [17]. Therefore, the extraction of type I collagen from scales may be beneficial in terms of both economic and environmental benefits, and it could possibly drive the development of new industries. Type I collagen from scales has gained increasing interest, and scales are widely regarded as a promising source of collagen [17]. Many successful extractions of collagen from scales have been reported, including tilapia scales collagen [18], gourami scales collagen [19], and miiuy croakers scales collagen [20]. Lizardfish (*Synodus macrops*) is a common economic fish species in China, and there have been no studies about lizardfish scales collagen.

Therefore, in this study, we isolated collagen from lizardfish scales by using acid and enzymatic extraction methods; characterized the physicochemical properties, structural properties, and thermal stability of acid-soluble collagen (ASC) and pepsin-soluble collagen (PSC), and investigated the rheological properties, and cell viability, all of which might provide useful information for the development and application of marine collagen.

## 2. Results

### 2.1. Collagen Yield

The collagen from lizardfish scales was prepared using acid extraction and enzymatic extraction separately. The yield of ASC and PSC was $4.2 \pm 0.2\%$ (based on a dry weight basis) and $4.7 \pm 0.1\%$ (dry weight), respectively.

### 2.2. Sodium Dodecyl Sulfate-Polyacrylamide Gel Electrophoresis (SDS-PAGE)

The electrophoretic patterns of ASC and PSC from lizardfish scales are illustrated in Figure 1. It is clear that ASC and PSC show similar electrophoretic patterns as both consist mainly of two different types of α-chains (α1 and α2) and dimeric β-chains. The molecular weight of collagen was analyzed using Quantity One 4.6.0 software (Bio-Rad Laboratories, Hercules, CA, USA); we found that the molecular weight of ASC (α1-MW, 137 kDa; α2-MW, 127 kDa) was slightly higher than that of PSC (α1-MW, 135 kDa; α2-MW, 123 kDa), which can be attributed to the removal of telopeptide regions of the PSC [21]. The protein patterns of ASC and PSC were similar to those of the collagen obtained from tilapia skin [18] and Pacific cod skin [22]. Although pepsin removed the cross-link-containing telopeptide, the electrophoresis patterns showed that PSC contained a higher intensity of β-chains than ASC, indicating that PSC has high molecular cross-linkages [23,24]. Moreover, the ratio of α1 and α2 was calculated by Image J software (VERSION 1.8.0, National Institute of Mental Health, Bethesda, MD, USA); specifically, the ratios of α1 and α2 for ASC and PSC were 1.86 and 2.23, respectively, both close to 2:1, implying that ASC and PSC extracted from lizardfish scales are type I collagen ($[\alpha 1]_2 \alpha 2$) [25].

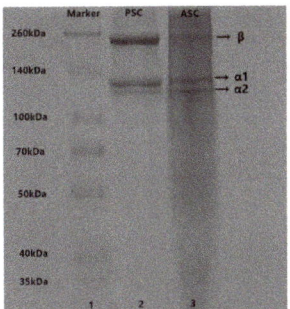

**Figure 1.** SDS-PAGE patterns of ASC and PSC from lizardfish scales. Lane 1: Marker standard; Lane 2: PSC; Lane 3: ASC. The experiment was conducted only once (n = 1).

### 2.3. Spectroscopy Characterization

#### 2.3.1. UV Absorption Spectrum

Generally, collagen has a maximum absorption peak in 210–240 nm range, which is attributed to the presence of C=O, –COOH, and $CONH_2$ groups in the polypeptide chains of collagen [23]. The UV absorption spectra of lizardfish scales collagen are shown in Figure 2a, namely, ASC and PSC showed sharp and intense maximum absorption peaks at 235 nm and 236 nm, respectively, which is consistent with the UV absorption characteristics of type I collagen [25]. The aromatic residues, including tyrosine and phenylalanine, have a maximum absorption peak at 280 nm. As shown in Figure 2a, ASC and PSC did not demonstrate a significant absorption peak at 280 nm.

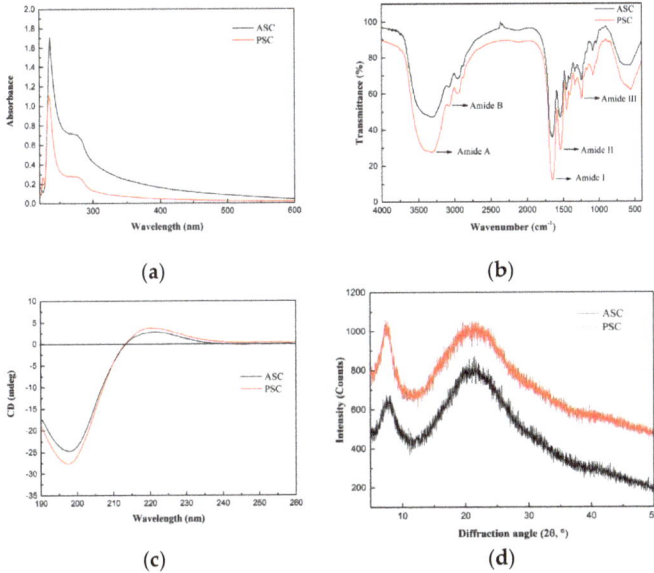

**Figure 2.** Spectroscopy properties of ASC and PSC. (**a**) UV absorption spectra, (**b**) Fourier transform infrared spectroscopy, (**c**) circular dichroism, and (**d**) X-ray diffraction. The experiment was conducted only once (n = 1).

#### 2.3.2. Fourier-Transform Infrared (FTIR) Spectrum

FTIR spectra of collagen from lizardfish scales are displayed in Figure 2b. ASC and PSC from lizardfish scales contained five major characteristic absorption bands, including

Amide A, Amide B, Amide I, Amide II, and Amide III. The Amide A band (3400–3440 cm$^{-1}$) is mainly associated with the stretching vibration of N–H [18]. However, the hydrogen bond formation leads to a change in wavenumber to a lower frequency [18]. The Amide A absorption bands of ASC and PSC were found at 3307 cm$^{-1}$ and 3324 cm$^{-1}$, respectively, indicating that N–H groups were involved in the formation of hydrogen bonds, which resulted in a shift of the Amide A band to the lower frequency. The Amide B band (3080 cm$^{-1}$) is linked to the asymmetrical stretch of –CH$_2$. We showed that the Amide B bands of ASC and PSC were located at 3080 cm$^{-1}$. In the present study, the positions of Amide I bands of ASC and PSC were found at wavenumbers of 1653 cm$^{-1}$ and 1654 cm$^{-1}$, respectively; Amide II bands of both ASC and PSC were located at 1542 cm$^{-1}$; and Amide III bands of ASC and PSC were observed at 1240 cm$^{-1}$ and 1241 cm$^{-1}$, respectively. Moreover, the ratios of absorption intensities between the Amide III band and 1450 cm$^{-1}$ band were approximately 1.0, confirming that the triple helical structures of ASC and PSC were well maintained [6].

### 2.3.3. Circular Dichroism (CD) Spectrum

CD is a simple and effective technique to identify whether the triple helical structure is intact [22]. The CD spectrum of native collagen with a triple-helix structure shows a positive peak at 221 nm (maximum positive cotton effect), a negative peak at 198 nm (maximum negative cotton effect), and a crossover point (zero rotation) at approximately 213 nm [10,22]. As shown in Figure 2c, the CD spectrum of lizardfish scales ASC and PSC exhibited weak positive absorption peaks at 221 nm and 220 nm, respectively, and negative absorption peaks were observed at 198 nm and 197 nm, respectively, both with a crossover point at 213 nm. Moreover, the Rpn values (the ratio of the positive to negative) of ASC and PSC were 0.12 and 0.14, respectively, indicating that the collagen extracted from lizardfish scales possess a triple-helix conformation [26,27].

### 2.3.4. X-ray Diffraction (XRD) Spectrum

The XRD patterns of ASC and PSC are shown in Figure 2d. We found that ASC and PSC consisted of two peaks, a sharp and a broad peak. The diffraction angles (2θ) of ASC were 7.86° and 21.25°, and those of PSC were 7.58° and 21.02°, which are consistent with the characteristic diffraction peaks of collagen [28]. The d value of the first sharp peak of ASC was 11.25 Å, and that of PSC was 11.66 Å, and this reflects the distance between the molecular chains [28]. The distance between the molecular chains of PSC was greater than that within ASC, indicating weaker molecular interactions in PSC. This may be related to the cleavage of the terminal peptide sequence of collagen [29]. The d value of the second relatively broad peak of ASC was 4.18 Å, and that of PSC was 4.23 Å, and this reflects the distance between their skeletons [22].

## 2.4. Amino Acid Composition

The amino acid compositions of the lizardfish scales ASC and PSC are shown in Table 1. It can be seen that glycine was the abundant amino acid in collagen, with ASC and PSC containing 35.1% and 34.9% of glycine, respectively. Similar results were found in the giant groaker skin collagen [30] and the Pacific cod skin collagen [22]. The results are consistent with glycine, which is identical in that in the collagen polypeptide chain, the repeating (Gly-X-Y)n assembles into a triple helix structure [30]. Alanine and proline accounted for 161 residues/1000 residues and 159 residues/1000 residues, and 158 residues/1000 residues and 157 residues/1000 residues in ASC and PSC, respectively. In addition, both the ASC and PSC were devoid of cysteine and tryptophan. Further, the amino acid (proline and hydroxyproline) contents of the ASC and PSC were 237 residues/1000 residues and 236 residues/1000 residues, respectively.

**Table 1.** Amino acid composition of the ASC and PSC from lizardfish scales. The results are expressed as residues/1000 total amino acid residues. Values represent the means ± standard deviations (SD) of duplicate assays (n = 3).

| Amino Acid | ASC | PSC |
|---|---|---|
| Aspartic acid | 15 ± 1 | 16 ± 2 |
| Glutamine acid | 13 ± 1 | 11 ± 1 |
| Serine | 50 ± 2 | 51 ± 2 |
| Histidine | 7 ± 1 | 7 ± 2 |
| Glycine | 351 ± 19 | 349 ± 21 |
| Threonine | 29 ± 2 | 30 ± 3 |
| Arginine | 15 ± 1 | 14 ± 1 |
| Alanine | 161 ± 11 | 159 ± 14 |
| Tyrosine | 5 ± 1 | 5 ± 1 |
| Valine | 25 ± 2 | 26 ± 1 |
| Methionine | 8 ± 1 | 7 ± 1 |
| Phenylalanine | 11 ± 2 | 12 ± 1 |
| Isoleucine | 8 ± 2 | 10 ± 2 |
| Leucine | 26 ± 3 | 25 ± 1 |
| Lysine | 35 ± 4 | 37 ± 2 |
| Proline | 158 ± 9 | 157 ± 7 |
| Hydroxylysine | 4 ± 1 | 5 ± 1 |
| Hydroxyproline | 79 ± 9 | 79 ± 7 |
| Total | 1000 | 1000 |
| Proline + Hydroxyproline | 237 ± 16 | 236 ± 14 |

### 2.5. Morphology Characterization

The morphology of collagen is vital for assessing its potential application in biomedicine [31]. The collagen solution obtained from lizardfish scales was lyophilized, and the morphology of collagen sponges was observed by scanning electron microscopy (SEM) (Figure 3). As shown in Figure 3a,a′, ASC and PSC were observed as white sponges with loose, uniform, and porous structures observed by the naked eye. ASC and PSC surfaces under SEM were partially wrinkled, which may be attributed to water being sublimated during the freeze-drying process [32]. The SEM images showed that ASC and PSC had a similar multilayer overlapping and porous microstructure. However, there were some differences in the structure between ASC and PSC under SEM observation. As observed at a magnification of 400×, ASC exhibited a compact sheet and porous structure (Figure 3b), while PSC had a loose and large sheet structure (Figure 3b′); ASC exhibited a more porous structure than PSC. It was clearly visible at higher magnifications (800×) that ASC had considerable fibrillary structure and a small number of sheet structures (Figure 3c), while PSC had large sheet-like film structures (Figure 3c′).

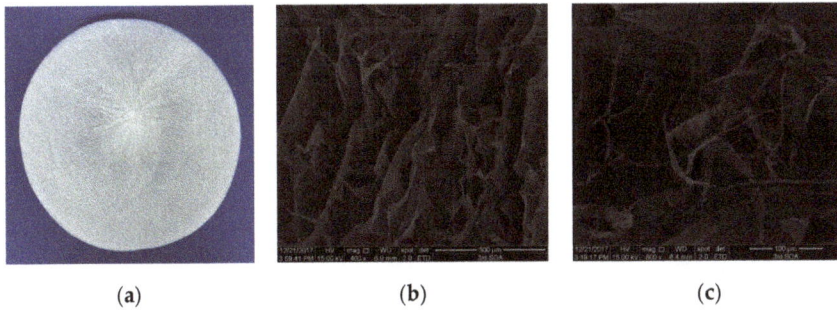

(a)        (b)        (c)

**Figure 3.** *Cont.*

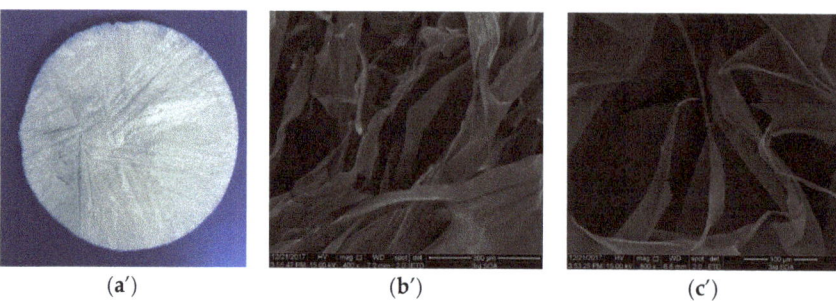

**Figure 3.** SEM images of ASC and PSC. (**a**) ASC, (**b**) ASC at 400× magnification, (**c**) ASC at 800× magnification, (**a′**) PSC, (**b′**) PSC at 400× magnification, and (**c′**) PSC at 800× magnification. The experiment was done only once (n = 1).

### 2.6. Thermal Stability

Differential scanning calorimetry (DSC) was used to measure the maximum transition temperature ($T_{max}$) of collagen. The DSC curves of collagen from the lizardfish scales are shown in Figure 4. It was observed that the $T_{max}$ of collagen from lizardfish scales was higher than that of rat tail collagen. The $T_{max}$ values of rat tail collagen, ASC, and PSC were 39.4 °C, 43.2 °C, and 42.5 °C, respectively. The $T_{max}$ of ASC was higher than PSC and the rat tail collagen, and the ΔH of ASC (0.981 J/g) was also higher than the PSC (0.711 J/g) and the rat tail collagen (0.680 J/g).

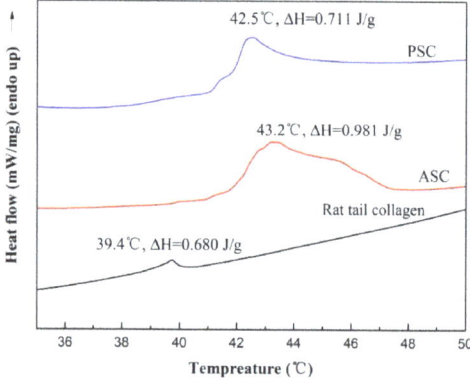

**Figure 4.** The DSC curve of ASC and PSC. The experiment was performed only once (n = 1).

### 2.7. Solubility

#### 2.7.1. The Influence of pH on the Solubility of Collagen Solutions

The relative solubility of ASC and PSC extracted from the scale of lizardfish at different pH showed similar trends, as shown in Figure 5a. ASC and PSC exhibited higher relative solubility in the very acidic pH range (1–4), and both ASC and PSC showed the maximum relative solubility at pH 2. The relative solubility of ASC and PSC decreased with increasing pH, and a sharp decrease in relative solubility of ASC and PSC occurred at pH above 5 and 4, and the minimum relative solubility was 11.09% and 7.70%, respectively. The isoelectric points (pI) of ASC and PSC were approximately around 7 and 8, respectively [33].

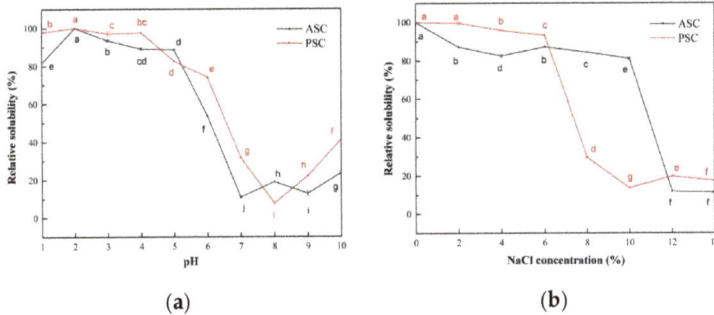

**Figure 5.** Relative solubility of ASC and PSC. (a) Effect of pH; (b) effect of NaCl concentration. Values represent the means ± standard deviations (SD) of duplicate assays (n = 3). Different letters indicated significant differences between the samples.

2.7.2. The Influence of NaCl Concentration on the Solubility of Collagen Solutions

The effect of NaCl concentration on the relative solubility of ASC and PSC from lizardfish scales is shown in Figure 5b. ASC and PSC showed high relative solubility at low NaCl concentrations, both above 80%. The relative solubility of ASC and PSC from lizardfish scales decreased with increasing NaCl concentrations, with the lowest values at 14% and 10% and 11.42% and 13.64% NaCl concentrations, respectively. Subsequently, as the NaCl concentration increased, the relative solubility of collagen remained relatively stable but very low (around 20%).

2.8. Rheological Properties

The frequency dependence of the rheological parameters elastic modulus (G′) and viscous modulus (G″) from lizardfish scales ASC and PSC was assessed using dynamic frequency scan tests. The G′ was defined as the elasticity of protein, and G″ was defined as the viscous behavior of the protein [34]. Figure 6 exhibits the dynamic frequency sweep tests of ASC and PSC, and the G′ and G″ values of ASC and PSC showed an increasing trend as the frequency increased from 0.01 to 10 Hz. The G′ and G″ values of PSC are higher than the corresponding G′ and G″ values of ASC between 0.01 and 10 Hz. As shown in Figure 6a, the increase in the G′ value of PSC was higher than that of ASC in the test frequency range 0.01–10 Hz.

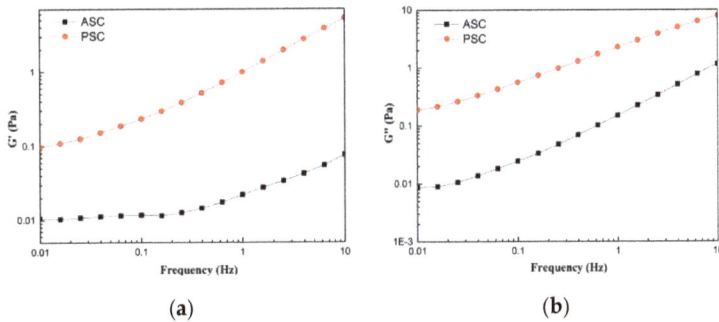

**Figure 6.** Rheological behavior of collagens solution (a) storage modulus (G′); (b) loss modulus (G″). The experiment was performed only once (n = 1).

2.9. Cell Compatibility

The cytotoxicity of the HaCaT (Cat No. CBP60331) and MC3T3-E1 (Cat No. CBP60946) cells lines on lizardfish scales collagen after 24 h and 48 h was investigated using a CCK-8 assay. The results of relative cell viability are shown in Figure 7. After 24 h of cell culture, the relative viability of the HaCaT cells on ASC and PSC were 107.18 ± 1.78% and 101.44 ± 3.62%, respectively, and for the MC3T3-E1 cells, 113.43 ± 2.40% and 105.95 ± 1.90%, respectively. Moreover, the relative viability of HaCaT cells on ASC and PSC were 111.78 ± 1.74% and 106.45 ± 1.89%, respectively, and for the MC3T3-E1 cells, 117.80 ± 1.65% and 110.64 ± 2.70%, respectively, after 48 h. The relative viability of the HaCaT and MC3T3-E1 cells on ASC and PSC increased during 48 h of cell culture. Moreover, the morphology of cells was observed under an inverted microscope, and there were no observable changes in the HaCaT and MC3T3-E1 cells compared to the control group (Figure 8).

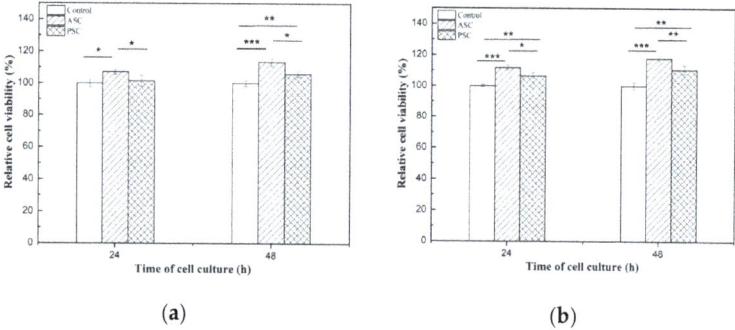

(a)          (b)

**Figure 7.** Relative cell viability of HaCaT and MC3T3-E1 cells after 24 h and 48 h of incubation in ASC and PSC. (**a**) is HaCaT cells; (**b**) is MC3T3-E1 cells. Values represent the means ± standard deviations (SD) of duplicate assays (n = 6). * $p < 0.5$, ** $p < 0.01$, *** $p < 0.001$.

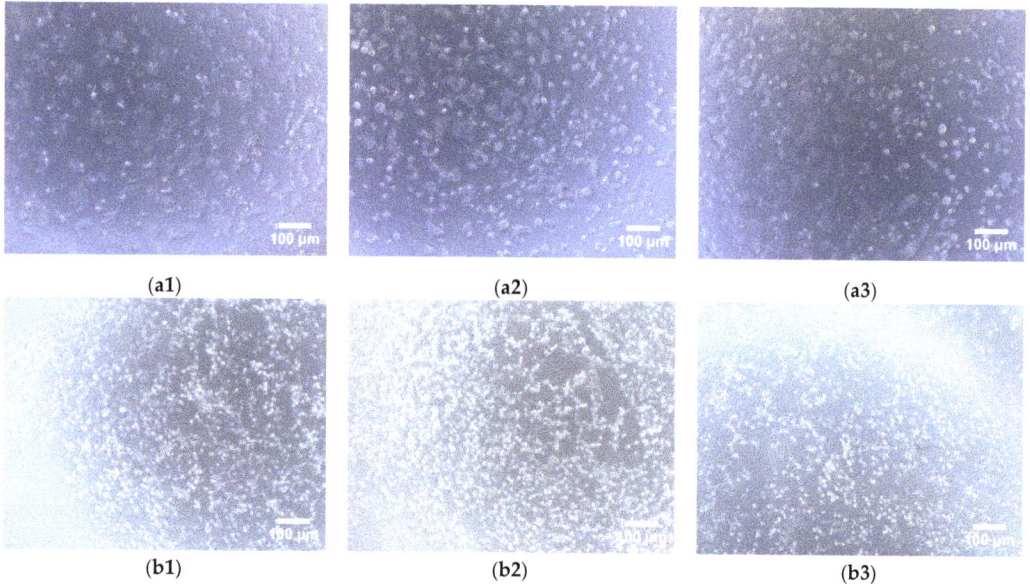

**Figure 8.** *Cont.*

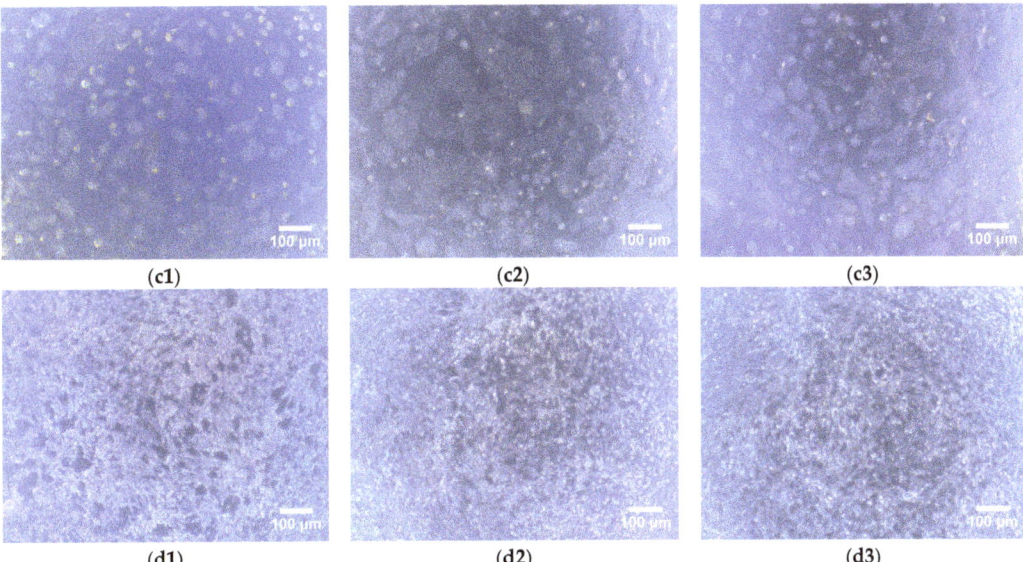

**Figure 8.** Morphology of HaCaT and MC3T3-E1 cells on lizardfish scales collagens (40× magnifications). (**a1–a3**) HaCaT cells for 24 h cell culture, (**a1**) is control, (**a2**) is ASC, and (**a3**) is PSC; (**b1–b3**) MC3T3-E1 cells for 24 h cell culture, (**b1**) is control, (**b2**) is ASC, (**b3**) is PSC; (**c1–c3**) HaCaT cells for 48 h cell culture, (**c1**) is control, (**c2**) is ASC, and (**c3**) is PSC; (**d1–d3**) MC3T3-E1 cells for 48 h cell culture, (**d1**) is control, (**d2**) is ASC, and (**d3**) is PSC.

## 3. Discussion

Collagen is an important and diverse biopolymer that has seen a significant increase in applications in food, medicine, cosmetics, and tissue engineering [35] with the highest structural order and the greatest stiffness, is widely used in materials for biomedical applications [36]. Marine collagen has been successfully isolated from marine by-products [1,37,38]. There are no reports on the use of lizardfish scales for collagen preparation.

In the present study, we isolated type I collagen from lizardfish scales by using acid and enzymatic extraction methods. It was found that the use of pepsin increased the yield of the collagen extraction, and this could be attributed to the fact that pepsin cleaves the cross-linked molecules in the telopeptide region, leading to further extraction with increased yield. This made the extraction yield of PSC higher than that of ASC. These results agreed with those of Keawdang et al. (2014), who reported that ASC and PSC from yellowfin tuna swim bladders were extracted with yields of 1.07% and 12.10%, respectively [38], and Matmaroh et al. (2011), who reported that ASC and PSC from spotted golden goatfish were extracted with yields of 0.46% and 1.20%, respectively [39]. The difference in the extraction yields could be attributed to the varying cross-linking of collagen fibrils in the different raw materials. In this study, the collagen yields from lizardfish scales were higher than that from bighead carp scales (2.7%) and spotted golden goatfish scales (ASC 0.46% and PSC 1.20%). Both the ASC and PSC had similar UV absorption spectra to those of soft-shelled turtle collagen [23], carp scales collagen [37], and red stingray skin collagen [25]. In addition, we also studied the infrared spectra of the ASC and PSC, and the infrared spectra of the ASC and PSC were similar to the spectra of type I collagen from tilapia skin and scales [18], giant salamander skin [33], and silver carp skin [6], where the Amide I band (1600–1700 cm$^{-1}$) typically corresponds to the stretching vibration of C=O along the protein polypeptide backbone. This can be used as a positive marker for peptide secondary structure, and therefore it is often used in the analysis [37]. The Amide II band (1500–1600 cm$^{-1}$) commonly arises from N–H bending coupled with C–N stretching vibrations [40]. The Amide III band (1200–1300 cm$^{-1}$) arises due to C–N stretching and

N–H in-plane bending from amide linkages, and this is the standard confirming presence of the triple-helical structures of collagen [17]. The absorption peaks of the Amide A band of PSC showed a higher wavenumber than those of the ASC, suggesting that fewer N–H groups in PSC were involved in hydrogen bonding in the polypeptide chain. Similar results were found in chicken feet collagen [41]. It has also been reported in the literature that the hydrolysis of telopeptide by pepsin might increase the free amino group, and this may have led to the higher wavenumber of PSC [40,42]. Moreover, the results of the CD spectrum obtained from the ASC and PSC was similar to the CD spectrum of gulf corvina collagen (positive absorption peaks at 221 nm and negative absorption peaks at 198 nm) [10], *Perinereis nuntia* cuticle collagen (positive absorption peaks at 221 nm and negative absorption peaks at 199 nm) [28], and Nile tilapia skin collagen (positive absorption peaks at 221 nm and negative absorption peaks at 197 nm) [16]. In addition, the XRD spectrum analysis showed that the distance between the molecular chains and the distance between their skeletons of the ASC and PSC were similar to the Pacific cod skin collagen [22] and the cuticle of the *Perinereis nuntia* collagen [28]. The results of the FTIR, CD, and XRD indicated that both the ASC and PSC had a native triple helix conformation, and that the acid and enzymatic extraction methods of collagen had no adverse effects on the molecular integrity of the collagen. The highly porous structure is an important feature of biomedical materials that can influence cell seeding, migration, growth, and other physiological activities [28]. The morphology results suggested that ASC and PSC from lizardfish scales have the potential for biomedical materials [41].

The pyrrolidone ring formed by the amino acids facilitates the strengthening of the triple helix structure of collagen, and this is directly linked to thermal stability and is one feature that determines the potential use of collagen. An analysis of the amino acid content showed that the ASC and PSC had higher amino acid contents than that of the grass carp skin collagen (186 residues/1000) [43], the spotted golden goatfish collagen (ASC 186 residues/1000 and PSC 189 residues/1000, respectively) [39], and the calf skin collagen (221 residues/1000) [44]. Therefore, collagen extracted from the lizardfish scales may have high thermal stability based on the amino acid analysis. Thus, we further characterized the thermal stability of the collagen. In general, collagen obtained from fish species that live in cold environments is often less thermal stable than collagen from fish species that live in warmer environments [39]. The lizardfish (*S. macrops*) is widely distributed in tropical and subtropical waters [45], and the $T_{max}$ of lizardfish scale collagen is similar to that of spotted golden goatfish scale collagen (ASC 41.58 °C, PSC 41.01 °C), a common and abundant species in tropical and sub-tropical regions [39]. In addition, it is higher than cold-water species arabesque greenling skin collagen (ASC 15.7 °C and PSC 15.4 °C, respectively) [46] and temperate-water fishes grass carp skin collagen (28.4 °C) [43]. These results were consistent with the results previously reported, indicating that the collagen obtained from the fish species living in cold environments often had lower hydroxyproline contents exhibited less thermal stability than collagen from fish species living in warmer environments [39]. These results were consistent with the amino acid composition of the above studies, with lizardfish scales collagen containing a higher total amino acid content (ASC 237 residues/1000 residues and 236 residues/1000 residues) than arabesque greenling skin collagen (ASC 159 residues/1000 and PSC 157 residues/1000, respectively) [46] and grass carp skin collagen (186 residues/1000 residues) [43]. Thermal stability is one of the most important properties that determine the potential applications of collagen, and it is related to the total amino acid content, habitat temperature, and body temperature [1]. In addition, the $T_{max}$ of lizardfish scale collagen was also higher than calf skin collagen (35.0 °C) [44], a collagen from terrestrial sources, and this indicated that collagen from lizardfish scales has the potential for use as an alternative source of terrestrial collagen.

The study of the effect of the NaCl concentration and pH on the relative solubility of collagen can provide useful information for collagen preparation as well as for processing and application. When collagen is used as a source in production in moisturizing cosmetics, solubility is a major determinant. This is because the hydrolyzed substances are used for cosmetic and medical cream formulations in this industry [47]. The ASC and PSC solutions exhibited the lowest solubility at pH 7 and pH 8, respectively, and this was attributed to the pI of protein with the total net charge of protein molecules being zero when the pH of the solution is equal to the pI [6,48]. In this case, the hydrophobic interaction between collagen molecules is enhanced, leading to aggregation and precipitation of the protein, thereby leading to the low solubility of the solution [21,37]. In contrast, as the solution pH increases above the pI, the net negatively charged residues of the protein increase, causing the ASC and PSC to display a slight increase in solubility at pH levels above 7 and 8, respectively. The differences in the relative solubility of collagen at varying pH levels are related to the molecular properties and conformation of collagen [38]. Kaewdang et al. (2014) [38] reported that the difference in the relative solubility of ASC and PSC at different pHs may be due to the removal of telopeptide regions that affect the protonation or deprotonation of charged amino and carboxyl groups, and this may affect the repulsion of molecules associated with different solubilities. Moreover, the effect of the NaCl concentration on the solubility of collagen solutions showed that the relative solubility of the PSC solutions decreased sharply above a 6% NaCl concentration, while the ASC solutions maintained a high relative solubility (greater than 80%). The relative solubility of the ASC solutions decreased sharply until the NaCl concentration was greater than 10%. The relative solubility of the collagen solutions decreased as the concentration of NaCl increased, and this may have been due to the protein precipitation and salting-out effect [21]. Jongjareonrak et al. (2005) [49] explained that the addition of salt increases the ionic strength and enhances the hydrophobic interaction between protein chains, resulting in a decrease in the solubility of collagen solutions. Thus, the ASC might be less susceptible to the "salting out" effect compared to the PSC [50]. A similar phenomenon has been found in giant croaker swim bladder collagen [48] and silver carp skin [6].

The results of the dynamic frequency scan test revealed that the preparation method markedly affects the rheological parameters, $G'$ and $G''$, of ASC and PSC extracted from lizardfish scales. An analysis of the frequency dependence of $G'$ and $G''$ suggested that the elasticity of the PSC had a greater dependence on frequency than that of the ASC, while the viscosity of the ASC had a greater dependence on frequency than that of the PSC. Moreover, it was noted that the $G'$ and $G''$ values of PSC were higher than the corresponding $G'$ and $G''$ values of ASC between 0.01 and 10 Hz (Figure 6), and these were similar to the collagen from chicken feet. In addition, the $G'$ and $G''$ of PSC were higher than those of ASC at a scan frequency range of 0.2–10 Hz [41], suggesting that the PSC exhibited good viscoelasticity. It was also observed that $G''$ was higher than $G'$ for all of the collagen, indicating a greater contribution of viscosity than elasticity in the ASC and PSC from lizardfish scales.

The CCK-8 assay was used to determine the viability of live cells. The relative viability of the HaCaT and MC3T3-E1 cells on the ASC and PSC were greater than 70% during the 48 h of cell culture, indicating that the ASC and PSC from lizardfish scales are not toxic to HaCaT and MC3T3-E1 cells [6]. However, the relative viability of the HaCaT and MC3T3-E1 cells increased during the 48 h of cell culture, suggesting that the lizardfish scales collagen had the ability to promote cell proliferation. And the relative viability of the HaCaT and MC3T3-E1 cells were both higher on ASC than PSC ($p < 0.05$). These results suggested that the ASC was associated with higher cell viability than PSC. Moreover, a morphological examination of the cells showed that both the HaCaT and MC3T3-E1 cells had similar cell growth patterns as the control groups over the culture period (Figure 8). Thus, the results suggested that lizardfish scales ASC and PSC can be used as non-toxic materials in the biomedical field.

## 4. Materials and Methods
### 4.1. Materials

Type I collagen from rat tail and protein markers (26,634) were purchased from Sigma Chemical Co. (St. Louis, MO, USA). Sodium dodecyl sulphate (SDS), Coomassie Brilliant

Blue R-250, and N,N,N',N'-tetramethylethylenediamine (TEMED) were obtained from Bio-Rad Laboratories (Hercules, CA, USA). HaCaT cell line (Cat No. CBP60331) and MC3T3-E1 cell line (Cat No. CBP60946) were provided by Cobioer (Nanjing, Chian). All chemicals were of analytical grade.

*4.2. Preparation of Collagen*

Collagen extraction from lizardfish scales was in accordance with the method of Chen et al. (2019) [29] with slight modifications. Lizardfish scales were purchased from a food processing factory in Zhangzhou, Fujian Province, China. The scales were cleaned several times with water to remove bones, spines, shellfish, shrimp feet, and offal, and then dried naturally indoors and stored at $-20\,^\circ$C until use. To remove noncollagenous proteins and pigments from the scales, the scales were soaked in 0.1 M NaOH at a ratio of 1:8 ($w/v$) at $4\,^\circ$C. The mixture was continuously stirred for 12 h (EUROSTAR 20 digital, IKA, Germany), with 0.1 M NaOH solution being changed every 6 h. The scales residues were washed with cold distilled water until the pH was neutral. Thereafter, the scales residues were treated with a ratio of 1:10 ($w/v$) of 0.5 M Na$_2$EDTA (pH 7.5) for 24 h under stirring, changing the solution at an interval of 6 h. The decalcified materials were washed with cold distilled water to achieve the neutral pH and dried, followed by crushing under liquid nitrogen. The samples were then stored at $-20\,^\circ$C until further processing of collagen extraction.

Pretreated scales' samples were extracted with 0.5 M acetic acid at ratio of 1:10 ($w/v$) for 24 h under stirring to obtain ASC, while PSC was obtained by extracting with 0.5 M acetic acid (1:10, $w/v$) containing 1% (pepsin 1:3000) pepsin for 24 h. The two suspensions were centrifuged at 14,334× $g$ for 30 min at $4\,^\circ$C using an Avanti J-26 XP centrifuge (Beckman Coulter, Inc., Brea, CA, USA), and the collagen in the supernatant was precipitated by adding NaCl to the final concentration of 2.5 M. After stirring for 2 h, the precipitates were collected by centrifugation at 14,334× $g$ for 30 min at $4\,^\circ$C. The precipitates were dissolved in 0.5 M acetic acid at a ratio of 1:20 ($w/v$) and dialyzed (molecular weight cutoff: 10 kDa, MD 77 MM, Viskase, Lombard, IL, USA) against 40 volumes of 0.1 M acetic acid for 24 h, and then dialyzed against 40 volumes of cold distilled water for 48 h; the dialysis water was changed every 6 h. All of the procedures were carried at $4\,^\circ$C. The dialyzed solution was freeze-dried (Telstar, lyoobeta-25, Spain) and stored at $-40\,^\circ$C.

The yield of collagen was calculated using the following equation:

$$\text{Yield (\%)} = \frac{m_1}{m_2} \times 100 \tag{1}$$

where $m_1$ is the weight of lyophilized collagen, and $m_2$ is the dry scales weight after pretreatment.

*4.3. SDS-PAGE Characterization*

The SDS-PAGE of the sample was conducted in accordance with the method of Laemmli (1970) [51] with slight modifications. The samples (2 mg/mL) were dissolved in cold distilled water and mixed at a 4:1 $v/v$ ratio with sample loading buffer (277.8 mM Tris-HCl, pH 6.8, 44.4% ($v/v$) glycerol, 4.4% SDS, and 0.02% bromophenol blue), followed by boiling for 10 min. Then, 10 µL of the samples' solution was loaded onto a gel consisting of 7.5% separating gel and 3% stacking gel at a constant voltage of 110 V for electrophoresis (Bio-Rad Laboratories, Hercules, CA, USA). After electrophoresis for 90 m, the gel was soaked using a solution consisting of 50% ($v/v$) methanol and 10% ($v/v$) acetic acid followed by staining with 0.125% Coomassie Brilliant Blue R-250 that contained 50% ($v/v$) methanol and 10% ($v/v$) acetic acid. The gel was finally destained with a mixture of 50% ($v/v$) ethanol and 10% ($v/v$) acetic acid for 30 m. The Marker of 46,634 was used to estimate the molecular weight of the collagen, and the type I collagen from rat tail was used as standard.

## 4.4. Spectral Characterization

### 4.4.1. UV Spectrum

The lyophilized collagen was dissolved in 0.5 M acetic acid to produce a 1 mg/mL sample solution, followed by centrifugation at 9729× $g$ for 5 min at 4 °C (Neofuge 15R, Shanghai Lishen Scientific Equipment Co., Ltd., Shanghai, China). The supernatant was analyzed by UV-visible spectrophotometer (UV-2550 Spectrophotometer, Shimadzu, Japan) at a wavelength range of 600–190 nm with a scan speed of 400 nm min$^{-1}$ with a data interval of 1 nm per point. The baseline was set with 0.5 M acetic acid.

### 4.4.2. FTIR

The infrared spectrum of the samples was obtained by using a Bruker FTIR spectrophotometer (VERTEX 70, Bruker, Karlsruhe, Germany) at room temperature. The samples (lyophilized collagen) were mixed with KBr by grinding at the ratio of 1:100 ($w/w$). The wavelength range was 4000–400 cm$^{-1}$, with a resolution of 4 cm$^{-1}$. The signals were collected automatically in 32 scans and ratioed against a background spectrum recorded from KBr.

### 4.4.3. CD

The samples were dissolved in precooled 0.5 M acetic acid to obtain a final concentration of 0.1 mg/mL. The sample solutions were centrifuged at 14,010× $g$ for 10 min at 4 °C (Neofuge 15R, Shanghai Lishen Scientific Equipment Co., Ltd., Shanghai, China), and then the supernatants were measured using a CD spectropolarimeter (Chirascan, Applied Photophysics Ltd., Leatherhead, UK). The spectrum was recorded at 260–190 nm wavelengths at 15 °C in 0.1 nm steps with a response time of 1 s.

### 4.4.4. XRD

The diffractograms of the samples were recorded by X-ray diffractometer (X'Pert Pro XRD, PANalytical, The Netherlands), which was operated at 40 kV and 40 mA with CuKα radiation (λ = 1.5406 Å). The data were collected at scanning speed of 4.5°·min$^{-1}$ and 2θ range of 5–50°. Bragg equation was used to calculate the d values of collagen:

$$d(\text{Å}) = \frac{\lambda}{2\sin\theta} \quad (2)$$

where λ is the X-ray wavelength (1.54°) and θ is the Bragg diffraction angle.

## 4.5. Amino Acid Analysis

The samples were hydrolyzed in 6 M HCl at 110 °C for 8 h. After being vaporized, the residue was dissolved in 100 mL of 0.1 M HCl [22]. Then 50 μL of the sample solution was analyzed using high-performance liquid chromatography (HPLC-MS/MS, Ultimate 3000-API 4000 Q TRAP, Thermo Fisher Scientific, Dreieich, Germany).

## 4.6. Microscopy Characterisation

The collagen solution (5–10 μL) without acetic acid was poured into a 12-cm-diameter lyophilization dish and then freeze-dried. The morphology of the sample was imaged using SEM (S-4800, HITACHI, Tokyo, Japan), with an accelerating voltage of 5 kV. After being coated with Pd, the samples were observed at 400× and 800× magnifications.

## 4.7. Thermal Stability

The thermal stability of the samples was measured using a differential scanning calorimeter (DSC2, Mettler-Toledo corp., Zurich, Switzerland) under a nitrogen atmosphere with a flow rate of 100 mL min$^{-1}$. The samples were dissolved in 0.4 M acetic acid at the ratio of 1:40 ($w/v$) for 48 h at 4 °C. The solution (5 mL–10 mL) was placed into aluminium crucible, and then scanned over the range of 20–70 °C at a heating rate of 1 °C/min. The empty aluminium crucible was used for reference. The maximum transition temperature

($T_{max}$) was obtained from the DSC thermogram, and the enthalpy of denaturation ($\Delta H$) was calculated from the area of the corresponding endothermic peak.

## 4.8. Solubility

### 4.8.1. Effect of pH

The effect of pH on collagen solubility was determined using the method described by Chen et al. (2016) [18], with bovine serum albumin (BSA) as the protein standard. The samples were dissolved in 0.5 M acetic acid at the final concentration of 0.2 mg/mL. The pH of the sample solution (5 mL) was adjusted from 2 to 10, with 6 M HCl or 6 M NaOH. Then, the sample solutions were mixed with distilled water of the same pH until the solution volume reached 10 mL. The relative solubility was calculated through comparison with the solubility obtained at the pH that exhibited the highest solubility.

Collagen solubility was determined at various pH levels using the method described by Chen et al. (2016) [18] with slight modifications. The samples were dissolved in 0.5 M acetic acid at a concentration of 0.3% ($w/v$) with gentle stirring at 4 °C for 12 h. The collagen solution (8 mL) was placed in a centrifuge tube. Then, the pH was adjusted to different levels, ranging from 2 to 10, using 6 M HCl or 6 M NaOH. The final volume was brought to 10 mL by distilled water previously adjusted to the same pH as the collagen solution tested. The solutions were gently stirred at 4 °C for 30 min and left overnight. Next, the supernatants were collected after centrifugation for 30 min at $10,000\times g$. Protein content in the supernatant was calculated using the Lowry method (1951) [52], with BSA as the protein standard. The relative solubility was determined in comparison with that obtained at the pH level that provided the highest solubility.

### 4.8.2. Effect of NaCl

The effect of NaCl on collagen solutions was measured in accordance with the method described by Chen et al. [18], BSA was used as standard. The samples were dissolved in 0.5 M acetic acid at a concentration of 0.2 mg/mL. The sample solution (5 mL) was mixed with 5 mL of a series of NaCl concentrations containing 0.5 M acetic acid to obtain the final solutions with NaCl concentrations of 0%, 2%, 4%, 6%, 8%, 10%, 12%, and 14%, $w/v$. The protein content was measured as described in Section 4.8.1, and the relative solubility was calculated using the solution with final NaCl concentrations of 0% ($w/v$) as a control.

## 4.9. Rheological Properties

The rheological properties of collagen were measured by a rheometer (MCR 302, Anton Paar, Graz, Austria) using a stainless-steel cone/plate geometry (0.5° cone angle, 60 mm cone diameter, gap of 57 µm). The sample (20 mg/mL) was dissolved in 0.5 M acetic acid and then assessed by dynamic frequency sweeps with a constant strain of 30%. The elastic modulus ($G'$) and viscous modulus ($G''$) of the sample were measured as functions of the frequency range of 0.01 to 10 Hz, at 25 °C [41]. Each sample was equilibrated for 10 min before measurement.

## 4.10. Cell Compatibility and Cell Morphology

The cytotoxicity of collagen to the HaCaT and MC3T3-E1 cells was evaluated using a CCK-8 assay with some modifications as described by Sripriya et al. (2015) [53]. The collagen samples were dissolved in distilled water at a concentration of 5 mg/mL. The bottom of the 96-well plates was coated with the collagen solutions (5 mg/mL) and dried under a laminar airflow hood followed by UV disinfection. The cells were seeded with a density of $1 \times 10^4$ cells per well and then incubated at 37 °C in a humidified atmosphere with 5% $CO_2$ for 24 h and 48 h. The CCK-8 solution was added to each well, and incubation was continued for 1.5 h. The absorbance values were measured at 450 nm (Mithras$^2$ LB 943, Berthold, Germany), and the uncoated wells were used as controls. The cell viability was calculated using Equation (2). Subsequently, the morphology of each group was observed under an inverted microscope (ECLIPSE Ti, Nikon, Japan).

$$\text{Cell viability (\%)} = \left(1 - \frac{\text{absorbance of treatment}}{\text{absorbance of control}}\right) \times 100\% \qquad (3)$$

*4.11. Statistical Analyses*

The analysis of variance (ANOVA) was performed using SPSS Version 17.0 software (IBM SPSS Statistics, Ehningen, Germany), and a value of $p < 0.05$ was used to indicate a significant deviation. The different letters indicate significant differences between the samples.

## 5. Conclusions

Collagen was successfully isolated from lizardfish by-product scales by using acid and pepsin extraction methods with yields of 4.2% and 4.7% (based on the dry weight). The analysis of SDS-PAGE and UV indicated that both ASC and PSC were type I collagen. The FTIR and CD spectra of ASC and PSC were similar; the collagen maintained the triple-helical structures well, indicating that the triple-helix structure of collagen was not disrupted by pepsin digestion. The two types of collagen exhibited multilayer overlapping and porous sheet-like microstructure under SEM. The analysis of the amino acid structure showed that the ASC and PSC had high amino acid contents at 237 residues/1000 residues and 236 residues/1000 residues, respectively. Solubility tests showed that ASC and PSC exhibited high solubility in the acidic pH ranges (pH 1–4) and low NaCl levels (1–6%, $w/v$). Moreover, the ASC from lizardfish scales exhibited higher $T_{max}$ (43.2 °C) compared to rat tail collagen (39.4 °C) and calf skin collagen (35 °C), indicating its potential as an alternative to collagen of terrestrial source. A dynamic rheological examination indicated that the preparation method may affect the viscoelasticity of the collagen, and that PSC exhibited better viscoelasticity than ASC. Both ASC and PSC were not toxic to the HaCaT and MC3T3-E1 cells, and the relative cell viability of ASC was higher than that of PSC during the 48 h of cell culture. Overall, the results suggest that lizardfish scales ASC may be considered a potential alternative to terrestrial collagen for further use in the biomedical area.

**Author Contributions:** J.C. conceptualization, validation, resources, writing—original draft preparation, writing—review and editing, supervision, project administration, funding acquisition; Y.L. conceptualization, methodology, formal analysis, data curation, writing—original draft preparation; G.W. conceptualization, methodology, software, formal analysis, data curation. All authors have read and agreed to the published version of the manuscript.

**Funding:** This research was funded by the National Natural Science Foundation of China, grant number 42076120, 41676129, 41106149; Scientific Research Foundation of the Third Institute of Oceanography, SOA, grant number 2019010; the Marine Economic Innovation & Development Project of Beihai, grant number Bhsfs008. The APC was funded by the National Natural Science Foundation of China, grant number 42076120.

**Institutional Review Board Statement:** Not applicable.

**Informed Consent Statement:** Not applicable.

**Data Availability Statement:** All data supporting the conclusions of this article are included in this article.

**Acknowledgments:** The authors would like to thank Jianlin He from the Third Institute of Oceanography, Ministry of Natural Resources, for his technical help for cell compatibility and cell morphology analysis.

**Conflicts of Interest:** The authors declare no conflict of interest.

## References

1. Ahmed, R.; Haq, M.; Chun, B.-S. Characterization of marine derived collagen extracted from the by-products of bigeye tuna (*Thunnus obesus*). *Int. J. Biol. Macromol.* **2019**, *135*, 668–676. [CrossRef]
2. Lee, J.M.; Suen, S.K.Q.; Ng, W.L.; Ma, W.C.; Yeong, W.Y. Bioprinting of Collagen: Considerations, Potentials, and Applications. *Macromol. Biosci.* **2021**, *21*, e2000280. [CrossRef]
3. Wang, S.; Zhao, J.; Chen, L.; Zhou, Y.; Wu, J. Preparation, isolation and hypothermia protection activity of antifreeze peptides from shark skin collagen. *LWT* **2014**, *55*, 210–217. [CrossRef]
4. Hong, H.; Fan, H.; Roy, B.C.; Wu, J. Amylase enhances production of low molecular weight collagen peptides from the skin of spent hen, bovine, porcine, and tilapia. *Food Chem.* **2021**, *352*, 129355. [CrossRef]
5. Davison-Kotler, E.; Marchall, W.S.; Garcia-Gareta, E. Sources of collagen for biomaterials in skin wound healing. *Bioengineering* **2019**, *6*, 56. [CrossRef]
6. Faralizadeh, S.; Rahimabadi, E.Z.; Bahrami, S.H.; Hasannia, S. Extraction, characterization and biocompatibility evaluation of collagen from silver carp (*Hypophthalmichthys molitrix*) skin by-product. *Sustain. Chem. Pharm.* **2021**, *22*, 100454. [CrossRef]
7. Bak, S.Y.; Lee, S.W.; Choi, C.H.; Kim, H.W. Assessment of the influence of acetic acid residue on type I collagen during iso-lation and characterization. *Materials* **2018**, *11*, 2518. [CrossRef]
8. Rastian, Z.; Pütz, S.; Wang, Y.J.; Kumar, S.; Fleissner, F.; Weidner, T.; Parekh, S.H. Type i collagen from jellyfish catostylus mosaicus for biomaterial applications. *ACS Biomater. Sci. Eng.* **2018**, *4*, 2115–2125. [CrossRef]
9. Subhan, F.; Ikram, M.; Shehzad, A.; Ghafoor, A. Marine Collagen: An Emerging Player in Biomedical applications. *J. Food Sci. Technol.* **2015**, *52*, 4703–4707. [CrossRef]
10. Cruz-López, H.; Rodríguez-Morales, S.; Enríquez-Paredes, L.M.; Villarreal-Gómez, L.J.; Olivera-Castillo, L.; Cortes-Santiago, Y.; YadiraLópez, L.M. Comparison of collagen characteristic from the skin and swim bladder of gulf corvina (*Cynoscion othonopterus*). *Tissue Cell* **2021**, *72*, 101593. [CrossRef]
11. Addad, S.; Exposito, J.-Y.; Faye, C.; Ricard-Blum, S.; Lethias, C. Isolation, Characterization and Biological Evaluation of Jellyfish Collagen for Use in Biomedical Applications. *Mar. Drugs* **2011**, *9*, 967–983. [CrossRef]
12. Tziveleka, L.-A.; Ioannou, E.; Tsiourvas, D.; Berillis, P.; Foufa, E.; Roussis, V. Collagen from the marine sponges Axinella can-nabina and Suberites carnosus: Isolation and morphological, biochemical, and biophysical characterization. *Mar. Drugs* **2017**, *15*, 152. [CrossRef]
13. Coppola, D.; Lauritano, C.; Esposito, F.P.; Riccio, G.; Rizzo, C.; de Pascale, D. Fish Waste: From problem to valuable resource. *Mar. Drugs* **2021**, *19*, 116. [CrossRef]
14. Jafari, H.; Lista, A.; Siekapen, M.M.; Ghaffari-Bohlouli, P.; Nie, L.; Alimoradi, H.; Shavandi, A. Fish Collagen: Extraction, characterization, and applications for biomaterials engineering. *Polymers* **2020**, *12*, 2230. [CrossRef]
15. Li, D.; Gao, Y.; Wang, Y.; Yang, X.; He, C.; Zhu, M.; Zhang, S.; Mo, X. Evaluation of biocompatibility and immunogenicity of micro/nanofiber materials based on tilapia skin collagen. *J. Biomater. Appl.* **2019**, *33*, 1118–1127. [CrossRef]
16. Caruso, G.; Floris, R.; Serangeli, C.; Di Paola, L. Fishery Wastes as a Yet Undiscovered Treasure from the Sea: Biomolecules Sources, Extraction Methods and Valorization. *Mar. Drugs* **2020**, *18*, 622. [CrossRef]
17. Liu, Y.; Ma, D.; Wang, Y.; Qin, W. A comparative study of the properties and self-aggregation behavior of collagens from the scales and skin of grass carp (*Ctenopharyngodon idella*). *Int. J. Biol. Macromol.* **2018**, *106*, 516–522. [CrossRef]
18. Chen, J.; Li, L.; Yi, R.; Xu, N.; Gao, R.; Hong, B. Extraction and characterization of acid-soluble collagen from scales and skin of tilapia (*Oreochromis niloticus*). *LWT* **2016**, *66*, 453–459. [CrossRef]
19. Tangguh, H.L.; Prahasanti, C.; Ulfah, N.; Krismariono, A. Characterization of pepsin-soluble collagen extracted from gourami (*Osphronemus goramy*) scales. *Niger. J. Clin. Pract.* **2021**, *24*, 89–92. [CrossRef]
20. Li, L.Y.; Zhao, Y.Q.; He, Y.; Chi, C.F.; Wang, B. Physicochemical and antioxidant properties of acid- and pepsin-soluble col-lagens from the scales of miiuy croaker (*Miichthys miiuy*). *Mar. Drugs* **2018**, *16*, 394. [CrossRef]
21. Pal, G.K.; Suresh, P.V. Physico-chemical characteristics and fibril-forming capacity of carp swim bladder collagens and ex-ploration of their potential bioactive peptides by in silico approaches. *Int. J. Biol. Macromol.* **2017**, *101*, 304–313. [CrossRef]
22. Sun, L.; Li, B.; Song, W.; Si, L.; Hou, H. Characterization of Pacific cod (*Gadus macrocephalus*) skin collagen and fabrication of collagen sponge as a good biocompatible biomedical material. *Process. Biochem.* **2017**, *63*, 229–235. [CrossRef]
23. Li, C.; Song, W.; Wu, J.; Lu, M.; Zhao, Q.; Fang, C.; Wang, W.; Park, Y.-D.; Qian, G.-Y. Thermal stable characteristics of acid- and pepsin-soluble collagens from the carapace tissue of Chinese soft-shelled turtle (*Pelodiscus sinensis*). *Tissue Cell* **2020**, *67*, 101424. [CrossRef]
24. Zhang, J.; Duan, R.; Ye, C.; Konno, K. Isolation and characterization of collagens from scale of silver carp (*hypophthalmichthys molitrix*). *J. Food Biochem.* **2010**, *34*, 1343–1354. [CrossRef]
25. Chen, J.; Li, M.; Yi, R.; Bai, K.; Wang, G.; Tan, R.; Sun, S.; Xu, N. Electrodialysis extraction of pufferfish skin (*Takifugu flavidus*): A promising source of collagen. *Mar. Drugs* **2019**, *17*, 25. [CrossRef]
26. Sun, L.; Hou, H.; Li, B.; Zhang, Y. Characterization of acid- and pepsin-soluble collagen extracted from the skin of Nile tilapia (*Oreochromis niloticus*). *Int. J. Biol. Macromol.* **2017**, *99*, 8–14. [CrossRef]
27. Zhu, S.C.; Yuan, Q.J.; Yang, M.T.; You, J.; Yin, T.; Gu, Z.P.; Hu, Y.; Xiong, S.B. A quantitative comparable study on multi-hierarchy conformation of acid and pepsin-solubilized collagens from the skin of grass carp (*Ctenopharyngodon idella*). *Mater. Sci. Eng. C* **2018**, *96*, 446–457. [CrossRef]

28. Liu, A.; Zhang, Z.; Hou, H.; Zhao, X.; Li, B.; Zhao, T.; Liu, L. Characterization of Acid- and Pepsin-Soluble Collagens from the Cuticle of Perinereis nuntia (*Savigny*). *Food Biophys.* **2018**, *13*, 274–283. [CrossRef]
29. Chen, J.; Li, J.; Li, Z.; Yi, R.; Shi, S.; Wu, K.; Li, Y.; Wu, S. Physicochemical and Functional Properties of Type I Collagens in Red Stingray (*Dasyatis akajei*) Skin. *Mar. Drugs* **2019**, *17*, 558. [CrossRef]
30. Tang, Y.; Jin, S.; Li, X.; Li, X.; Hu, X.; Chen, Y.; Huang, F.; Yang, Z.; Yu, F.; Ding, G. Physicochemical properties and biocompatibility evaluation of collagen from the skin of giant croaker (*Nibea japonica*). *Mar. Drugs* **2018**, *16*, 222. [CrossRef]
31. Sun, B.; Li, C.; Mao, Y.; Qiao, Z.; Jia, R.; Huang, T.; Xu, D.; Yang, W. Distinctive characteristics of collagen and gelatin extracted from Dosidicus gigas skin. *Int. J. Food Sci. Technol.* **2021**, *56*, 3443–3454. [CrossRef]
32. Song, Z.; Liu, H.; Chen, L.; Chen, L.; Zhou, C.; Hong, P.; Deng, C. Characterization and comparison of collagen extracted from the skin of the Nile tilapia by fermentation and chemical pretreatment. *Food Chem.* **2021**, *340*, 128139. [CrossRef]
33. Chen, X.H.; Jin, W.G.; Chen, D.J.; Dong, M.R.; Xin, X.; Li, C.Y.; Xu, Z. Collagens made from giant salamander (*Andrias da-vidianus*) skin and their odorants. *Food Chem.* **2021**, *361*, 130061. [CrossRef]
34. Akram, A.N.; Zhang, C. Effect of ultrasonication on the yield, functional and physicochemical characteristics of collagen-II from chicken sternal cartilage. *Food Chem.* **2020**, *307*, 125544. [CrossRef]
35. Ma, Y.H.; Teng, A.G.; Zhang, K.X.; Zhang, K.; Zhao, H.Y.; Duan, S.M.; Liu, S.Z.; Guo, Y.; Wang, W.H. A top-down approach to improve collagen film's performance: The comparisons of macro, micro and nano sized fibers-sciencedirect. *Food Chem.* **2020**, *309*, 125624. [CrossRef]
36. Guo, S.J.; He, L.L.; Yang, R.Q.; Chen, B.Y.; Xie, X.D.; Jiang, B.; Tian, W.D.; Ding, Y. Enhanced effects of electrospun collagen-chitosan nanofiber membranes on guided bone regeneration. *J. Biomater. Sci. Polym. Ed.* **2020**, *31*, 155–168. [CrossRef]
37. Pal, G.K.; Suresh, P. Comparative assessment of physico-chemical characteristics and fibril formation capacity of thermostable carp scales collagen. *Mater. Sci. Eng. C* **2017**, *70*, 32–40. [CrossRef]
38. Kaewdang, O.; Benjakul, S.; Kaewmanee, T.; Kishimura, H. Characteristics of collagens from the swim bladders of yellowfin tuna (*Thunnus albacares*). *Food Chem.* **2014**, *155*, 264–270. [CrossRef]
39. Matmaroh, K.; Benjakul, S.; Prodpran, T.; Encarnacion, A.B.; Kishimura, H. Characteristics of acid soluble collagen and pepsin soluble collagen from scale of spotted golden goatfish (*Parupeneus heptacanthus*). *Food Chem.* **2011**, *129*, 1179–1186. [CrossRef]
40. Wang, S.-S.; Yu, Y.; Sun, Y.; Liu, N.; Zhou, D.-Q. Comparison of physicochemical characteristics and fibril formation ability of collagens extracted from the skin of farmed river puffer (*Takifugu obscurus*) and Tiger Puffer (*Takifugu rubripes*). *Mar. Drugs* **2019**, *17*, 462. [CrossRef]
41. Zhou, C.S.; Li, Y.H.; Yu, X.J.; Yang, H.; Ma, H.L.; Yagoub, A.E.A.; Cheng, Y.; Hu, J.L.; Otu, P.N.Y. Extraction and characterization of chicken feet soluble collagen. *LWT-Food Sci. Technol.* **2016**, *74*, 145–153. [CrossRef]
42. Chuaychan, S.; Benjakul, S.; Kishimura, H. Characteristics of acid- and pepsin-soluble collagens from scale of seabass (*Lates calcarifer*). *LWT Food Sci. Technol.* **2015**, *63*, 71–76. [CrossRef]
43. Zhang, Y.; Liu, W.; Li, G.; Shi, B.; Miao, Y.; Wu, X. Isolation and partial characterization of pepsin-soluble collagen from the skin of grass carp (*Ctenopharyngodon idella*). *Food Chem.* **2007**, *103*, 906–912. [CrossRef]
44. Zhong, M.; Chen, T.; Hu, C.Q.; Ren, C.H. Isolation and characterization of collagen from the body wall of sea cucumber sti-chopus monotuberculatus. *J. Food Sci.* **2015**, *80*, C671–C679. [CrossRef] [PubMed]
45. Chen, J.; Liu, Y.; Wang, G.; Sun, S.; Liu, R.; Hong, B.; Gao, R.; Bai, K. Processing optimization and characterization of angiotensin-I-converting enzyme inhibitory peptides from lizardfish (*Synodus macrops*) scale gelatin. *Mar. Drugs* **2018**, *16*, 228. [CrossRef]
46. Nalinanon, S.; Benjakul, S.; Kishimura, H. Collagens from the skin of arabesque greenling (*Pleurogrammus azonus*) solubilized with the aid of acetic acid and pepsin from albacore tuna (*Thunnus alalunga*) stomach. *J. Sc. Food Agr.* **2010**, *90*, 1492–1500. [CrossRef]
47. Oliveira, V.D.M.; Assis, C.R.D.; Costa, B.D.A.M.; Neri, R.C.D.A.; Monte, F.T.D.; Freitas, H.M.S.D.C.V.; França, R.C.P.; Santos, J.F.; Bezerra, R.D.S.; Porto, A.L.F. Physical, biochemical, densitometric and spectroscopic techniques for characterization collagen from alternative sources: A review based on the sustainable valorization of aquatic by-products. *J. Mol. Struct.* **2021**, *1224*, 129023. [CrossRef]
48. Chen, Y.; Jin, H.; Yang, F.; Jin, S.; Liu, C.; Zhang, L.; Huang, J.; Wang, S.; Yan, Z.; Cai, X.; et al. Physicochemical, antioxidant properties of giant croaker (*Nibea japonica*) swim bladders collagen and wound healing evaluation. *Int. J. Biol. Macromol.* **2019**, *138*, 483–491. [CrossRef]
49. Jongjareonrak, A.; Benjakul, S.; Visessanguan, W.; Nagai, T.; Tanaka, M. Isolation and characterisation of acid and pep-sin-solubilised collagens from the skin of brownstripe red snapper (*Lutjanus vitta*). *Food Chem.* **2005**, *93*, 475–484. [CrossRef]
50. Kiew, P.L.; Mashitah, M.D. Isolation and characterization of collagen from the skin of Malaysian catfish (*Hybrid Clarias sp.*). *J. Korean Soc. Appl. Biol. Chem.* **2013**, *56*, 441–450. [CrossRef]
51. Laemmli, U.K. Cleavage of structural proteins during the assembly of the head of bacteriophage T4. *Nature* **1970**, *227*, 680–685. [CrossRef] [PubMed]
52. Lowry, O.H.; Rosebrough, N.J.; Farr, A.L.; Randall, R.J. Protein measurement with the Folin phenol reagent. *J. Biol. Chem.* **1951**, *193*, 265–275. [CrossRef]
53. Sripriya, R.; Kumar, R. A Novel Enzymatic Method for Preparation and Characterization of Collagen Film from Swim Bladder of Fish Rohu (*Labeo rohita*). *Food Nutr. Sci.* **2015**, *6*, 1468–1478. [CrossRef]

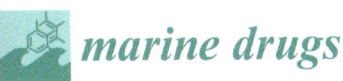

Article

# Comparison of Physicochemical and Structural Properties of Acid-Soluble and Pepsin-Soluble Collagens from Blacktip Reef Shark Skin

Baolin Ge [1], Chunyu Hou [1], Bin Bao [1], Zhilin Pan [1], José Eduardo Maté Sánchez de Val [2], Jeevithan Elango [1,2,*] and Wenhui Wu [1,*]

[1] Department of Marine Pharmacology, College of Food Science and Technology, Shanghai Ocean University, Shanghai 201306, China; 13561936983@163.com (B.G.); ytxiaoyu@163.com (C.H.); bbao@shou.edu.cn (B.B.); zlpan4869@163.com (Z.P.)

[2] Department of Biomaterials Engineering, Faculty of Health Sciences, UCAM-Universidad Católica San Antonio de Murcia, Guadalupe, 30107 Murcia, Spain; jemate@ucam.edu

* Correspondence: srijeevithan@gmail.com or jelango@ucam.edu (J.E.); whwu@shou.edu.cn (W.W.)

**Abstract:** Fish collagen has been widely used in tissue engineering (TE) applications as an implant, which is generally transplanted into target tissue with stem cells for better regeneration ability. In this case, the success rate of this research depends on the fundamental components of fish collagen such as amino acid composition, structural and rheological properties. Therefore, researchers have been trying to find an innovative raw material from marine origins for tissue engineering applications. Based on this concept, collagens such as acid-soluble (ASC) and pepsin-soluble (PSC) were extracted from a new type of cartilaginous fish, the blacktip reef shark, for the first time, and were further investigated for physicochemical, protein pattern, microstructural and peptide mapping. The study results confirmed that the extracted collagens resemble the protein pattern of type-I collagen comprising the $\alpha_1$, $\alpha_2$, $\beta$ and $\gamma$ chains. The hydrophobic amino acids were dominant in both collagens with glycine and hydroxyproline as major amino acids. From the FTIR spectra, α helix (27.72 and 26.32%), β-sheet (22.24 and 23.35%), β-turn (21.34 and 22.08%), triple helix (14.11 and 14.13%) and random coil (14.59 and 14.12%) structures of ASC and PSC were confirmed, respectively. Collagens retained their triple helical and secondary structure well. Both collagens had maximum solubility at 3% NaCl and pH 4, and had absorbance maxima at 234 nm, respectively. The peptide mapping was almost similar for ASC and PSC at pH 2, generating peptides ranging from 15 to 200 kDa, with 23 kDa as a major peptide fragment. The microstructural analysis confirmed the homogenous fibrillar nature of collagens with more interconnected networks. Overall, the preset study concluded that collagen can be extracted more efficiently without disturbing the secondary structure by pepsin treatment. Therefore, the blacktip reef shark skin could serve as a potential source for collagen extraction for the pharmaceutical and biomedical applications.

**Keywords:** blacktip skin collagens; amino acid profile; protein pattern; microstructure

## 1. Introduction

Marine organisms cover three-fourths of the land surface, claiming to be a treasure for many biologically active substances, especially proteins and carbohydrates. The extraction of proteins from marine sources has been increasing at a tremendous rate due to their distinct environment and biological activity. For instance, collagens from fish species have been explored by researchers for many years to sort-out the suitable materials for biomaterial fabrication in tissue engineering applications. It is well-known that collagen, the most abundant structural protein in the extracellular matrix (ECM), is the main component of various connective tissues in the body [1,2]. Based on the structure, molecular composition and distribution, collagens are classified according to at least 29 different types [3]. However, the main backbone of most of the collagens is composed of chains of polypeptides with the repeating sequence (Gly-X-Y)n, where X and Y are commonly occupied by proline and hydroxyproline [1]. Collagen from the skins of several fish species such as tilapia [4], horse mackerel, yellow sea bream, and tiger puffer [5], black ruff (*Centrolophus niger*) [6], and Parang-Parang (*Cirocentrus dorab*) [7] were reported earlier.

Much empirical evidence proved the adaptability of fish collagen for the fabrication of different biomaterials for artificial tissue implants. For instance, different types of scaffolds were fabricated using collagens from tilapia [8,9], *Trachicephalus uranoscopus* [10], bigeye snapper *Priacanthus hamrur* [11], etc. Fish collagen has been used as an alternative to mammalian counterparts for food, biomedical and pharmaceutical uses due to safety reasons and religious constraints [12]. In addition, fish processing industries produce large quantities of byproducts, in which most of the sources such as skin, bones, and scales are poorly utilized [13].

The blacktip reef shark (*Carcharhinus melanopterus*) belongs to the Carcharhinidae family, a species of requiem shark which is commonly found in Pacific regions like southern Asia, the Philippines and northern Australia. Shark is commonly used for shark fin and fillet production. During shark processing, the generated wastes, particularly skin and cartilage, can be ultimately used as potential source material for collagen extraction [14,15]. Unfortunately, none of the studies has used blacktip reef shark skin for collagen extraction and, therefore, it is important to understand the properties of collagens extracted from blacktip reef sharks, due to its potential value. Hence, this study is intended to accomplish the above objectives to extract the collagens using acetic acid and pepsin. It is important to investigate the physicochemical and functional properties of collagens that are extracted in two different ways: with and without enzymatic digestion. Therefore, in the present study, we tried to extract and characterize acid-soluble and pepsin soluble collagen from Blacktip reef shark (*Carcharhinus melanopterus*) skin, and provided a simultaneous comparison of collagens. Accordingly, the present results would be useful in developing a viable alternative collagen material for further biomedical and pharmaceutical applications.

## 2. Results

### 2.1. Protein Pattern of Collagens

The protein pattern between ASC and PSC was compared by using the SDS-PAGE method. ASC and PSC had similar molecular patterns, having $\alpha_1$, $\alpha_2$, $\beta$ and $\gamma$ chains, which confirm that both collagens belong to the type I category (Figure 1).

By comparing the standard molecular weight marker and standard analysis, the molecular weights of $\alpha 1$, $\alpha 2$, and $\beta$ were about 135, 120 and 250 kDa, respectively. As expected, increasing collagen concentration from 0.5 mg/mL to 1 mg/mL had increased the bandwidth. Specifically, the pepsin treatment increased $\alpha$ and $\beta$ band thickness compared to ASC, which claims the efficiency of pepsin in collagen extraction. As evidence, the final yield of PSC was higher (17.78% ± 0.64%) than ASC (15.46% ± 0.42%) (data are shown as mean ± standard deviation, $n = 3$, $p < 0.05$). However, the intact structure of collagen was more stable in ASC than in PSC, since the pepsin treatment had triggered the strong hydrolysis of collagen; as a result, many smaller peptide fractions were generated in PSC compared to ASC. From the gel image, it was clear that the higher molecular weight of collagen $\beta$ and $\gamma$ could be disintegrated into smaller fractions in PSC, which was not obvious in ASC.

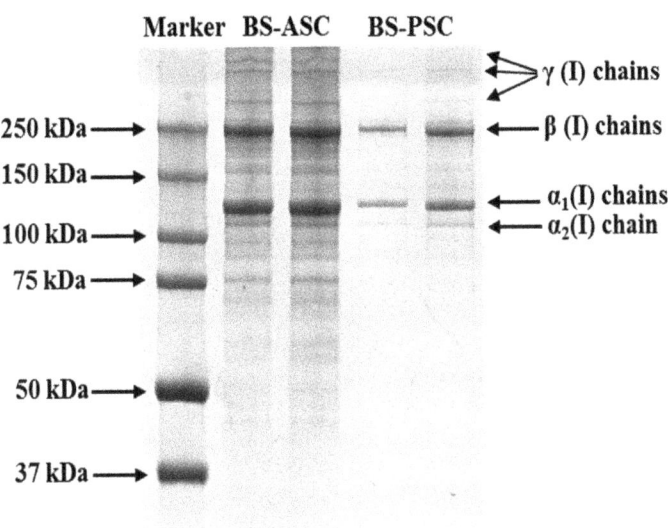

**Figure 1.** SDS-PAGE patterns of ASC and PSC from the skin of blacktip reef shark on 7.5% gel. Lane 1: protein markers; lane 2: BS-ASC (0.5 mg/mL); lane 3: BS-ASC (1 mg/mL); lane 4: BS-PSC (0.5 mg/mL); lane 5: BS-PSC (1 mg/mL).

## 2.2. Amino Acid Composition of Collagens

The total amino acid residues present in collagens were determined to understand the pattern of amino acid composition in ASC and PSC. In general, the pattern of the amino acid profile was similar between ASC and PSC. For instance, both collagens had a higher content of glycine as a major amino acid, only the percentage varies in between collagens, having higher content in PSC (293 residue/1000 residues) than ASC (283 residue/1000 residues) (Table 1). The second major amino acid was hydroxyproline (195 and 202 amino acid residue/1000 residues for ASC and PSC, respectively), followed by alanine, proline and glutamic acid, respectively.

**Table 1.** Amino acid composition of acid-soluble and pepsin soluble collagens from blacktip reef shark skin (residues/1000 residues).

| Amino Acid | Acid Soluble Collagen | Pepsin Soluble Collagen |
|---|---|---|
| Leucine (Leu) | 23.24 ± 0.13 [a] | 20.52 ± 0.41 [b] |
| Isoleucine (Ile) | 18.05 ± 0.70 [a] | 17.24 ± 0.01 [b] |
| Phenylalanine (Phe) | 11.07 ± 0.34 [a] | 10.73 ± 0.16 [a] |
| Valine (Val) | 21.53 ± 1.04 [a] | 19.45 ± 0.09 [b] |
| Methionine (Met) | 3.37 ± 0.16 [a] | 3.21 ± 0.15 [a] |
| Tyrosine (Tyr) | 1.69 ± 0.32 [a] | 1.06 ± 0.14 [b] |
| Alanine (Ala) | 103.94 ± 0.07 [a] | 105.04 ± 0.05 [b] |
| Threonine (Thr) | 20.46 ± 0.53 [a] | 19.91 ± 0.27 [b] |
| Glutamic acid (Glu) | 66.63 ± 0.29 [a] | 64.74 ± 0.06 [b] |
| Glycine (Gly) | 292.95 ± 0.46 [a] | 283.86 ± 0.19 [b] |
| Serine (Ser) | 38.49 ± 0.15 [a] | 36.22 ± 0.15 [b] |
| Aspartic acid (Asp) | 38.30 ± 0.28 [a] | 36.43 ± 0.10 [b] |

Table 1. Cont.

| Amino Acid | Acid Soluble Collagen | Pepsin Soluble Collagen |
| --- | --- | --- |
| Arginine (Arg) | 43.86 ± 0.2 [a] | 43.00 ± 0.15 [b] |
| Lysine (Lys) | 21.13 ± 0.54 [a] | 20.41 ± 0.34 [b] |
| Histidine (His) | 7.14 ± 0.32 [a] | 6.50 ± 0.20 [b] |
| Proline (Pro) | 195.84 ± 0.47 [a] | 202.22 ± 0.37 [b] |
| Hydroxyproline (Hyp) | 92.3 ± 0.16 [a] | 109.46 ± 0.13 [b] |
| Total | 1000.00 | 1000.00 |
| Imino acid | 288.14 ± 0.31 [a] | 311.68 ± 0.24 [b] |

All values are shown as mean ± standard deviation ($n = 3$, [a] and [b] in the same row indicate significant differences, $p < 0.05$).

There was no sulfur-containing amino acid observed in either collagen. From the results, it was clear that the hydrophobic amino acids such as glycine, proline, alanine, valine, leucine, isoleucine, and phenylalanine were more dominant than hydrophilic amino acids such as serine and threonine in both collagens. Compared to ASC, the content of amino acid was in general higher in PSC, which also supports the higher yield and liberation of peptide fragments in PSC (Figure 1). The content of imino acids such as proline and hydroxyproline in PSC (311.68 residues/1000 residues) was much higher than in ASC (288.14 residues/1000 residues).

2.3. Maximum Absorption of Collagens

This experiment was performed to investigate the two characteristic features of collagens: (1) to identify the maximum absorption (nm) of collagen and (2) to verify the contamination of non-collagenous protein presence in extracted collagens. The results showed that the collagens had maximum absorbance at 234 nm, respectively (Figure 2A). The absorption intensity was more in PSC at 230 nm than in ASC. There was no absorbance at 280 nm that usually corresponds to a sulfur-containing amino acid, cysteine, which is normally absent in collagen. From the above finding, it was further confirmed that the extracted collagen was pure.

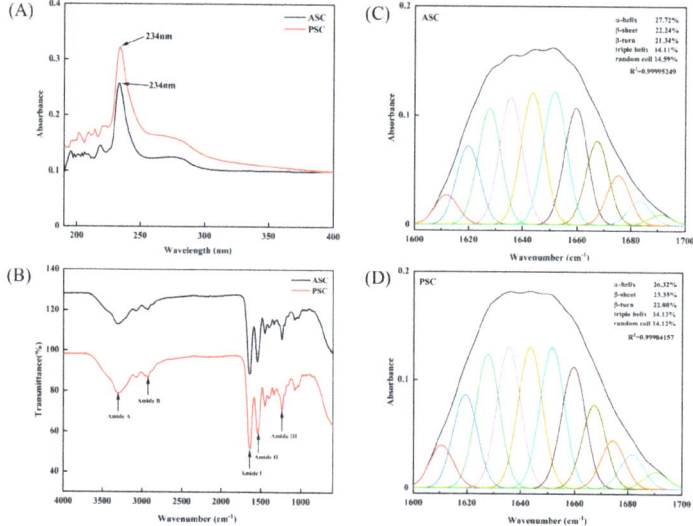

Figure 2. (A) UV–Vis spectrum of ASC and PSC made from the skin of the blacktip reef shark. (B) Fourier transform infrared spectra of BS-ASC and BS-PSC. Secondary structure analysis of ASC (C) and PSC (D) through the deconvolution of amide I band (between 1600 and 1700 cm$^{-1}$).

## 2.4. Secondary Structure Analysis

The structural changes of collagens were investigated by using FTIR spectra. FTIR transmission spectra of ASC and PSC were shown in Figure 2B and Table 2. Both collagens had general transmission patterns in major amide bands such as amide A, amide B, amide I, amide II and amide III, respectively. The maximum transmission wave numbers of amide A and amide B (which represent N-H stretch and $CH_2$ asymmetric stretch, respectively), were at 3298 and 2926 cm$^{-1}$, and 3298 and 2930 cm$^{-1}$ for ASC and PSC, respectively. ASC and PSC had maximum transmission for amide I at 1639 cm$^{-1}$, amide II at 1542 and 1546 cm$^{-1}$ and amide III at 1237 cm$^{-1}$, respectively. There were not many differences observed in amide I, II and III bands between ASC and PSC. The IR absorption ratios of two collagens were 1.11 (ASC), and 1.03 (PSC), respectively.

**Table 2.** FTIR spectra peak position and assignments for blacktip reef shark acid-soluble collagen (ASC) and pepsin-soluble collagen (PSC).

| Region | Wavenumber (cm$^{-1}$) | | Assignment | References |
|---|---|---|---|---|
| | ASC | PSC | | |
| Amide A | 3298 | 3298 | N-H stretch | Doyle et al. [16] |
| Amide B | 2926 | 2930 | $CH_2$ asymmetrical stretch | Abe and Krimm [17] |
| Amide I | 1639 | 1639 | C=O stretch | Muyonga et al. [18] |
| Amide II | 1542 | 1546 | N-H bend coupled with C-N stretch | Jackson et al. [19] |
| Amide III | 1237 | 1237 | N-H in-plane bend | Jackson et al. [19] |

In addition, the secondary structural pattern of collagen was determined by using PeakFit Version 4.12 software and the Gaussian peak fitting algorithm. The data showed that ASC and PSC contained 27.72 and 26.32% of α helix, 22.24 and 23.35% of β-sheet, 21.34 and 22.08% of β-turn, 14.11 and 14.13% of triple helix and 14.59 and 14.12% of the random coil, respectively (Figure 2C).

## 2.5. Solubility against pH and Salt

The functional behavior of collagen is generally investigated by determining pH and salt solubilities. For this intention, collagen was solubilized with different salt concentrations (ranging from 0–6%) and pH (ranging from 1 to 11), respectively. In general, increasing salt concentration from 0–6% decreased the solubility of collagen from 100% to 70% (Figure 3A). Both collagens reach the exponential phase (optimum) at 3% NaCl; after that, a sudden decrease in the solubility of collagens was observed. On the other hand, a typical sigmoid curve was observed in a collagen solubility pattern against pH (Figure 3B). Similar to salt, both collagens had no significant changes in solubility against pH, and the maximum solubility was obtained at pH 4.

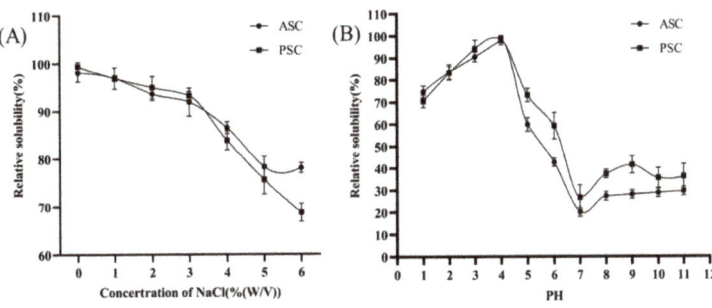

**Figure 3.** Relative solubility (%) at different pH values (**A**) and NaCl concentrations (**B**) of ASC and PSC isolated from blacktip reef shark skin extracted using different methods.

## 2.6. Peptide Mapping

Peptide mapping was used to understand the hydrolysis pattern of collagen by proteolytic enzymes. Based on the earlier protocol, the collagen was hydrolyzed by trypsin with two different pHs at 2.5 and 7.8 for 3 h and 3 min. Due to the higher activity of trypsin at neutral or slightly basic pH (6–7.5), the reaction was carried-out at pH 7.8 for a shorter time. As shown in Figure 4A, the peptide map was not so obvious in all the collagens hydrolyzed by trypsin at pH 2.5 and 7.8, except ASC at pH 2.5. The hydrolytic pattern of ASC was significantly different from PSC, which had no peptide bands, unlike ASC (Figure 4A). The unseen peptide bands of collagens were visible as the gel concentration increased from 7.5 to 12% (Figure 4B). The data showed that proteolytic hydrolysis of ASC released the low MW peptide fragments ranging from 200 to 5 kDa MW at 2.5 pH, whereas the peptide fragments from 55 to 23 kDa MW were observed at pH 7.8 for ASC (Figure 4B). In general, all the collagens had a major peptide fragment at 23 kDa, both collagens had similar peptide fragments ranging from 55 to 23 kDa at pH 7.8, and no higher molecular component was seen in any of the groups.

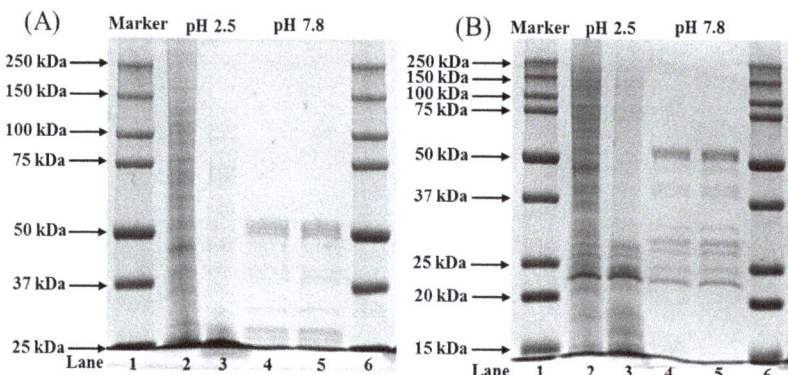

**Figure 4.** Peptide maps of ASC and PSC from the skin of blacktip reef shark digested by trypsin using 7.5% (**A**) and 12% (**B**) gels. Lanes 1 and 6: protein markers; lanes 2 and 4: ASC; lanes 3 and 5: PSC. Lanes 2 and 3: peptide fragments of collagens with trypsin digestion at pH 2.5; lanes 4 and 5: peptide fragments of collagens with trypsin digestion at pH 7.8.

## 2.7. Microstructural Analysis

The microstructural features of collagens were determined by using SEM at different magnifications (100, 50 and 10 μm). It was seen that both collagens had a fibrillary and more condensed network-like structure (Figure 5). The distribution of fiber was more homogeneous and alveolate porous. There were more interconnected filaments with varying thicknesses in both collagens. As seen, there were not many changes in the microstructural characteristics of either collagen. The fibril bundle structure of collagen was further confirmed by the AFM experiment. Similar to SEM, the fibril bundle structure was denser and more condensed in nature in both ASC and PSC (Figure 6). However, the AFM image of PSC showed longer filaments with loosely connected intra-structure than ASC, where the filaments were shorter and more connected to each other.

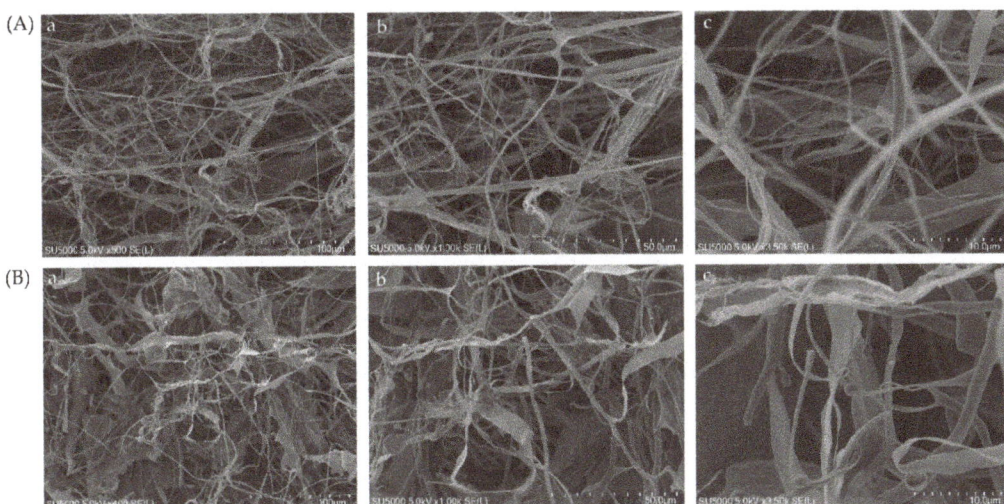

**Figure 5.** Scanning electron microscopic structure of ASC (**A**) and PSC (**B**) from blacktip reef shark skin. SEM image with different magnifications: (**a**) (100 μm), (**b**) (50 μm), (**c**) (10 μm).

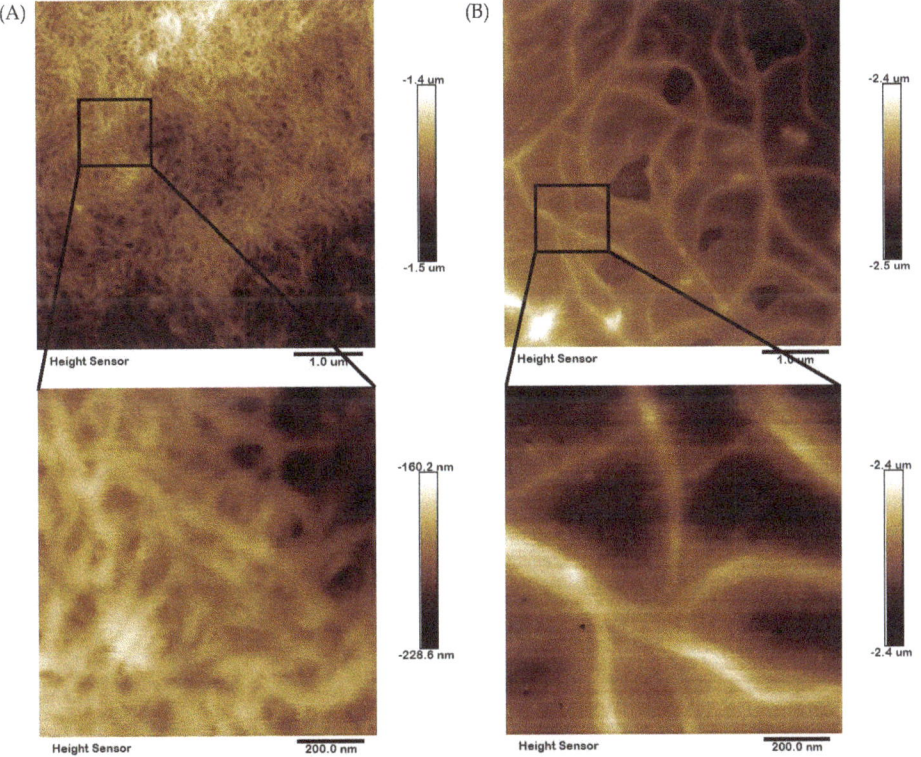

**Figure 6.** High-resolution AFM image of blacktip reef shark skin collagen fiber bundle. The ASC (**A**) and PSC (**B**) fibril display the natural structure.

## 3. Discussion

From the protein pattern, we confirm that the extracted collagens were characterized as type-I collagen due to the presence of α1, α2, β and γ chains. To support this finding, earlier reports dealing with fish skin type-I collagens had a similar molecular pattern of proteins [20–22]. The SDS-PAGE protein profile further confirmed that the extracted collagen was pure and had no presence of other proteins. The pattern of the amino acid composition of blacktip reef shark skin collagen was very similar to the earlier reported fish collagens [22]. The higher amount of amino acid content in PSC was related to the extensive hydrolysis process of raw materials by pepsin, which ultimately facilitated the solubilization process of collagen in raw material and thereby releases many smaller fractions.

The maximum absorbance of collagen at 234 nm was due to higher amounts of glycine (which absorbs maxima at 216.8 nm) and peptide bonds (at 230 nm) [23]. In addition, the liberation of more peptides (which tend to absorb UV maxima at 230 nm) by pepsin treatment might be the actual reason for the higher absorption of PSC at 234 nm than ASC. Interestingly, no absorbance peak of collagens at 280 nm further confirmed that the extracted collagens were pure.

FTIR analysis confirmed that the secondary structure of collagen was not significantly altered by the different extraction procedures with acid and pepsin. Only $CH_2$ asymmetric stretch and N-H bend coupled with C-N stretch were more pronounced in PSC than ASC, which was due to the extensive hydrolysis of collagen by pepsin. The IR absorption ratio indicated that the triple helix and high molecular structure of the two collagens were intact [24]. The amide I band in the wavelength range from 1600 to 1700 cm$^{-1}$ was used to calculate the collagen secondary structure [25,26]. Using the Gaussian peak fitting algorithm, we confirmed that neither collagen had any significant changes in α helix, β-sheet, β-turn, triple helix and random coil, which confirms that the pepsin treatment had not significantly altered the secondary and triple helical structure of collagen and only improved the production yield. A recent study also reported a similar finding in the secondary structures of α helix, β-sheet, β-turn and triple helix by pepsin soluble collagen [27]. This finding reveals the compatibility of pepsin use in collagen extraction from blacktip reef shark skin.

Increasing ion concentration on the surface reduces the free functional groups and the hydrophilic nature, thereby reducing the solubility of collagens [28]. The maximum solubility of collagen against pH was observed at 4, which corresponded to the isoionic point of collagens; for instance, it was reported that the isoionic point of collagen ranged from pH 3 to 5 [29,30].

In the present study, the collagens were hydrolyzed at pH 7.8 by trypsin for a shorter duration (3 min) unlike pH 2.5 (3 h), due to the higher proteolytic activity of trypsin at pH 7.8 [31]. The peptide fragments observed in the present study were similar to the peptide maps generated in earlier studies [32,33]. At pH 2.5, the peptide fragments were derived from higher MW components; as evidence, the intensity of high MW bands such as α, β and γ was decreased significantly and almost absent in collagens treated at pH 7.8. To support this finding, earlier studies reported similar findings with the absence of a higher MW component after trypsin hydrolysis [34–36]. The lower amount of peptide bands observed in PSC at pH 2.5 compared to ASC was mainly attributed to the earlier hydrolysis of collagen by pepsin during extraction, which makes them more susceptible to consecutive hydrolysis by another proteolytic enzyme, trypsin, to liberate peptides less than the measurable range (below 15 kDa). In contrast, the lower amount of peptide fragments in collagens treated at pH 7.8 than at pH 2.5 were due to the extensive hydrolysis of collagen by trypsin at an optimum pH of 7.5 and thereby smaller peptides could be obtained (less than 15 kDa). To support this finding, earlier studies reported a similar observation of peptide mapping of collagens (ASC and PSC) extracted from fresh Spanish mackerel [31], and largefin longbarbel catfish [37]. The similar microstructural properties of ASC and PSC proved that the pepsin treatment did not contribute to any major changes in the microstructure, as evidenced by FTIR data earlier (Figure 3).

## 4. Materials and Methods

### 4.1. Chemicals

Sodium hydroxide (NaOH), acetic acid, sodium chloride (NaCl), hydrochloric acid (HCl), ethanol, and potassium bromide (KBr) were purchased from Sinopharm Chemical Reagent Co., Ltd. (Shanghai, China). Pepsin from porcine stomach mucosa (EC 3.4.23.1; 1:3000 U) was purchased from Beijing Solarbio Science & Technology Co., Ltd. (Beijing, China). Trypsin (EC 3.4.21.4, 1:250), dithiothreitol (DTT), and Coomassie brilliant blue R-250 were purchased from Sigma-Aldrich Corporation (St. Louis, MO, USA). Dual Color protein standard marker with MW of 37–250 kDa (Catalog No. 1610374), 4× Laemmli Sample Buffer (Catalog No. 1610747), 10× Tris/Glycine/SDS (Catalog No. 1610732) were purchased from Bio-Rad Laboratories Inc. (Hercules, CA, USA). All reagents were used at an analytical grade unless otherwise specified.

### 4.2. Raw Materials and Pre-Treatment

The skin of the blacktip reef shark (*Carcharhinus melanopterus*) was purchased from M/s. Yueqing Ocean Biological Health Care Product Co., Ltd. Zhejiang, China. The skins were washed thoroughly with tap-water and cut into small pieces, then stored in plastic bags in the freezer at $-80\ °C$ until further use. The skin pieces of blacktip reef shark were mixed with 0.1 M NaOH at a sample-to-solution ratio of 1:10 ($w/v$) at 4 °C with stirring for 24 h to remove water-soluble substances and non-collagenous protein, respectively, and the alkali solution was refreshed every 8 h. The samples were then repeatedly washed with distilled water until a neutral pH of washing water was obtained.

### 4.3. Preparation of Acid-Soluble and Pepsin-Soluble Collagen

All procedures were carried out at 4 °C with stirring. Acid-soluble (ASC) and pepsin-soluble collagens (PSC) were extracted from blacktip reef shark skin according to our earlier method with some modifications [38]. For extraction of acid-soluble collagen, the cleaned skins were soaked with 0.5 M acetic acid in a ratio of 1:20 ($w/v$) for 48 h. The mixture was then centrifuged at 20,000× $g$ for 30 min at 4 °C using a Himac CR 21G High-speed floor centrifuge (Hitachi, Tokyo, Japan).

At the same time, the centrifugation pellet from the first extraction was redissolved in 0.5 M acetic acid for second extraction for 48 h, and then the supernatant was combined with the earlier extraction. After centrifuge, the collagen was precipitated by mixing the supernatant with 1.0 M NaCl. The salting-out precipitates were redissolved in 10 volumes of 0.5 M acetic acid and dialyzed using dialysis membranes (MWCO: 10 kDa) against distilled water until a neutral pH was obtained. The dialyzed sample was lyophilized using a freeze-dryer (Labconco Freezone 2.5L, Kansas City, MO, USA), and concentrates were stored at $-80\ °C$. The procedure for the extraction of pepsin soluble collagen was the same as the extraction of acid-soluble collagen by using 1% pepsin in 0.5 M of acetic acid. A detailed flow chart of the blacktip reef shark skin collagen preparation procedure is presented in Figure 7.

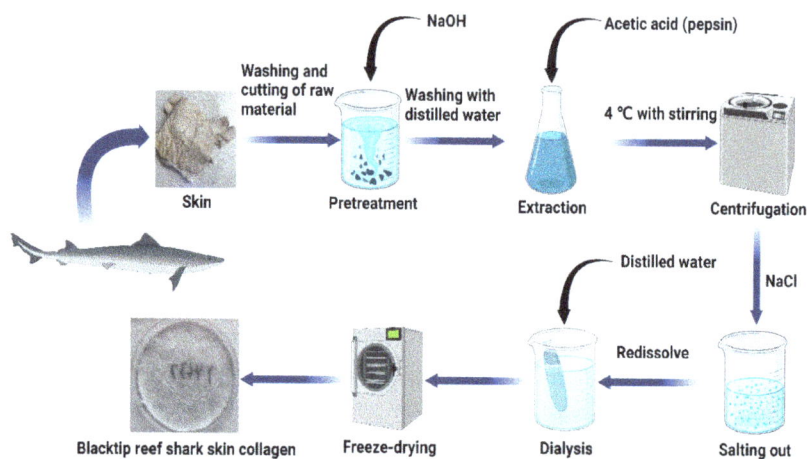

**Figure 7.** Schematic representation of steps involved in collagen extraction.

*4.4. Molecular Pattern*

The molecular pattern of purified collagen was determined by using sodium dodecyl sulfate-polyacrylamide gel electrophoresis (SDS-PAGE) according to Laemmli's method [39]. The ASC and PSC samples were prepared with SDS to obtain 0.5 mg/mL and 1 mg/mL, respectively. The collagen samples were mixed with (3:1) 4 × Laemmli Sample Buffer (SDS, Tris-HCl, bromophenol blue, glycerol, and DTT) and oscillated slightly with a scroll oscillator (TianGen Biotech Co, Ltd., Beijing, China). The samples were boiled for 5 min and the boiled mixture was briefly centrifuged at 1890 g. The test samples and standard protein standard marker (MW ranging from 37 kDa to 250 kDa) (Bio-Rad Laboratories Inc., Hercules, CA, USA) were loaded onto 4.5% stacking polyacrylamide gel with 7.5% separating gel (Cat# PG112, EpiZyme Biotechnology, Shanghai, China). The electrophoresis unit was set at a constant voltage of 200V in order to efficiently separate the collagen samples using a mini-PROTEAN Tetra Cell (Bio-Rad Laboratories Inc., Richmond, CA, USA). After the electrophoresis, the gel was stained with 0.25% Coomassie brilliant blue R-250 solution for 30 min and discolored with the mixture of 20% ($v/v$) ethanol and 10% ($v/v$) acetic acid twice, each for 1 h until clear protein bands were observed. The protein bands were then captured using the gel documentation system (Clinx GenoSens 2100(T), Shanghai, China).

*4.5. Amino Acid Composition*

The amino acid content of collagen samples was analyzed by using an amino acid analyzer (Hitachi LA-8080, Tokyo, Japan) [14]. The freeze-dried collagens were completely hydrolyzed in 6M HCl at 110 °C for 24 h. The excess amount of solvent was evaporated under the vacuum incubator until the dried sample then dissolved in distilled water and the drying process was repeated three to four times. In the end, the dried sample was dissolved with a minimum amount of sodium citrate buffer solution (pH 2.2) and filtered through a 0.45 nm hydrophilic membrane. The amino acid analyzer was calibrated with a standard reagent, and a positive control of all amino acids was run as a reference before analyzing the test sample. The retention time of each amino acid peak was equalized with the respective positive control amino acid peak and the content of amino acid is expressed as the number of residues/1000 residues.

*4.6. UV Absorption*

The maximum absorption of collagen in the UV range was determined using a UV-vis spectrophotometer in order to confirm the purity and contamination of other proteins [33].

The ultraviolet absorption spectra of blacktip reef shark skin collagens were recorded by a spectrophotometer (MAPADA UV-3000PC, Shanghai, China). Freeze-dried collagen was dissolved in 0.5 M acetic acid and the absorption from 190 to 400 nm was measured at a scan speed of 2 nm/s with an interval of 1 nm. An aliquot of 0.5 M acetic acid was used as blank.

*4.7. Fourier Transform Infrared Spectroscopy (FTIR)*

The structural and amide differences between ASC and PSC were determined by using the Spotlight 400 FT-IR Imaging System (PerkinElmer, Waltham, MA, USA) equipped with a deuterated triglycine sulfate detector. The 2 mg freeze-dried sample was mixed with dried KBr (100 mg) in order to make a 13 × 1 mm thin transparent disk by subjecting a pressure of approximately $5 \times 10^6$ Pa. The transparent disk was then placed in a sample holder in FTIR and the spectra in a range of 4000 to 600 $cm^{-1}$, with automatic signal gain collected in 32 scans at a resolution of 2 $cm^{-1}$. The absorption intensity of the peaks was calculated using the baseline method. The resultant spectra were analyzed using Origin Pro 2021 software. The secondary structures of the collagen were analyzed through the areas of 1600–1700 $cm^{-1}$ in the amide I region using PeakFit Version 4.12 software (SeaSolve software Inc., Framingham, USA) and the Gaussian peak fitting algorithm. Finally, the secondary structure percentage was calculated by dividing the peak area of the secondary structure by the whole peak area of all the secondary structures.

*4.8. Relative Solubility*

The relative solubility of collagen was determined by varying NaCl and pH by following our previous protocol [40]. The freeze-dried collagen sample (10 mg/mL) was prepared with 0.5 M acetic acid with gentle stirring at 4 °C for 12 h and used for solubility experiments.

4.8.1. Effect of pH

The collagen solution (5 mL) was transferred into a series of centrifuge tubes, adjusted to pH values ranging from 1 to 11 by the addition of the appropriate amount of 6 M NaOH or 6 M HCl. The resulting sample solution totaled 10 mL of distilled water. The solution was stirred gently for 30 min at 4 °C and centrifuged at 5000× $g$ for 30 min. An aliquot (1 mL) of the supernatant was collected from each tube and the protein content was measured. The relative solubility of collagen was calculated compared with the pH rendering the highest solubility.

4.8.2. Effect of NaCl

The collagen solution (5 mL) was mixed with 5 mL of cold NaCl in acetic acid of various concentrations (0–12%, $w/v$) to obtain final concentrations of 1–6% ($w/v$). The mixture was stirred gently at 4 °C for 30 min and centrifuged at 10,000× $g$ for 30 min at 4 °C. The relative solubility was calculated compared with that of the salt concentration exhibiting the highest solubility.

*4.9. Peptide Mapping*

The peptide mapping pattern of collagen against the proteolytic enzyme, trypsin, was determined by following the method of Li et al., with some modification [31]. The freeze-dried collagen sample was dissolved in 0.5 M acetic acid, pH 2.5, at a concentration of 1.5 mg/mL. In parallel, another set of collagen samples was dissolved in a 0.2 M sodium phosphate buffer, pH 7.8, at a concentration of 1.5 mg/mL. After the addition of trypsin with an enzyme/substrate ratio of 1/2 ($w/w$) to collagen solutions, the reaction mixtures were incubated at 37 °C for 3 h (pH 2.5) and 3 min (pH 7.8), respectively. The SDS-PAGE sample buffer was added to the digestion samples, and the mixtures were boiled for 5 min to terminate the reaction. Using 4.5% stacking gel, 7.5% and 12.5% separating gels, SDS-PAGE was performed to separate peptides generated by the protease digestion and compared.

### 4.10. Microstructural Analysis

The changes in the structural properties between ASC and PSC were determined by scanning electron microscopy (SEM). The freeze-dried collagen samples were pasted on an aluminum plate with conductive adhesive tape in the desired orientation and placed in an ion coater for the gold coating to increase the electrical conductivity. The metalized collagen samples on the SEM sample holder (20-s glow discharged carbon support adhesive films) were mounted and then introduced into the specimen chamber for analysis. The surface morphology of collagen was captured with different magnifications of 100 μm, 50 μm and 10μm by using SEM (Hitachi SU5000, Tokyo, Japan) at an accelerating voltage of 15 kV.

### 4.11. Atomic Force Microscope Analysis

In order to evaluate the surface morphology, collagen fiber alignment, topography and superficial properties of the collagen, an atomic force microscope (AFM, Bruker Corporation, Billerica, MA, USA) was carried-out with collagen samples by following the standard operating procedure [41]. SNL-series silicon 1 cantilevers with a normal spring cantilever of 0.35 N/m were used. The nominal AFM tip radius is 2 nm and the maximized tip radius is 12 nm. 10 μL collagen aqueous solution was cast on freshly cleaved muscovite mica and was allowed to dry in ambient air for 60 min. Images were obtained using a multimode scanning probe microscope with NanoScope Analysis software (version 1.80, Bruker Corporation, Billerica, MA, USA) operating in the tapping mode, in air, at room temperature. Surface images were acquired at fixed resolution (512 × 512 data points) with a scan rate of 1.0 Hz.

### 4.12. Statistical Analysis

Each experiment was replicated three times. Data were expressed as mean ± standard deviation and mentioned in the figure legends. Statistical analysis was performed using GraphPad Prism 9 software (GraphPad Inc, San Diego, CA, USA) using two-way ANOVA with Fisher's LSD test multiple comparison analysis. The values identified as outliers were excluded from statistical analysis. Results were considered statistically significant if the $p$-value < 0.05.

## 5. Conclusions

In this study, the structural and functional changes in ASC and PSC were investigated, and it was found that the use of pepsin had contributed to the increase in the collagen yield; however, it produced many smaller protein fragments after extraction. Therefore, the functional and structural properties were investigated in ASC and PSC, and no significant differences were observed in both collagens, which directly revealed that the pepsin treatment did not affect the secondary structures such as α helix, β-sheet, β-turn, and triple helix. Therefore, the physicochemical, structural and functional properties of collagens indicate that the PSC could be an appropriate material for biomaterial fabrication in tissue regeneration applications.

**Author Contributions:** Conceptualization, J.E. and W.W.; validation, J.E.M.S.d.V.; formal analysis, B.G.; investigation, B.G. and C.H.; resources, W.W.; writing—original draft preparation, J.E. and B.G.; writing—review and editing, B.B. and Z.P.; supervision, J.E.; project administration, W.W.; funding acquisition, J.E. and W.W. All authors have read and agreed to the published version of the manuscript.

**Funding:** The research work was financially supported by the National Natural Science Foundation of China (Grant No. 82173731), the Research Fund for International Young Scientists (Grant No. 81750110548), the Natural Science Foundation of Shanghai (Grant No. 21ZR1427300) and Internal funding from UCAM- Universidad Católica San Antonio de Murcia, (Grant No. PMAFI-27/21), Murcia, Spain.

**Institutional Review Board Statement:** Not applicable.

**Data Availability Statement:** Not applicable.

**Acknowledgments:** We are thankful and acknowledge the College of Food Science and Technology, Shanghai Ocean University, China for providing the proper facilities to carry-out this work.

**Conflicts of Interest:** The authors declare that they have no conflict of interest.

# References

1. Jafari, H.; Lista, A.; Siekapen, M.M.; Ghaffari-Bohlouli, P.; Nie, L.; Alimoradi, H.; Shavandi, A. Fish Collagen: Extraction, Characterization and Applications for Biomaterials Engineering. *Polymers* **2020**, *12*, 2230. [CrossRef] [PubMed]
2. Rahman, M.A. Collagen of Extracellular Matrix from Marine Invertebrates and Its Medical Applications. *Mar. Drugs* **2019**, *17*, 118. [CrossRef] [PubMed]
3. Lim, Y.-S.; Ok, Y.-J.; Hwang, S.-Y.; Kwak, J.-Y.; Yoon, S. Marine Collagen as a Promising Biomaterial for Biomedical Applications. *Mar. Drugs* **2019**, *17*, 467. [CrossRef] [PubMed]
4. Zhang, J.; Jeevithan, E.; Bao, B.; Wang, S.; Gao, K.; Zhang, C.; Wu, W. Structural characterization, in-vivo acute systemic toxicity assessment and in-vitro intestinal absorption properties of tilapia (*Oreochromis niloticus*) skin acid and pepsin solublilized type I collagen. *Process Biochem.* **2016**, *51*, 2017–2025. [CrossRef]
5. Wang, S.-S.; Yu, Y.; Sun, Y.; Liu, N.; Zhou, D.-Q. Comparison of Physicochemical Characteristics and Fibril Formation Ability of Collagens Extracted from the Skin of Farmed River Puffer (*Takifugu obscurus*) and Tiger Puffer (*Takifugu rubripes*). *Mar. Drugs* **2019**, *17*, 462. [CrossRef] [PubMed]
6. Bhuimbar, M.V.; Bhagwat, P.K.; Dandge, P.B. Extraction and characterization of acid soluble collagen from fish waste: Development of collagen-chitosan blend as food packaging film. *J. Environ. Chem. Eng.* **2019**, *7*, 102983. [CrossRef]
7. Wijaya, H.; Putriani, S.; Safithri, M.; Tarman, K. Isolation and allergenicity of protein collagen from parang-parang fish skin (*Cirocentrus dorab*). In Proceedings of the 2nd International Conference on Food and Agriculture (ICoFA), Bali, Indonesia, 2–3 November 2019.
8. Li, J.; Wang, M.; Qiao, Y.; Tian, Y.; Liu, J.; Qin, S.; Wu, W. Extraction and characterization of type I collagen from skin of tilapia (*Oreochromis niloticus*) and its potential application in biomedical scaffold material for tissue engineering. *Process Biochem.* **2018**, *74*, 156–163. [CrossRef]
9. Suzuki, A.; Kodama, Y.; Miwa, K.; Kishimoto, K.; Hoshikawa, E.; Haga, K.; Sato, T.; Mizuno, J.; Izumi, K. Manufacturing micropatterned collagen scaffolds with chemical-crosslinking for development of biomimetic tissue-engineered oral mucosa. *Sci. Rep.* **2020**, *10*, 22192. [CrossRef]
10. Selvakumar, G.; Kuttalam, I.; Mukundan, S.; Lonchin, S. Valorization of toxic discarded fish skin for biomedical application. *J. Clean. Prod.* **2021**, *323*, 129147. [CrossRef]
11. Radhika Rajasree, S.R.; Gobalakrishnan, M.; Aranganathan, L.; Karthih, M.G. Fabrication and characterization of chitosan based collagen/gelatin composite scaffolds from big eye snapper *Priacanthus hamrur* skin for antimicrobial and anti-oxidant applications. *Mater. Sci. Eng. C* **2020**, *107*, 110270. [CrossRef]
12. Nurilmala, M.; Suryamarevita, H.; Hizbullah, H.H.; Jacoeb, A.M.; Ochiai, Y. Fish skin as a biomaterial for halal collagen and gelatin. *Saudi J. Biol. Sci.* **2022**, *29*, 1100–1110. [CrossRef] [PubMed]
13. Xu, N.; Peng, X.-L.; Li, H.-R.; Liu, J.-X.; Cheng, J.-S.-Y.; Qi, X.-Y.; Ye, S.-J.; Gong, H.-L.; Zhao, X.-H.; Yu, J.; et al. Marine-Derived Collagen as Biomaterials for Human Health. *Front. Nutr.* **2021**, *8*, 493. [CrossRef] [PubMed]
14. Kittiphattanabawon, P.; Benjakul, S.; Visessanguan, W.; Shahidi, F. Isolation and characterization of collagen from the cartilages of brownbanded bamboo shark (*Chiloscyllium punctatum*) and blacktip shark (*Carcharhinus limbatus*). *LWT-Food Sci. Technol.* **2010**, *43*, 792–800. [CrossRef]
15. Kittiphattanabawon, P.; Benjakul, S.; Visessanguan, W.; Kishimura, H.; Shahidi, F. Isolation and Characterisation of collagen from the skin of brownbanded bamboo shark (*Chiloscyllium punctatum*). *Food Chem.* **2010**, *119*, 1519–1526. [CrossRef]
16. Doyle, B.B.; Bendit, E.G.; Blout, E.R. Infrared spectroscopy of collagen and collagen-like polypeptides. *Biopolymers* **1975**, *14*, 937–957. [CrossRef]
17. Abe, Y.; Krimm, S. Normal vibrations of crystalline polyglycine I. *Biopolymers* **1972**, *11*, 1817–1839. [CrossRef]
18. Muyonga, J.H.; Cole, C.G.B.; Duodu, K.G. Characterisation of acid soluble collagen from skins of young and adult Nile perch (*Lates niloticus*). *Food Chem.* **2004**, *85*, 81–89. [CrossRef]
19. Jackson, M.; Choo, L.P.; Watson, P.H.; Halliday, W.C.; Mantsch, H.H. Beware of Connective Tissue Proteins: Assignment and Implications of Collagen Absorptions in Infrared Spectra of Human Tissues. *Biochim. Biophys. Acta-Mol. Basis Dis.* **1995**, *1270*, 1–6. [CrossRef]
20. Ogawa, M.; Moody, M.W.; Portier, R.J.; Bell, J.; Schexnayder, M.A.; Losso, J.N. Biochemical properties of black drum and sheepshead seabream skin collagen. *J. Agric. Food Chem.* **2003**, *51*, 8088–8092. [CrossRef]
21. Tian, M.; Xue, C.; Chang, Y.; Shen, J.; Zhang, Y.; Li, Z.; Wang, Y. Collagen fibrils of sea cucumber (*Apostichopus japonicus*) are heterotypic. *Food Chem.* **2020**, *316*, 126272. [CrossRef]
22. Nalinanon, S.; Benjakul, S.; Kishimura, H.; Osako, K. Type I collagen from the skin of ornate threadfin bream (*Nemipterus hexodon*): Characteristics and effect of pepsin hydrolysis. *Food Chem.* **2011**, *125*, 500–507. [CrossRef]

23. Reategui-Pinedo, N.; Salirrosas, D.; Sanchez-Tuesta, L.; Quinones, C.; Jauregui-Rosas, S.R.; Barraza, G.; Cabrera, A.; Ayala-Jara, C.; Martinez, R.M.; Baby, A.R.; et al. Characterization of Collagen from Three Genetic Lines (Gray, Red and F1) of *Oreochromis niloticus* (Tilapia) Skin in Young and Old Adults. *Molecules* **2022**, *27*, 1123. [CrossRef] [PubMed]
24. Chen, J.; Li, L.; Yi, R.; Xu, N.; Gao, R.; Hong, B. Extraction and characterization of acid-soluble collagen from scales and skin of tilapia (*Oreochromis niloticus*). *LWT-Food Sci. Technol.* **2016**, *66*, 453–459. [CrossRef]
25. Petibois, C.; Gouspillou, G.; Wehbe, K.; Delage, J.-P.; Deleris, G. Analysis of type I and IV collagens by FT-IR spectroscopy and imaging for a molecular investigation of skeletal muscle connective tissue. *Anal. Bioanal. Chem.* **2006**, *386*, 1961–1966. [CrossRef] [PubMed]
26. Muyonga, J.H.; Cole, C.G.B.; Duodu, K.G. Fourier transform infrared (FTIR) spectroscopic study of acid soluble collagen and gelatin from skins and bones of young and adult Nile perch (*Lates niloticus*). *Food Chem.* **2004**, *86*, 325–332. [CrossRef]
27. Chen, S.; Hong, Z.; Wen, H.; Hong, B.; Lin, R.; Chen, W.; Xie, Q.; Le, Q.; Yi, R.; Wu, H. Compositional and structural characteristics of pepsin-soluble type I collagen from the scales of red drum fish, *Sciaenops ocellatus*. *Food Hydrocoll.* **2022**, *123*, 107111. [CrossRef]
28. Usha, R.; Ramasami, T. Influence of hydrogen bond, hydrophobic and electrovalent salt linkages on the transition temperature, enthalpy and activation energy in rat tail tendon (RTT) collagen fibre. *Thermochim. Acta* **1999**, *338*, 17–25. [CrossRef]
29. Highberger, J.H. The isoelectric point of collagen. *J. Am. Chem. Soc.* **1939**, *61*, 2302–2303. [CrossRef]
30. Ballantyne, A.D.; Davis, S. Modelling charge across pH and the isoelectric point of bovine collagen during leather manufacture. In Proceedings of the IULTCS Congress 2019: "Benign by Design"-Leather, the Future through Science and Technology, Dresden, Germany, 25–28 June 2019.
31. Li, Z.-R.; Wang, B.; Chi, C.-f.; Zhang, Q.-H.; Gong, Y.-d.; Tang, J.-J.; Luo, H.-y.; Ding, G.-f. Isolation and characterization of acid soluble collagens and pepsin soluble collagens from the skin and bone of Spanish mackerel (*Scomberomorous niphonius*). *Food Hydrocoll.* **2013**, *31*, 103–113. [CrossRef]
32. Abedin, M.Z.; Karim, A.A.; Ahmed, F.; Latiff, A.A.; Gan, C.-Y.; Ghazali, F.C.; Sarker, M.Z.I. Isolation and characterization of pepsin-solubilized collagen from the integument of sea cucumber (*Stichopus vastus*). *J. Sci. Food Agric.* **2013**, *93*, 1083–1088. [CrossRef]
33. Veeruraj, A.; Arumugam, M.; Ajithkumar, T.; Balasubramanian, T. Isolation and characterization of collagen from the outer skin of squid (*Doryteuthis singhalensis*). *Food Hydrocoll.* **2015**, *43*, 708–716. [CrossRef]
34. Jongjareonrak, A.; Benjakul, S.; Visessanguan, W.; Tanaka, M. Isolation and characterization of collagen from bigeye snapper (*Priacanthus macracanthus*) skin. *J. Sci. Food Agric.* **2005**, *85*, 1203–1210. [CrossRef]
35. Mizuta, S.; Yamada, Y.; Miyagi, T.; Yoshinaka, R. Histological changes in collagen related to textural development of prawn meat during heat processing. *J. Food Sci.* **1999**, *64*, 991–995. [CrossRef]
36. Cui, F.-x.; Xue, C.-h.; Li, Z.-j.; Zhang, Y.-q.; Dong, P.; Fu, X.-y.; Gao, X. Characterization and subunit composition of collagen from the body wall of sea cucumber *Stichopus japonicus*. *Food Chem.* **2007**, *100*, 1120–1125. [CrossRef]
37. Zhang, M.; Liu, W.; Li, G. Isolation and characterisation of collagens from the skin of largefin longbarbel catfish (*Mystus macropterus*). *Food Chem.* **2009**, *115*, 826–831. [CrossRef]
38. Elango, J.; Lee, J.W.; Wang, S.; Henrotin, Y.; Mate Sanchez de Val, J.E.; Regenstein, J.M.; Lim, S.Y.; Bao, B.; Wu, W. Evaluation of Differentiated Bone Cells Proliferation by Blue Shark Skin Collagen via Biochemical for Bone Tissue Engineering. *Mar. Drugs* **2018**, *16*, 350. [CrossRef]
39. Laemmli, U.K. Cleavage of structural proteins during the assembly of the head of bacteriophage T4. *Nature* **1970**, *227*, 680–685. [CrossRef]
40. Jeevithan, E.; Wu, W.; Wang, N.; Lan, H.; Bao, B. Isolation, purification and characterization of pepsin soluble collagen isolated from silvertip shark (*Carcharhinus albimarginatus*) skeletal and head bone. *Process Biochem.* **2014**, *49*, 1767–1777. [CrossRef]
41. Shi, C.; Bi, C.; Ding, M.; Xie, J.; Xu, C.; Qiao, R.; Wang, X.; Zhong, J. Polymorphism and stability of nanostructures of three types of collagens from bovine flexor tendon, rat tail, and tilapia skin. *Food Hydrocoll.* **2019**, *93*, 253–260. [CrossRef]

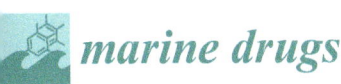

Article

# Preparation and Characterization of Tilapia Collagen-Thermoplastic Polyurethane Composite Nanofiber Membranes

Sijia Wu [1,2,†], Longhe Yang [1,†] and Junde Chen [1,*]

1 Technical Innovation Center for Utilization of Marine Biological Resources, Third Institute of Oceanography, Ministry of Natural Resources, Xiamen 361005, China; gagasaid@163.com (S.W.); longheyang@tio.org.cn (L.Y.)
2 College of Materials, Xiamen University, Xiamen 361005, China
* Correspondence: jdchen@tio.org.cn; Tel.: +86-592-215527
† These authors contributed equally to the work.

**Abstract:** Marine collagen is an ideal material for tissue engineering due to its excellent biological properties. However, the limited mechanical properties and poor stability of marine collagen limit its application in tissue engineering. Here, collagen was extracted from the skin of tilapia (*Oreochromis nilotica*). Collagen-thermoplastic polyurethane (Col-TPU) fibrous membranes were prepared using tilapia collagen as a foundational material, and their physicochemical and biocompatibility were investigated. Fourier transform infrared spectroscopy results showed that thermoplastic polyurethane was successfully combined with collagen, and the triple helix structure of collagen was retained. X-ray diffraction and differential scanning calorimetry results showed relatively good compatibility between collagen and TPU.SEM results showed that the average diameter of the composite nanofiber membrane decreased with increasing thermoplastic polyurethane proportion. The mechanical evaluation and thermogravimetric analysis showed that the thermal stability and tensile properties of Col-TPU fibrous membranes were significantly improved with increasing TPU. Cytotoxicity experiments confirmed that fibrous membranes with different ratios of thermoplastic polyurethane content showed no significant toxicity to fibroblasts; Col-TPU fibrous membranes were conducive to the migration and adhesion of cells. Thus, these Col-TPU composite nanofiber membranes might be used as a potential biomaterial in tissue regeneration.

**Keywords:** collagen; Col-TPU composite nanofiber membranes; electrospinning; thermal stability; mechanical properties

Citation: Wu, S.; Yang, L.; Chen, J. Preparation and Characterization of Tilapia Collagen-Thermoplastic Polyurethane Composite Nanofiber Membranes. *Mar. Drugs* 2022, 20, 437. https://doi.org/10.3390/md20070437

Academic Editor: Sik Yoon

Received: 29 May 2022
Accepted: 29 June 2022
Published: 30 June 2022

**Publisher's Note:** MDPI stays neutral with regard to jurisdictional claims in published maps and institutional affiliations.

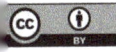

**Copyright:** © 2022 by the authors. Licensee MDPI, Basel, Switzerland. This article is an open access article distributed under the terms and conditions of the Creative Commons Attribution (CC BY) license (https://creativecommons.org/licenses/by/4.0/).

## 1. Introduction

As accidents and diseases lead to tissue damage, natural tissue repair materials are a popular area of research [1]. Collagen has good biocompatibility and can promote cell proliferation and differentiation [2]. What is more, fabricated collagen nanofiber membranes have high-density pores and network structures from micro- to macro-length scales via non-thermal electrospinning. Thus, collagen electrospinning nanofiber membranes enable biomaterials to simulate the extracellular matrix (ECM) environment in vitro [3]. This, in turn, acts as a source of foundation materials for the repair of natural tissue and provides an environment for cell adhesion and proliferation. These collagen-based natural tissue repair materials are frequently used in skin, tendons, blood vessels, as well as nerve and bone regeneration [4,5]. The risk of disease transmission and religious factors have limited traditional collagen such as bovine and pig collagen [6]. Therefore, researchers have focused on searching for marine collagen. Wang et al. separated types I and V collagens from the skin of deep-sea redfish by chromatographic techniques [7]. Chen et al. separated type I collagen from the scales of the lizardfish and maintained the triple-helical structures with no cytotoxicity [8]. Recently, some Japanese scholars extracted collagen from the scales of barramundi (*Lates calcarifer*), which was found to be comparable to that of mammals and showed potential for three-dimensional cell cultivation [9]. Tilapia is a kind of freshwater and saltwater fish promoted by the FAO for aquaculture all around the world, and the production of tilapia is increasing year after year [10]. Marine tilapia collagens have also received significant attention in recent years [11–13]. However, marine collagen, without specific shape, structure, or function, cannot be directly applied. Collagen can be compounded with other materials to prepare nanofiber membranes endowed with high-density pores and a network structure with micro- to macro-lengths in scale. Researchers have developed a series of collagen-polymer nanofibrous membranes. Shue et al. fabricated a series of composite fibrous membranes incorporated with fish collagen, nanohydroxyapatite, and poly (lactic-co-glycolic acid) (PLGA) to guide bone regeneration [14]. He et al. prepared collagen-polycaprolactone (PCL) nanofiber membranes, which had diameters of at least 150 nm [15]. However, marine composite fibrous membranes often have limited mechanical properties and poor thermal stability, which hampers their use in tissue repair [16].

Thermoplastic polyurethane (TPU) is an elastomeric polymer with excellent mechanical properties, wear resistance, good elasticity, and toughness [17]. TPU also has good degradability when hydrolyzed, oxidized, or enzymatically degraded in vivo [18]. Routes to degradation of TPU can combine materials in the degradation process to retain $CO_2$ and water and modulate changes in pH and chemical stability of the surrounding tissues [19]. Therefore, TPU promotes a stable environment for tissue regeneration; it has good mechanical properties and is environmentally friendly [20]. However, there are few reports of the micromorphology, microstructure, thermal stability, mechanical properties, and biocompatibility of collagen-thermoplastic polyurethane (Col-TPU) composite fiber membranes.

For this reason, the aim of this study was to develop collagen-based nanofibrous membranes that are suitable for the growth of fiber cells and have balanced mechanical properties, good thermal stability, and the potential to become fundamental materials for tissue repair. First, collagen was extracted from tilapia skin. Then, collagen and TPU fundamental materials were used to electrospin a series of Col-TPU nanofiber membranes. The compatibility, micromorphology, microstructure, thermal stability, mechanical properties, and biocompatibility of Col-TPU composite fiber membranes were then studied.

## 2. Results and Discussion
### 2.1. Collagen Structure Identification

The sodium dodecyl sulfate-polyacrylamide gel electrophoresis (SDS-PAGE) analysis showed three main bands, as seen in Figure 1. Tilapia skin collagen showed similar electrophoretic patterns to type I rat tail collagen consisting of two different α-chains (α1 and α2), dimeric β-chains, and γ-chains. Tilapia collagen was also consistent with rainbow trout (*Onchorhynchus mykiss*) [21] and black sea gilthead bream (*Sparus aurata*) [22]. Herein, the molecular weight of collagen was analyzed using Quantity One 4.6.0 software (Bio-Rad Laboratories, Hercules, CA, USA). Two bands had molecular weights of 130 and 121 kDa. They were assigned to two α-chains of collagen: α1 and α2 [23]. The two high-molecular-weight components had weights over 200 kDa. These were identified as a β-chain consisting of two α-chains and a γ-chain consisting of three α-chains, respectively [24]. In addition, the ratio of α1 and α2 was calculated with Image J software (VERSION 1.8.0, National Institute of Mental Health, Bethesda, MD, USA); specifically, approximately 2:1 was consistent with the molecular structure of type I collagen [α1]$_2$α2, thus indicating that the prepared TSC was type I collagen.

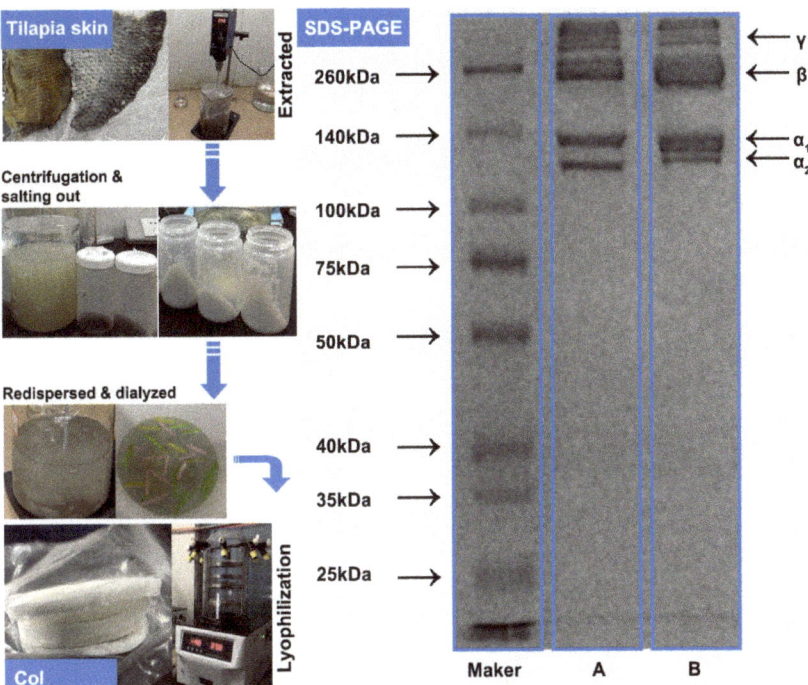

**Figure 1.** Preparation and characterization of collagen. (**A**) Type I rat tail collagen, (**B**) Tilapia skin collagen.

### 2.2. Structural Analysis of Col-TPU Composite Nanofiber Membranes

#### 2.2.1. Scanning Electron Microscope (SEM) Analysis

SEM (Figure 2) revealed that Col-TPU composite nanofiber membranes (Col95, Col90, Col80, Col60) are uniform and continuous with no beads and better straightness than pure TPU. They range in diameter from 112 nm to 858 nm. The porosity increased with increasing TPU ratios. The average diameters of Col100, Col95, Col90, Col80, and Col60 decreased from 379.96 ± 134.28 nm to 378.40 ± 151.87 nm, 316.80 ± 94.51 nm, 313.80 ± 102.88 nm, and 232.94 ± 87.82 nm, respectively (Table 1). The average diameters of the nanofibers decreased gradually with the increasing compound ratio of TPU. The porosity of all composite nanofiber membranes was higher than 45%, which benefits water and oxygen permeability. The appropriate porosity also facilitates cell migration and cell attachment in the resulting pore structure.

**Table 1.** SEM results of Col-TPU composite nanofiber membranes.

| Ratio (Col:TPU) | Abbreviation | Average Diameter (nm) | Porosity (%) |
|---|---|---|---|
| 100:0 | Col00 | 379.96 ± 134.28 | 46.59 |
| 95:5 | Col95 | 378.40 ± 151.87 | 47.29 |
| 90:10 | Col90 | 316.80 ± 94.51 | 48.81 |
| 80:20 | Col80 | 313.80 ± 102.88 | 49.15 |
| 60:40 | Col60 | 232.94 ± 87.82 | 52.89 |

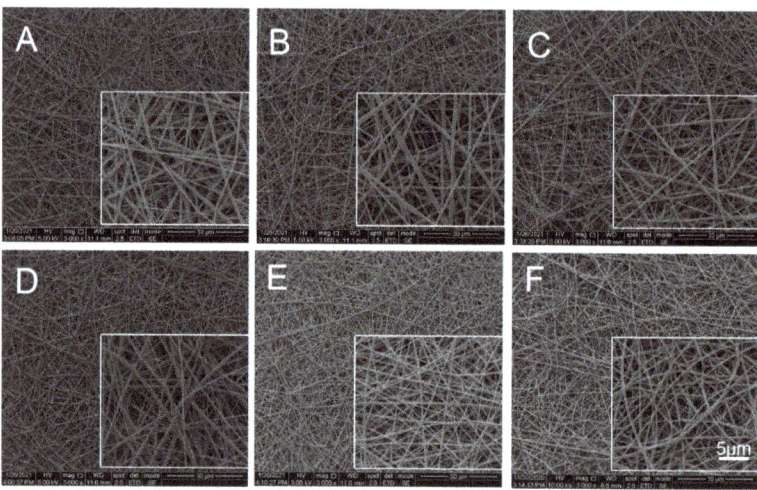

**Figure 2.** SEM analysis. (**A**) Col100. (**B**) Col95. (**C**) Col90. (**D**) Col80. (**E**) Col60. (**F**) TPU.

2.2.2. FTIR

Main Characteristic Peak

All Col-TPU composite nanofiber membranes have five characteristic peaks that were similar to collagen peaks (Figure 3A,B). The amide A band of collagen was near 3315 cm$^{-1}$, the amide B band was at 2920–2944 cm$^{-1}$, the amide I was at 1625–1690 cm$^{-1}$, the amide II band was at 1500–1600 cm$^{-1}$, and the amide III band was oriented at 1200–1300 cm$^{-1}$. Figure 3B and Table S1 shows that the amide A band of Col100 was oriented at 3311 cm$^{-1}$, and the Col-TPU composite nanofiber membranes were blue-shifted from 3307 cm$^{-1}$ to 3309 cm$^{-1}$ with increasing TPU, which may be caused by the N-H vibration (3310 cm$^{-1}$) coupling effect of the group in TPU. The amide B band reflects the ubiquitinated coupling between the amide A band and the amide II band. Col100 was oriented at 2932 cm$^{-1}$, and Col-TPU composite nanofiber membranes were blue-shifted to 2939 cm$^{-1}$ with increasing TPU. This affected the asymmetric stretching of the C-H group (2942 cm$^{-1}$) in TPU, thus indicating that collagen and TPU were prepared successfully. The amide I and II bands of Col100 were oriented at 1655 cm$^{-1}$ and 1655 cm$^{-1}$. The amide I and II bands of Col-TPU composite nanofiber membranes were ultimately red-shifted to 1554 cm$^{-1}$ and 1534 cm$^{-1}$ with increasing TPU ratios. This may be due to the combination of collagen and TPU, thus showing the characteristic peak of TPU and resulting in a red-shift of the hydroxyl peak. The C=C stretching vibration absorption peak (1532 cm$^{-1}$) of TPU in the Col-TPU composite nanofiber membranes approached the N-H out-of-plane vibration absorption peak at 1537 cm$^{-1}$ in collagen, thus leading to two peaks that expanded into one wide absorption peak on the surface of Col-TPU composite nanofiber membranes [25].

The amide III band of Col100 was oriented at 1223 cm$^{-1}$, and the Col-TPU composite nanofiber membranes were blue-shifted to 1230 cm$^{-1}$ upon the addition of TPU, which may affect the vibration of C-C-N in the ethyl carbamate bond (-NHCOO-) in TPU near 1240 cm$^{-1}$. Moreover, the absorption peaks in the region of 1100 cm$^{-1}$ (stretching vibration of C-O-C) in TPU were blue-shifted from 1000 cm$^{-1}$ to 1100 cm$^{-1}$ when the ratio is 60:40 (collagen:TPU). This suggests that TPU combined with collagen to form Col-TPU composite nanofiber membranes during the interfacial interaction between collagen and TPU [26]. The absorption ratio of the amide III band to 1450 cm$^{-1}$ (amide III/A1450) is an important index to determine the integrity of the collagen triple helix structure. When the ratio is <0.5, collagen unwinds the triple helix structure due to denaturation. The absorption ratio of amide III/A1450 in Col100 was 1.114. After adding TPU, and the absorbance ratios of Col-TPU composite nanofiber membranes were 1.131 (Col95), 1.127 (Col90), 1.036 (Col80), and 0.948 (Col60). These data indicate the presence of triple-helical structures of collagen in Col-TPU composite nanofiber membranes [27].

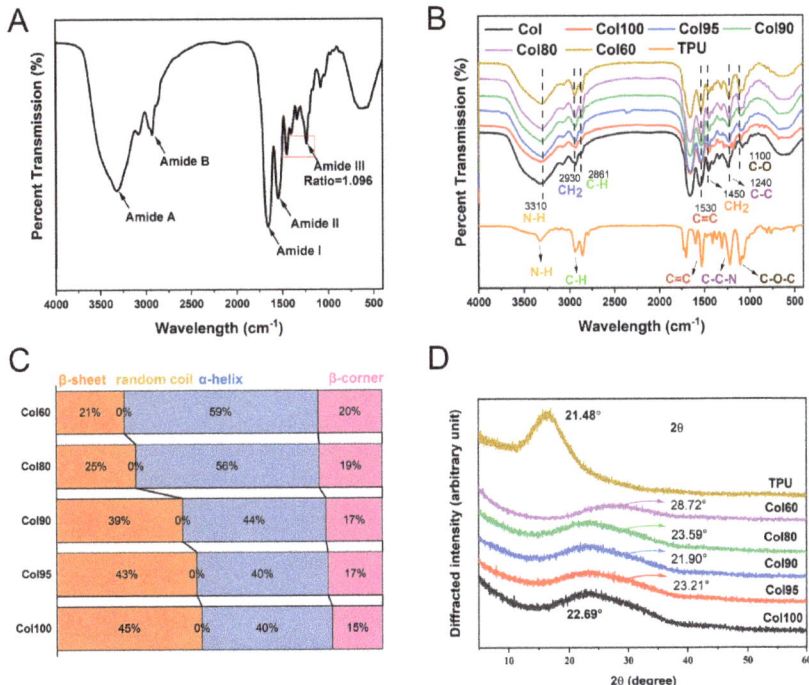

**Figure 3.** Spectroscopy analysis. (**A**) FTIR of collagen; (**B**) FTIR of Col-TPU composite nanofiber membranes; (**C**) Conformation relative content of amide I band in Col-TPU composite nanofiber membranes; (**D**) XRD of Col-TPU composite nanofiber membranes.

Secondary Structure

The secondary structure ratios of Col-TPU composite nanofiber membranes were associated with the amide I band including an α-helix structure, a β-sheet structure, and a β-turn structure. Figure 3C shows that the ratio of β-sheet for collagen decreased from 45% to 21% with increasing TPU ratios, thus suggesting that a more compact structure of the composite nanofiber membrane was formed due to the interactions from larger volumes of side-chain amino acids between collagen and TPU [28]. All Col-TPU composite nanofiber membranes lacked a random collagen structure, suggesting that TPU would not destroy the overall conformation of the secondary structure of collagen. The α-helix ratio of composite nanofiber membranes increased from 40% to 59% with increasing TPU, thus suggesting that the addition of TPU makes sense for the formation of the α-helix. The ratio of the β-turn of Col100 is 14.18%. With increasing TPU ratio, the β-turn of Col-TPU composite nanofiber membranes increased from 15% to 20%. The β-turn mostly transformed into a β-sheet resulting from more -NH groups forming hydrogen bonds, thus indicating that the composite reaction between collagen and TPU is conducive to the formation of an ordered secondary structure leading to a stable collagen structure [29].

2.2.3. XRD

The tertiary structure of the Col-TPU composite nanofiber membranes is shown in Figure 3D. Each Col-TPU composite nanofiber membrane has only one characteristic peak at about 20° in the XRD pattern. This represents the distance between collagen frameworks associated with the diffuse scattering of collagen fibers [30]. These data indicate that the collagen phase does not change upon the addition of TPU. TPU is an amorphous polymer, and there is a wide diffraction peak from 16° to 26° caused by the polyether chain segment in its amorphous structure [31].

Figure 3D shows that the wide peak of the Col-TPU composite nanofiber membranes increased to a TPU diffraction peak with an increasing TPU ratio. No obvious characteristic TPU peaks were observed in the pattern. These results indicate that TPU and collagen have high compatibility, and the mixed-membrane matrix can accommodate TPU without affecting its crystal shape. However, 2θ was at 28.72° when the ratio of TPU shifted to almost 40° while maintaining the wide amorphous peak. This suggests that when the ratio of collagen and TPU was lower than 6:4, the tertiary structure of the Col-TPU nanofibrous membrane resulted in a wider diffraction peak. This result was caused by the strong hydrogen bond action between groups of collagen and the secondary amine groups of TPU, which is beneficial in improving the toughness of Col-TPU composite nanofiber membranes [32].

### 2.3. Differential Scanning Calorimetry (DSC)

The DSC curves of the Col-TPU composite nanofiber membranes are shown in Figure 4. The changes in disappearance of the endothermic peak, the emergence of new peaks, and the change in the enthalpy potentially indicate the components are incompatible [33]. From Figure 4, the endothermic peak of Col100 is 70 °C. There was no obvious peak in TPU because it belongs to the elastomer. Therefore, it does not contain boundaries between soft and hard phases. According to the peaks of collagen-based composites, the addition of TPU in collagen did not generate a new crest, indicating the two had good compatibility. Due to the uniformity of compatibility, the summits of the endothermic peak will be in close proximity to each other if the two phases are compatible [34]. The endothermic peaks of Col95, Col90, and Col80 were 72.1 °C, 74.4 °C, and 73.7 °C, respectively. When the ratio of TPU to composite nanofiber membranes increased to 20, the endothermic peak began to decrease. When the ratio of TPU doubled (60:40), the peak appeared at 65.5 °C. Thus, at the appropriate TPU proportion, the compatibility could be maintained. In addition, the melting enthalpy (ΔH$_f$) of Col100, Col95, Col90, Col80, and Col60 was 49.5 J/g, 47.5 J/g, 46.4 J/g, 41.3 J/g, and 31.8 J/g, respectively. The decrease in enthalpy, in association with the changes in the temperature transition, may indicate there is a limited consistency in the boundary of the two phases [35].

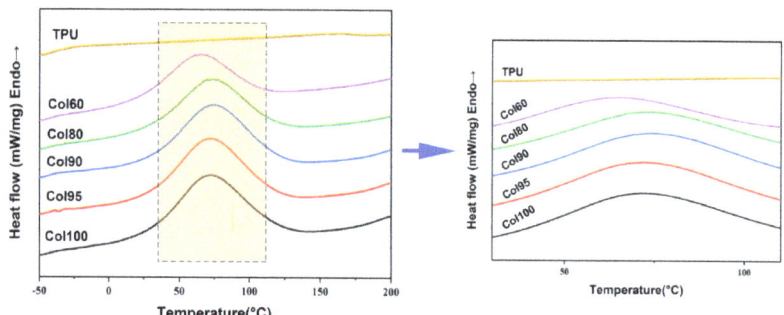

**Figure 4.** The DSC curves of Col-based composite nanofiber membranes.

### 2.4. TGA

The thermal stability of Col-TPU nanofibrous membranes was evaluated by thermogravimetric analysis (TGA). The thermogain-loss trend of all samples can be divided into two stages (Figure 5A–F). In stage one, the temperature leading to a 5% weight reduction is caused by the evaporation of free water in the sample defined as T5% (Table S2). The T5% of the Col-TPU composite nanofiber membranes with different ratios are roughly the same. When the ratio of TPU increased to 40, the weight loss temperature of Col-TPU nanofibrous membranes increased from 65.0 °C to 75.7 °C, which implied enhanced water retention of nanofibrous membranes. Col100 and Col-TPU composite nanofiber membranes have weight loss caused by thermal decomposition in stage two. The temperature of the maximum decomposition rate (Tp) was used to characterize this thermal decomposition temperature [36]. The weight-loss curves of all Col-TPU composite nanofiber membranes were higher than those of Col100. Table S2 shows that the Tp in Col100 is at 314 °C. With increasing TPU, the Tp of Col-TPU composite nanofiber membranes gradually reached 314 °C, 320.5 °C, 320.7 °C, and 321.8 °C, respectively. These data indicate that the thermal stability of Col-TPU composite nanofiber membranes improved versus collagen with increasing TPU. We also investigated the weight-loss stage when the weight dropped by half (with the decomposition temperature defined as $T_{50\%}$). This was a good metric of thermal stability. When the ratio of TPU increased, the $T_{50\%}$ of Col100 changed from 327.0 °C to 331.0 °C, 342.3 °C, 343.0 °C, and 353.7 °C. These further indicated that the addition of TPU led to better heat resistance with improved decomposition temperatures. At the same decomposition temperature, the residual Col-TPU composite nanofiber membranes were 5% higher than that in Col100 after heating. The Col-TPU composite nanofiber membranes had less decomposition at high temperatures. These data indicate that TPU might slow the decomposition of the collagen matrix and prevent external diffusion and release, thus improving the thermal stability of Col-TPU composite nanofiber membranes.

*2.5. Water Contact Angle (WCA)*

The hydrophilicity of Col-TPU composite nanofiber membranes was assessed with the WCA. Figure 6A shows that the WCA of Col100 was 87.1 ± 0.6°, thus indicating that collagen is hydrophilic [37]. When the ratio of TPU increased, the WCA of Col-TPU composite nanofiber membranes increased to 96.7 ± 0.0°, 95.5 ± 0.1, and 91.1 ± 0.5°. The diameter of fibers, the surface roughness, and the pore structure of the membrane affect the hydrophilicity of the material [14]. TPU decreased the diameters of the nanofiber membrane so that the surface of the membranes had more visible pores. This further weakened the barrier properties of the composite material, making it easy for water to penetrate and leading to a lower water contact angle [38]. Moreover, Col-TPU composite nanofiber membranes are hydrophobic, which may be caused by electrospinning disrupting the hydrophilic balance and producing a higher WCA. When the ratio of TPU increased to 40, the WCA of the Col-TPU composite nanofiber membrane (Col60) was 79.1 ± 1.4°, thus indicating that the wetting behavior of Col-TPU composite nanofiber membranes gradually changed from hydrophobic to hydrophilic. These data indicate that the hydrophilic groups on the TPU molecular chain gap and collagen microfiber were transferred to the side of the low-moisture section after absorbing water at the high-moisture section when TPU reached a certain ratio [39]; this, in turn, increased the hydrophilic groups in the Col-TPU composite nanofiber membranes and greatly increased the water absorption performance of the composite nanofiber membranes. These observations were consistent with the FTIR results.

Appropriate hydrophilicity has great significance for biomaterials, and improved surface hydrophilicity is expected to promote cell adhesion and proliferation [40]. Thus, the proper addition of TPU can lead to stable hydrophilicity of Col-TPU composite nanofiber membranes. This, in turn plays an important role in improving the adhesion and growth of cells on the surface of nanofibers.

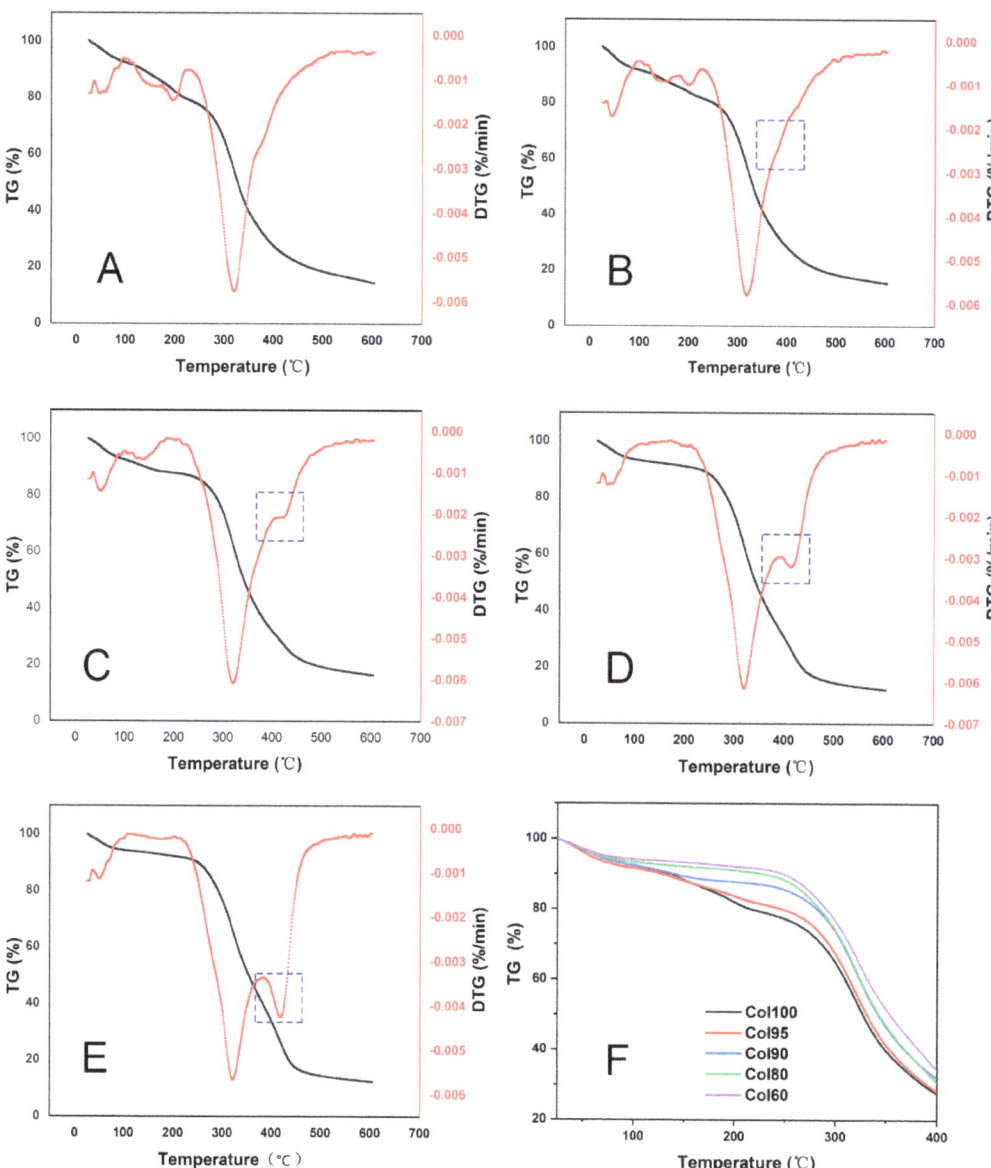

**Figure 5.** TG-DTA thermogravimetric curve. (**A**) Col100; (**B**) Col95; (**C**) Col90; (**D**) Col80; (**E**) Col60; (**F**) Local enlarged view of TG curve.

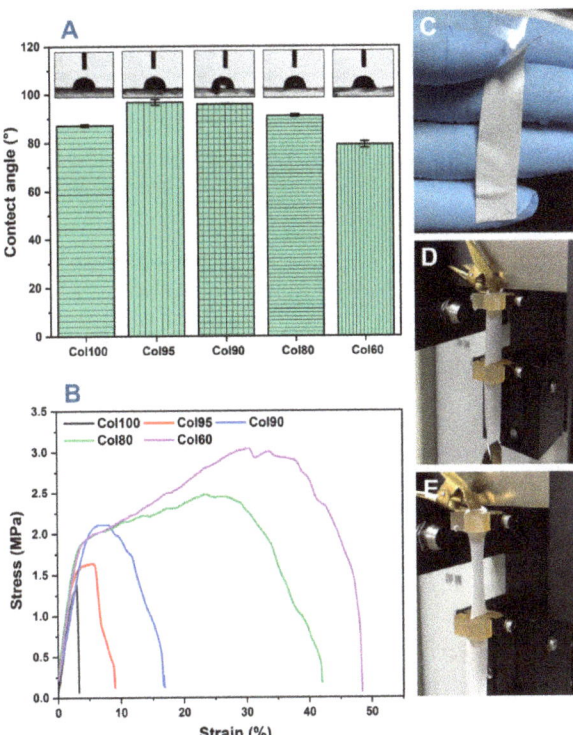

**Figure 6.** Properties of Col based composite nanofiber membranes. (**A**) WCA; (**B**) Stress–stain curve; (**C**) Prepared Col-TPU composite nanofiber membrane; (**D**) Before tensile test; (**E**) After tensile test.

## 2.6. Mechanical Properties

The mechanical properties of Col-TPU composite nanofiber membranes were evaluated as shown in Figure 6B and Table 2. The breaking strength reflects the anti-aging ability of the material [41]. The breaking strength of Col100 is 36.21 cN, which is lower than all Col-TPU composite nanofiber membranes. With an increase in the TPU ratio, the breaking strength gradually increases from 43.26 cN (Col95) to 56.28 cN (Col60), thus indicating that the Col-TPU composite nanofiber membranes had better wear resistance and mechanical durability. Elongation at breaking reflects the toughness and elasticity of the composites' mechanical properties. The elongation at the breaking of Col100 is 3.20%, which has tensile mechanical properties caused by the relaxation process immediately after fiber formation. However, during the relaxation process, the poor deformation ability of the collagen molecular chain and the loss of molecular orientation generate poor tensile properties.

**Table 2.** Properties of Col-TPU composite nanofiber membranes.

| Samples | Thickness (mm) | Width (mm) | Breaking Strength (cN) | Tensile Strain (%) | Tensile Strength (MPa) |
|---|---|---|---|---|---|
| Col100 | 10.50 | 0.0242 | 36.21 | 3.20 | 1.40 |
| Col95 | 9.80 | 0.0264 | 43.26 | 8.90 | 1.64 |
| Col90 | 10.20 | 0.0200 | 44.06 | 16.50 | 2.12 |
| Col80 | 10.60 | 0.0190 | 51.10 | 41.90 | 2.49 |
| Col60 | 10.40 | 0.0174 | 56.28 | 48.30 | 3.05 |

TPU is an elastic body with excellent elasticity and wear resistance. It is very soft and flexible with a low modulus. After adding TPU, the values for elongation at break of

Col95, Col90, Col80, and Col60 were 8.90%, 16.50%, 41.90%, and 48.30%, respectively. The elongation at break of Col-TPU composite nanofiber membranes increased significantly with increasing TPU content. Tensile strength is commonly used to describe the external force that the composite material can bear, which in turn depends on the maximum external force for each fiber in the unit area; Col100 was 1.40 MPa. As TPU increased gradually, the tensile strength of Col95, Col90, Col80, and Col60 increased to 1.64 MPa, 2.12 MPa, 2.49 MPa, and 3.05 MPa, respectively. The tensile strengths of Col90, Col80, and Col60 were similar to the tensile strength of human tissues [42]. For instance, the native blood vessel structures in the human body, such as the left internal mammary artery (4.1–4.3 MPa), saphenous vein (1 MPa), and femoral artery (1–2 MPa), limit the burst strength to prevent rupture due to variation in blood pressure [43]. Similarly, stiffness of ECM in vivo was verified in the approximate range of 0.1 kPa (brain tissues) to 100 GPa (bone tissues) [38].

Ideal tissue repair materials are expected to have sufficient long-term mechanical properties to support tissue growth—especially scaffold materials such as tissue-engineered cartilage, bone, muscle legs, and ligaments [44]. Furthermore, the excellent elastic properties can withstand repeated dynamic loads and maintain structural stability to simulate human tissues; these properties are needed for tissue engineering applications in the heart, skin, blood vessels, and cartilage [45]. The ratio of TPU in Col-TPU composite nanofiber membranes significantly affected the mechanical properties. Col-TPU composite nanofiber membranes give the material better flexibility and can lead to close contact with the surrounding tissues after implanting the chosen tissue repair material [39]. Col-TPU composite nanofiber membranes have high strength, good anti-aging ability, and suitable flexibility in comprehensive mechanical properties. As such, Col-TPU composite nanofiber membranes can theoretically contribute to a stable environment for tissue regeneration.

*2.7. Cytocompatibility*

2.7.1. Cell Proliferation and Cytotoxicity

To evaluate the biocompatibility of Col-based composite nanofiber membranes, a CCK-8 assay was used to investigate the proliferation of MC3T3-E1 cells on Col100 and Col-TPU composite nanofiber membranes for 1, 2, and 3 days (Tables S3 and S4 as well as Figure 7G). After culturing for 3 days, all samples showed a significant difference compared to the control group with higher absorbance. The proliferation rate of all samples was higher than 164% after 3 days of culture, which was higher than that of polycaprolactone/poly composite nanofiber membranes (approximately 111%), polycaprolactone/poly/hydroxyapatite composite nanofiber membranes (approximately 112%), and silk fibroin nanofiber membranes (ranged from 83% to 90%) [46,47]. The cytotoxicity assay is also an important index reflecting the biocompatibility of fabricated materials. Specifically, the cytotoxicity of composite nanofiber membranes was grade 0, according to the ISO standard (ISO10993.12-2004). The presence of collagen on composite nanofiber membrane surfaces improved the tendency of cells to adhere to the scaffolds [48]. Col-TPU composite nanofiber membranes support cell growth.

2.7.2. Cell Morphology

The morphology of MC3T3-E1 cells cultured on Col100 and Col-TPU composite nanofiber membrane surfaces was preliminarily evaluated by SEM analysis; the cell morphology can be observed in Figure 7A–F. After 3 days of culture, the cells grew well on Col00 and Col-TPU composite nanofiber membranes and showed a natural spindle shape. Similar changes in morphology were found in Liu's research [49]. These Col-TPU composite nanofiber membranes were well distributed with increased pseudopodia and spreading area. Compared to the control group (Figure 7A), cells adhered to fibers well, thus indicating that Col-based composite nanofiber membranes can support cell adhesion and diffusion.

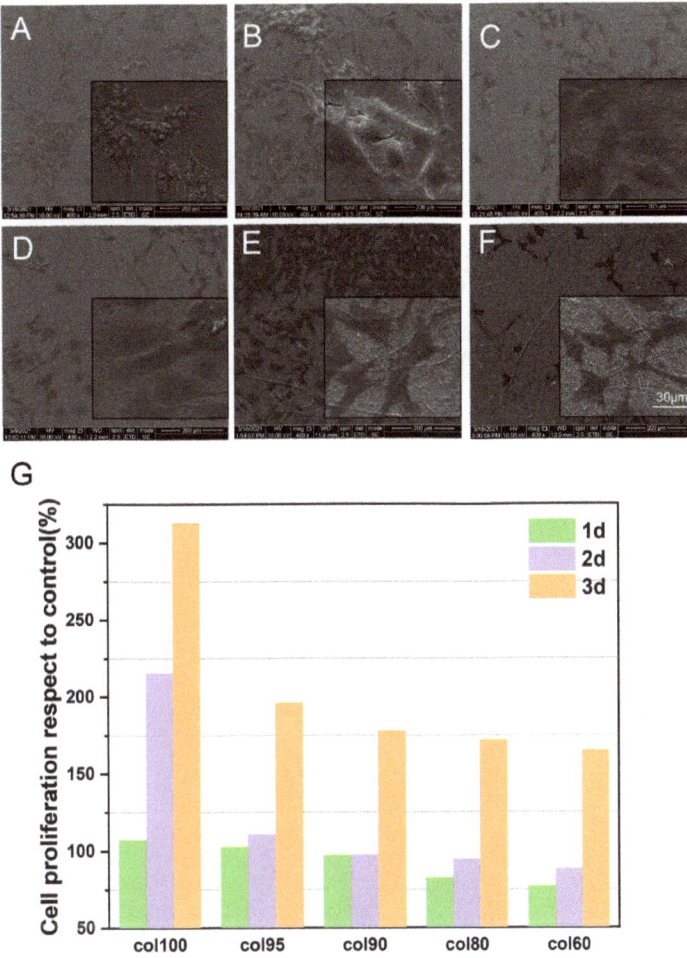

**Figure 7.** Growth of MC3T3-E1 cells on collagen-based composite nanofiber membranes. (**A**) Control; (**B**) Col100; (**C**) Col95; (**D**) Col90; (**E**) Col80; (**F**) Col60; (**G**) Cell proliferation rate.

2.7.3. Cell Adhesion

Figure 8 shows that MC3T3-E1 fibroblasts adhered and diffused evenly along the fibers inside and on the surface of the Col100 and Col-TPU composite nanofiber membranes. The cells adhered firmly with a normal and round shape, thus presenting a dense amount along the length of the fiber edges. The number of high-density cells was observed over time. There were more cells at 3 days than at 1 day, which is consistent with the CCK-8 cell proliferation assay. Few apoptotic nuclei were observed on Col100 membranes, which indicated that collagen may affect intracellular signaling and cellular responses [50]. As the collagen ratio decreased, fewer cells adhered to Col-TPU composite nanofiber membranes.

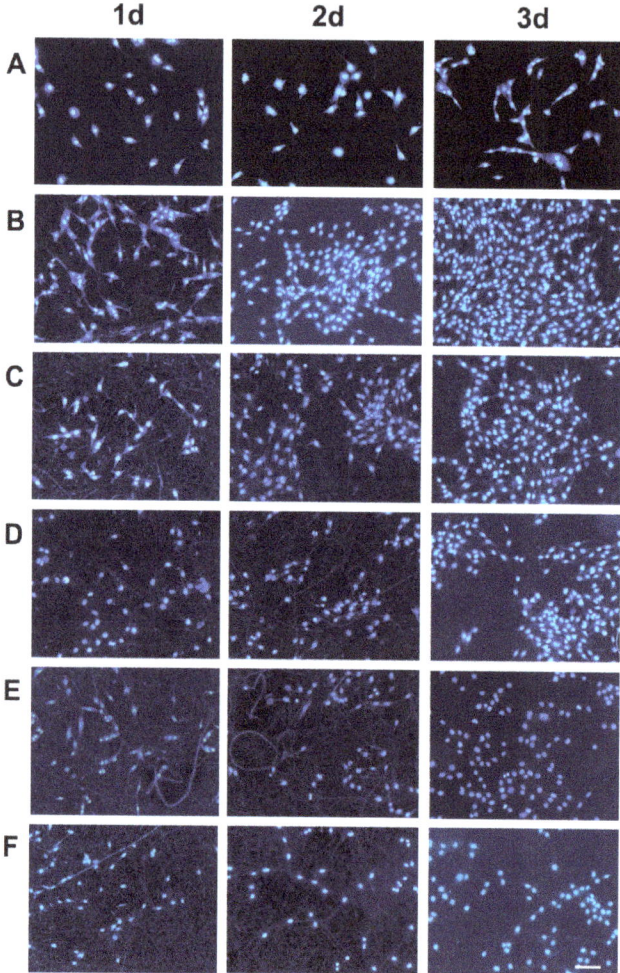

**Figure 8.** Positive fluorescence microscope scan of MC3T3-El cells on Col-based composite nanofiber membranes; scale bar is 150 μm. (**A**) Control; (**B**) Col100; (**C**) Col95; (**D**) Iol90; (**E**) Col80; (**F**) Col60.

Figures 9 and S2 show similar trends. After 3 days, there were many viable cells filled with MC3E3-E1 fibroblasts on the material's surface. Col100 was significantly better than the Col-TPU composite nanofiber membranes. The number of adherents decreased with reduced collagen proportion in the Col-TPU composite nanofiber membranes. Identifying the appropriate ratios between collagen and TPU is key to the success of the material. As a result, processed tissue engineering materials can be developed with the desired properties and biocompatibility.

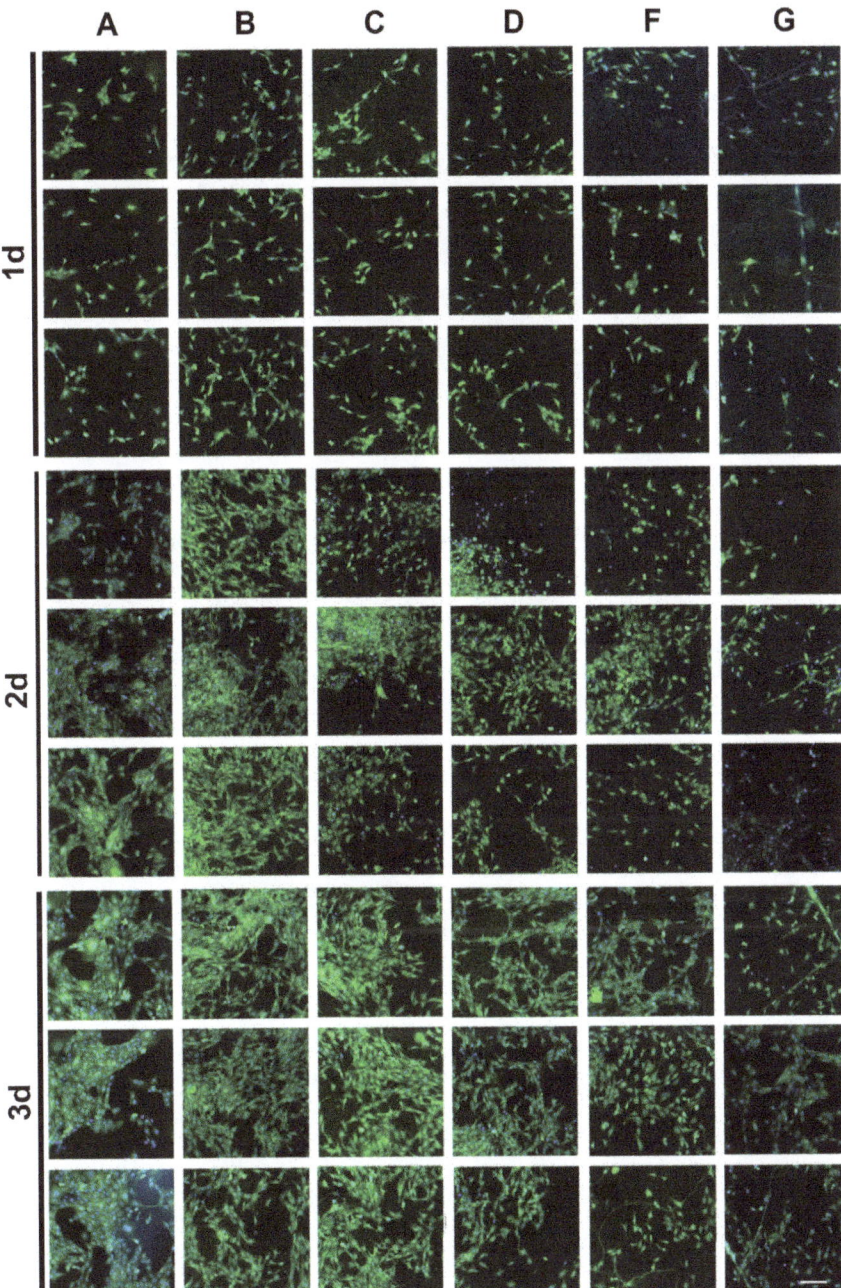

**Figure 9.** HCA scan of MC3T3-E1 cells on control and samples (green: cytoplasm; blue: nucleus); scale bar is 150 μm. (**A**) Control; (**B**) Col100; (**C**) Col95; (**D**) Col90; (**F**) Col80; (**G**) Col60.

Overall, the Col-TPU composite nanofiber membranes promoted migration and adhesion of MC3T3-E1 cells on the surface of the materials and also supported the proliferation of MC3T3-E1 cells on the surface. This result was consistent with the conclusions of similar experiments [51], thus indicating that the Col-TPU composite nanofiber membranes have good biocompatibility.

## 3. Materials and Methods

### 3.1. Materials

Tilapia (*Oreochromis nilotica*) skin was obtained from Beihai Quality Aquatic Products Co., Ltd. (Beihai, China). Type I collagen from rat tail and protein markers (26634) were purchased from Thermo Fisher Scientific (St. Louis, MO, USA). TPU was purchased from Dongguan Jiayang New Material Technology Co., Ltd (Dongguan, China). The 1,1,1,3,3,3-hexafluoro-2-propanol (HFIP) was from Sigma-Aldrich (Shanghai, China) Trading Co., Ltd. (Shanghai, China). The separating gel buffer (pH = 8.8), stacking gel buffer (pH = 6.8), sodium dodecyl sulfate (SDS), and loading buffer (5×, with DTT) were purchased from Beijing Solarbio Science & Technology Co., Ltd. (Beijing, China). Coomassie Brilliant Blue R-250 and N,N,N′,N′-tetramethylethylenediamine (TEMED) were obtained from Bio-Rad Laboratories (Hercules, CA, USA). Coomassie Brilliant Blue (CBB, R-250) was purchased from Sinopharm Chemical Reagent Co. Ltd. (Shanghai, China). Phosphate buffer solution (PBS, pH = 7.4) was purchased from Wuhan Servicebio Technology (Wuhan, China) Co. Ltd., and potassium bromide (KBr, spectral pure) powder was purchased from PIKE (Mount Airy, NC, USA). Mouse embryo osteoblast precursor (MC3T3-E1) cells (Cat No. CBP60946) were provided by Cobioer (Nanjing, China). The pression vector (LV-GFP) was synthesized by Amer Genomics Biotechnology Co., Ltd. (Xiamen, China). The cell counting kit-8 (CCK-8) was obtained from Dojindo (Beijing, China). In addition, 4′,6-diamino-2-phenylindole (DAPI) and paraformaldehyde (POM, pH = 7.4) were purchased from Solarbio (Beijing, China). All reagents were of analytical grade.

### 3.2. Preparation and Characterization of Collagen

Collagen was prepared by acid treatment according to the methods described by Li et al. [52] with slight modifications. Before preparation, the adhering residue tissues of skins were removed manually. Then, the non-collagenous proteins and pigments of skins were removed by treatment with 10 volumes of 0.1 mol/L $NaHCO_3$ for 6 h. As shown in Figure 1, the pretreated skins were soaked in 0.5 M acetic acid with a sample-to-solvent ratio of 1:40 ($w/v$) for 24 h. The extracted liquid was then centrifuged at 9000× $g$ for 30 min. The supernatant was precipitated by adding 4% NaCl, salted out for 30 min, and allowed to rest for 30 min. The resulting precipitate was collected using a freezing high-speed centrifuge (J-26 XP, Beckman Coulter Inc., Miami, FA, USA) at 9000× $g$ for 30 min. The supernatant was then discarded, and the precipitate was removed until no precipitate remained. The collection was then dissolved and redispersed at a 1:9 ($w/v$) ratio in 0.5 M acetic acid and dialyzed against 20 volumes of 0.1 M acetic acid for 24 h, followed by 24 h of dialysis with distilled water five times. Thereafter, the tilapia skin collagen was lyophilized and stored at −20 °C until further use. All of these steps were conducted at temperatures below 4 °C.

The SDS-PAGE of the sample was conducted in accordance with the method of Chen et al. [53] with slight modifications. The samples were dissolved in cold distilled water and mixed at a 4:1 $v/v$ ratio with sample loading buffer (277.8 mM Tris-HCl, pH 6.8, 44.4% ($v/v$) glycerol, 4.4% SDS, and 0.02% bromophenol blue) followed by boiling for 10 min. Next, 10 μL of samples were loaded onto a gel consisting of 8% separating gel and 3% stacking gel at a constant voltage of 110 V for electrophoresis (Bio-Rad Laboratories, Hercules, CA, USA). After electrophoresis for 90 min, the gel was soaked in 50% ($v/v$) methanol and 10% ($v/v$) acetic acid followed by staining with 0.125% CBB R-250 containing 50% ($v/v$) methanol and 10% ($v/v$) acetic acid. The gel was finally destained with a mixture of 50% ($v/v$) ethanol and 10% ($v/v$) acetic acid for 30 m. Marker 46634 was used to estimate the molecular weight of collagen, and type I collagen from rat tail was used as a standard.

## 3.3. Collagen-Based Composite Electrospun Fiber Membranes

The 4% collagen and 3% TPU were dissolved in HFIP separately in accordance with Jiang et al. [54]. A series of collagen-based composite spinning solutions were prepared with collagen and TPU solutions in different ratios (100:0, 95:5, 90:10, 80:20, 60:40) at room temperature. The spinning solutions were stirred using a magnetic stirrer (RCT digital S025, IKA, Staufen, Germany) until the solution was uniform and free of bubbles after mixing for 1 h. The mixture was then placed in a 2.5 mL syringe. The collagen-based composite electrospun fiber membranes were fabricated using an electrospinning apparatus (WL-2, Beijing Albizhi Ion Technology Co. Ltd., Beijing, China) with an applied voltage of 20 kV. The distance from the needle to the collector plate was 15 cm, and the propelling rate of the pump was 0.1 mL/h. The entire electrospinning process was conducted at room temperature at a relative humidity of 30–50%. The samples obtained from electrospinning were dried in a desiccator overnight to remove any residual organic solvent until use.

## 3.4. Structural Analysis of Col-TPU Nanofiber Membranes

### 3.4.1. SEM

The morphology of the collagen-based composite electrospun fiber membranes was visualized using a scanning electron microscope (Quanta 450, FEI, Hillsboro, OR, USA). The sample was fixed on the sample platform with conductive adhesive, and sputtered with a gold coating for 30 s. The images were captured with SEM, with an accelerating voltage of 5–10 kV. The average nanofiber diameter of each sample was randomly measured using ImageJ (version 1.8.0, National Institute of Health, Bethesda, OR, USA) software in parallel three times by calculating the average and standard deviation per micrograph with more than 50 counts per image.

### 3.4.2. FTIR

The infrared spectra of the samples were obtained with a Bruker FTIR spectrophotometer (Tensor27, Bruker, Madison, Germany) at room temperature. The samples were mixed with KBr by grinding at the ratio of 1:100 ($w/w$). The wavelength range was 4000-400 cm$^{-1}$ with a resolution of 4 cm$^{-1}$. The signals were collected automatically over 32 scans and ratioed against a background spectrum recorded from KBr. The secondary structure of the samples was then analyzed with OMNIC$^{TM}$ software (Version 8.2, Thermo Nicolet Corporation, Madison, WI, USA) and PeakFit software (Version 4.12, Systat Software Inc., San Jose, CA, USA).

### 3.4.3. XRD

The diffractograms of the samples were recorded with an X-ray diffractometer (X'Pert Pro XRD, PANalytical, The Netherlands) operating at 40 kV and 25 mA with CuKα radiation ($\lambda$ = 1.5418 Å). The data were collected at a scanning speed of $10°·\text{min}^{-1}$ and a 2θ range of 5–90°.

## 3.5. DSC

The DSC curves were obtained using a DSC instrument (DSC 204 F1, Netzsch, Selb, Bavaria, Germany) and the method reported by Kun et al. [55]. A certain amount of the samples (approximately 2–5 mg) were loaded into the bottom of an aluminum crucible and pressed with a lid. The samples were then transferred to the DSC instrument. During DSC scanning, the sample was cooled quickly with liquid nitrogen to $-60\ °C$ from room temperature and then heated to 200 °C at a heating rate of 10 °C/min in nitrogen atmosphere (purge flow of 50 mL/min and protective flow of 70 mL/min). Indium metal standard was used for temperature calibration.

## 3.6. Thermal Stability

The thermogravimetric analysis was conducted according to the methods described by Krishnakumar et al. [56] with some modifications. Thermogravimetric analysis (TGA2,

Mettler Toledo Co. Ltd., Shanghai, China) used continuous nitrogen (flow rate 50 mL/min) in the sample chamber. Approximately 1 mg of the sample was placed in a crucible and pressed to create complete contact followed by sequential heating from 20 °C to 600 °C at a constant heating rate of 10 °C/min; the thermogravimetric data at the first heating curve were then recorded.

### 3.7. WCA

The static water contact angle was recorded following the protocol reported by Lalia et al. [57]. The WCA of all samples was studied with a video optical contact angle measurement instrument (OCA15EC, DataPhysics, Filderstadt, Germany) and the sessile drop method. The samples were fixed on a glass slide, and deionized water (2 µL) was dispensed slowly onto the surface with a water rate of 5 µL/s. The water contact angle was measured at 3 s, and five different sites were measured from each sample to determine the uniform distribution of the samples. The images and calculation of the angle of the drop contact surface on both sides were recorded and analyzed with SCA20 (DataPhysics, Filderstadt, Germany) software.

### 3.8. Mechanical Properties

Sample mechanical properties were measured using a uniaxial tensile test according to the methods described by Zhu et al. [58]. Samples were trimmed into 1 cm × 5 cm strips, and both ends (1 cm on each side) of the samples were gripped by the fiber tensile tester (XQ−1C, New Fiber Instrument Co. Ltd., Shanghai, China). Material stress–strain curves were obtained through load deformation. The data were recorded by measuring the tensile strength and elongation at break at a tensile speed of 20 mm/min.

### 3.9. Cytocompatibility

#### 3.9.1. Cell Proliferation

The proliferation evaluation of samples on MC3T3-E1 (Cat No. CBP60946) cells lines used a CCK-8 assay as reported by Yuan et al. [59] with slight modifications. The Col-TPU composite nanofiber membranes were spun on 14 mm-diameter round coverslips. Before culturing, samples were soaked in 75% ethanol for 30 min and UV-sterilized for 1 h. Subsequently, the samples were placed in a 24-well culture plate. After sterilization with 75% ethanol for 30 min, cells were rinsed three times with sterilized PBS solution (0.1 M) and cultured in Roswell Park Memorial Institute (RPMI)−1640 medium (Gibco, CA, USA) containing 10% fetal bovine serum (FBS) and 1% penicillin-streptomycin mixture (100 unit/mL penicillin, 100 µg/mL streptomycin) (Solarbio, Beijing, China). The cell density of MC3T3-E1 cells was adjusted to $1 \times 10^4$ cells/well and seeded onto the samples cultured in the 24-well plate. The cells were cultured in a cell incubator with an atmosphere of 5% $CO_2$ at 37 °C (HERAcell 150i, Thermo Scientific, Waltham, MA, USA). The CCK-8 solution was added to each well at 1, 2, and 3 days after culture. The optical densities of each well were measured using a multi-function microporous plate analyzer (Mithras2 LB 943, Berthold, Germany). The 14 mm-diameter round coverslips with no samples were used as the control; wells with no samples or coverslips were used as the blank; and the cell proliferation was calculated as follows:

$$\text{Cell proliferation (\%)} = A_s - A_0/A_c - A_0 \times 100\%, \tag{1}$$

where $A_c$, $A_s$, and $A_b$ were the absorbance at 450 nm of the control group, the experimental group, and the blank group, respectively.

#### 3.9.2. Cell Morphology

Samples containing cultured MC3T3-E1 were immobilized in 2.5% POM for 3 days after inoculation. Before observation, the samples were washed with PBS and then washed with distilled water at least three times. Finally, all samples were gold-sputtered before cell morphologies were examined using SEM.

### 3.9.3. Cell Adhesion

After 1, 2, and 3 days of cell inoculation, the MC3T3-E1 cells were fixed with 2.5% glutaraldehyde at pH = 7.4. During observation, the sample was washed with PBS three times for 5 min each, and the excess water was absorbed by the filter paper. After removal, the cells were inverted with 10 μL of DAPI and stained for 5 min. The adhesion of cells was observed with a laser scanning confocal microscope (LSCM) (TCSSP5, Leica Microsystems, Heerbrugg, Germany) or a positive fluorescence microscope (Axio Imager A2, ZEISS, Oberkochen, Germany). After 3 days of cell inoculation, the cells were fixed in 5% POM, and cell growth was observed using an automatic Cellomics Arrayscan (VTI-HCS, Thermo Scientific, Waltham, MA, USA).

### 3.10. Statistical Analyses

The analysis of variance was calculated using SPSS Version 17.0 software (IBM SPSS Statistics, Ehningen, Germany), and a value of $p < 0.05$ was used to indicate a significant deviation. Different letters indicate significant differences between samples.

## 4. Conclusions

In this study, collagen was extracted from tilapia fish skin and identified as type I collagen by SDS-PAGE. A series of Col-TPU composite nanofiber membranes (Col95, Col90, Col80, and Col60) were prepared via electrospinning and shown to be stable and have a nanostructure. There was relatively good compatibility between collagen and TPU. Besides maintaining the triple-helical structures of collagen, the addition of TPU enhanced the porosity, thermal stability, and mechanical properties of the composite. Thus, it was found to be more suitable for human tissue environments for long-term growth. In vitro fibroblast culture demonstrated a high cell proliferation rate with no cytotoxicity. The Col-TPU composite nanofiber membrane allowed the proliferation and migration of MC3T3-E1 cells and promoted fibrogenesis of cells; there was good biocompatibility. These results suggested that Col-TPU composite materials with different ratios of TPU were candidate biomaterials for tissue repair.

**Supplementary Materials:** The following supporting information can be downloaded at: https://www.mdpi.com/article/10.3390/md20070437/s1, Figure S1: HCA scan of Col-TPU composite nanofiber membranes, scale bar is 150 μm; Table S1: Comparison of Col-TPU composite nanofiber membranes different spectral peak positions in FTIR spectra; Table S2: The thermogravimetric analysis of Col-TPU composite nanofiber membranes; Table S3: CCK-8 assay $OD_{450}$ of Col-TPU composite nanofiber membranes. The sequence of letters a–d represents the size of the mean value ($a > b > c > d$). The same letter indicates no statistically significant difference ($p < 0.05$, $n = 4$); Table S4: Cell proliferation and cytotoxicity evaluation of Col-TPU composite nanofiber membranes respect to control, % and grade.

**Author Contributions:** J.C. conceptualization, validation, resources, writing—review and editing, supervision, project administration, funding acquisition; S.W. conceptualization, methodology, formal analysis, data curation, writing—original draft preparation; L.Y. conceptualization, methodology, software, formal analysis, data curation. All authors have read and agreed to the published version of the manuscript.

**Funding:** This research was funded by the National Natural Science Foundation of China, grant number 42076120, 41676129, 41106149; Scientific Research Foundation of the Third Institute of Oceanography, SOA, grant number 2019010, 2019016; The APC was funded by the Scientific Research Foundation of the Third Institute of Oceanography, SOA, grant number 2019016.

**Institutional Review Board Statement:** Not applicable.

**Data Availability Statement:** Data is contained within the article or Supplementary Materials.

**Conflicts of Interest:** The authors declare no conflict of interest.

## References

1. Hart, D.A.; Nakamura, N.; Shrive, N.G. Perspective: Challenges presented for regeneration of heterogeneous musculoskeletal tissues that normally develop in unique biomechanical environments. *Front. Bioeng. Biotechnol.* **2021**, *9*, 760273. [CrossRef] [PubMed]
2. Shekhter, A.B.; Fayzullin, A.L.; Vukolova, M.N.; Rudenko, T.G.; Osipycheva, V.D.; Litvitsky, P.F. Medical applications of collagen and collagen-based materials. *Curr. Med. Chem.* **2019**, *26*, 506–516. [CrossRef]
3. Mohammadalizadeh, Z.; Bahremandi-Toloue, E.; Karbasi, S. Synthetic-based blended electrospun scaffolds in tissue engineering applications. *J. Mater. Sci.* **2022**, *57*, 4020–4079. [CrossRef]
4. Dorthe, E.W.; Williams, A.B.; Grogan, S.P.; D'Lima, D.D. Pneumatospinning biomimetic scaffolds for meniscus tissue engineering. *Front. Bioeng. Biotechnol.* **2022**, *10*, 810705. [CrossRef] [PubMed]
5. Law, J.X.; Liau, L.L.; Saim, A.; Yang, Y.; Idrus, R. Electrospun collagen nanofibers and their applications in skin tissue engineering. *Tissue Eng. Regener. Med.* **2017**, *14*, 699–718. [CrossRef] [PubMed]
6. Acheson, D.; MacKnight, C. Clinical implications of bovine spongiform encephalopathy. *Clin. Infect. Dis.* **2019**, *32*, 1726–1731. [CrossRef]
7. Wang, L.; Zou, Y.F.; Jiang, S.; Xu, J.M.; Jiang, S.H.; Hu, Q.H. Chromatographic separation and physicochemical properties of collagen species in the skin of deep-sea redfish (*Sebastes mentella*). *Food Hydrocoll.* **2011**, *25*, 1134–1138. [CrossRef]
8. Chen, J.D.; Wang, G.Y.; Li, Y.S. Preparation and characterization of thermally stable collagens from the scales of lizardfish (*Synodus macrops*). *Mar. Drugs* **2021**, *19*, 597. [CrossRef]
9. Yunoki, S.; Hatayama, H.; Ohyabu, Y.; Kobayashi, K. Fibril matrices created with collagen from the marine fish barramundi for use in conventional three-dimensional cell culture. *Int. J. Biol. Macromol.* **2022**, *203*, 361–368. [CrossRef]
10. Huang, R.Q.; Chen, S.W.; Ma, G.Z.; Yang, B.W.; Guo, R.J.; Li, Q.X.; Zhong, J.Y. Research on the extraction of collagen from scales of tilapia. *Adv. Mater. Res.* **2011**, *295–297*, 796–799. [CrossRef]
11. Liu, C.W.; Hsieh, C.Y.; Chen, J.Y. Investigations on the wound healing potential of tilapia piscidin (TP)2-5 and TP2-6. *Mar. Drugs* **2022**, *20*, 205. [CrossRef] [PubMed]
12. Ge, B.S.; Wang, H.N.; Li, J.; Liu, H.H.; Yin, Y.H.; Zhang, N.L.; Qin, S. Comprehensive assessment of nile tilapia skin (*Oreochromis niloticus*) collagen hydrogels for wound dressings. *Mar. Drugs* **2020**, *18*, 178. [CrossRef] [PubMed]
13. Jin, L.; Zheng, D.X.; Yang, G.Y.; Li, W.; Yang, H.; Jiang, Q.; Chen, Y.J.; Zhang, Y.X.; Xie, X. Tilapia skin peptides ameliorate diabetic nephropathy in STZ-induced diabetic rats and HG-induced GMCs by Improving mitochondrial dysfunction. *Mar. Drugs* **2020**, *18*, 363. [CrossRef]
14. Jin, S.; Sun, F.; Zou, Q.; Huang, J.H.; Zuo, Y.; Li, Y.B.; Wang, S.P.; Cheng, L.; Man, Y.; Yang, F.; et al. Fish collagen and hydroxyapatite reinforced poly(lactide-co-glycolide) fibrous membrane for guided bone regeneration. *Biomacromolecules* **2019**, *20*, 2058–2067. [CrossRef]
15. He, X.L.; Wang, L.; Lv, K.N.; Li, W.J.; Qin, S.; Tang, Z.H. Polyethylene oxide assisted fish collagen-poly-epsilon-caprolactone nanofiber membranes by electrospinning. *Biomacromolecules* **2022**, *12*, 900. [CrossRef]
16. Zhou, T.; Sui, B.Y.; Mo, X.M.; Sun, J. Multifunctional and biomimetic fish collagen/bioactive glass nanofibers: Fabrication, antibacterial activity and inducing skin regeneration in vitro and in vivo. *Int. J. Nanomed.* **2017**, *12*, 3495–3507. [CrossRef] [PubMed]
17. Xu, Z.C.; Wang, X.Y.; Huang, H. Thermoplastic polyurethane–urea elastomers with superior mechanical and thermal properties prepared from alicyclic diisocyanate and diamine. *J. Appl. Polym. Sci.* **2020**, *137*, 49575. [CrossRef]
18. Tatai, L.; Moore, T.G.; Adhikari, R.; Malherbe, F.; Jayasekara, R.; Griffiths, I.; Gunatillake, P.A. Thermoplastic biodegradable polyurethanes: The effect of chain extender structure on properties and in-vitro degradation. *Biomaterials* **2007**, *28*, 5407–5417. [CrossRef]
19. Enayati, M.; Eilenberg, M.; Grasl, C.; Riedl, P.; Kaun, C.; Messner, B.; Walter, I.; Liska, R.; Schima, H.; Wojta, J.; et al. Biocompatibility assessment of a new biodegradable vascular graft via in vitro co-culture approaches and in vivo model. *Ann. Biomed. Eng.* **2016**, *44*, 3319–3334. [CrossRef]
20. Xu, C.C.; Hong, Y. Rational design of biodegradable thermoplastic polyurethanes for tissue repair. *Bioact. Mater.* **2022**, *15*, 250–271. [CrossRef]
21. Lee, J.K.; Kang, S.I.; Kim, Y.J.; Kim, M.J.; Heu, M.S.; Choi, B.D.; Kim, J.S. Comparison of collagen characteristics of sea- and freshwater-rainbow trout skin. *Food Sci. Biotechnol.* **2016**, *25*, 131–136. [CrossRef] [PubMed]
22. Gaspar-Pintiliescu, A.; Anton, E.D.; Iosageanu, A.; Berger, D.; Matei, C.; Mitran, R.A.; Negreanu-Pirjol, T.; Craciunescu, O.; Moldovan, L. Enhanced wound healing activity of undenatured type I collagen isolated from discarded skin of black sea gilthead bream (*Sparus aurata*) conditioned as 3d porous dressing. *Chem. Biodivers.* **2021**, *18*, e2100293. [CrossRef] [PubMed]
23. Abbas, A.A.; Shakir, K.A.; Walsh, M.K. Functional properties of collagen extracted from catfish (*Silurus triostegus*) waste. *Foods* **2022**, *11*, 633. [CrossRef] [PubMed]
24. Sun, L.C.; Du, H.; Wen, J.X.; Zhong, C.; Liu, G.M.; Miao, S.; Cao, M.J. Physicochemical properties of acid-soluble collagens from different tissues of large yellow croaker (*Larimichthys crocea*). *Int. J. Food Sci. Technol.* **2021**, *56*, 5371–5381. [CrossRef]
25. Fang, H.; Zhang, L.J.; Chen, A.L.; Wu, F.J. Improvement of mechanical property for PLA/TPU blend by adding pla-tpu copolymers prepared via in situ ring-opening polymerization. *Polymers* **2022**, *14*, 1530. [CrossRef]

26. Džunuzović, J.V.; Stefanović, I.S.; Džunuzović, E.S.; Dapčević, A.; Šešlija, S.I.; Balanč, B.D.; Lama, G.C. Polyurethane networks based on polycaprolactone and hyperbranched polyester: Structural, thermal and mechanical investigation. *Prog. Org. Coat.* **2019**, *137*, 105305. [CrossRef]
27. Chen, J.D.; Li, L.; Yi, R.Z.; Xu, N.H.; Gao, R.; Hong, B.H. Extraction and characterization of acid-soluble collagen from scales and skin of tilapia (*Oreochromis niloticus*). *LWT-Food Sci. Technol.* **2016**, *66*, 453–459. [CrossRef]
28. Jalan, A.; Kastner, D.W.; Webber, K.G.I.; Smith, M.S.; Price, J.L.; Castle, S.L. Bulky dehydroamino acids enhance proteolytic stability and folding in beta-hairpin peptides. *Org. Lett.* **2017**, *19*, 5190–5193. [CrossRef]
29. Lin, T.A.; Lin, J.-H.; Bao, L. A study of reusability assessment and thermal behaviors for thermoplastic composite materials after melting process: Polypropylene/thermoplastic polyurethane blends. *J. Clean. Prod.* **2021**, *279*, 123473. [CrossRef]
30. Pei, Y.; Jordan, K.E.; Xiang, N.; Parker, R.N.; Mu, X.; Zhang, L.; Feng, Z.B.; Chen, Y.; Li, C.M.; Guo, C.C.; et al. Liquid-exfoliated mesostructured collagen from the bovine achilles tendon as building blocks of collagen membranes. *ACS Appl. Mater. Interfaces* **2021**, *13*, 3186–3198. [CrossRef]
31. Fang, C.Q.; Yang, R.; Zhang, Z.S.; Zhou, X.; Lei, W.Q.; Cheng, Y.L.; Zhang, W.; Wang, D. Effect of multi-walled carbon nanotubes on the physical properties and crystallisation of recycled PET/TPU composites. *RSC Adv.* **2018**, *8*, 8920–8928. [CrossRef] [PubMed]
32. Liu, J.; Zhang, L.; Ci, M.Y.; Sui, S.Y.; Zhu, P. Study on the rheological properties of regenerated cellulose/thermoplastic polyurethane blend spinning solutions. *Ferroelectrics* **2020**, *562*, 104–113. [CrossRef]
33. Lopes, M.S.; Catelani, T.A.; Nascimento, A.L.; Garcia, J.S.; Trevisan, M.G. Ketoconazole: Compatibility with pharmaceutical excipients using DSC and TG techniques. *J. Therm. Anal. Calorim.* **2019**, *141*, 1371–1378. [CrossRef]
34. Yehia, A.A.; Mansour, A.A.; Stoll, B. Detection of compatibility of some rubber blends by DSC. *J. Therm. Anal. Calorim.* **1997**, *48*, 1299–1310. [CrossRef]
35. Frick, A.; Rochman, A. Characterization of TPU-elastomers by thermal analysis (DSC). *Polym. Test.* **2004**, *23*, 413–417. [CrossRef]
36. Saha, P.; Khomlaem, C.; Aloui, H.; Kim, B.S. Biodegradable polyurethanes based on castor oil and poly (3-hydroxybutyrate). *Polymers* **2021**, *13*, 1387. [CrossRef]
37. Bacakova, L.; Filova, E.; Parizek, M.; Ruml, T.; Svorcik, V. Modulation of cell adhesion, proliferation and differentiation on materials designed for body implants. *Biotechnol. Adv.* **2011**, *29*, 739–767. [CrossRef]
38. Jing, X.; Li, X.; Jiang, Y.F.; Zhao, R.H.; Ding, Q.J.; Han, W.J. Excellent coating of collagen fiber/chitosan-based materials that is water- and oil-resistant and fluorine-free. *Carbohydr. Polym.* **2021**, *266*, 118173. [CrossRef]
39. Chen, L.; Yan, C.; Zheng, Z. Functional polymer surfaces for controlling cell behaviors. *Mater. Today* **2018**, *21*, 38–59. [CrossRef]
40. Cui, Y.; Yang, Y.; Qiu, D. Design of selective cell migration biomaterials and their applications for tissue regeneration. *J. Mater. Sci.* **2020**, *56*, 4080–4096. [CrossRef]
41. Arhant, M.; Gall, M.L.; Gac, P.-Y.L. Fracture test to accelerate the prediction of polymer embrittlement during aging-case of PET hydrolysis. *Polym. Degrad. Stab.* **2022**, *196*, 109848. [CrossRef]
42. Hasan, A.; Memic, A.; Annabi, N.; Hossain, M.; Paul, A.; Dokmeci, M.R.; Dehghani, F.; Khademhosseini, A. Electrospun scaffolds for tissue engineering of vascular grafts. *Acta Biomater.* **2014**, *10*, 11–25. [CrossRef] [PubMed]
43. Assanah, F.; Khan, Y. Cell responses to physical forces, and how they inform the design of tissue-engineered constructs for bone repair: A review. *J. Mater. Sci.* **2018**, *53*, 5618–5640. [CrossRef]
44. Hasan, A.; Ragaert, K.; Swieszkowski, W.; Selimovic, S.; Paul, A.; Camci-Unal, G.; Mofrad, M.R.; Khademhosseini, A. Biomechanical properties of native and tissue engineered heart valve constructs. *J. Biomech.* **2014**, *47*, 1949–1963. [CrossRef] [PubMed]
45. Richardson, B.M.; Walker, C.J.; Maples, M.M.; Randolph, M.A.; Bryant, S.J.; Anseth, K.S. Mechanobiological interactions between dynamic compressive loading and viscoelasticity on chondrocytes in hydrazone covalent adaptable networks for cartilage tissue engineering. *Adv. Healthc. Mater.* **2021**, *10*, 2002030. [CrossRef] [PubMed]
46. Fang, R.; Zhang, E.W.; Xu, L.; Wei, S.C. Electrospun PCL/PLA/HA based nanofibers as scaffold for osteoblast-like cells. *J. Nanosci. Nanotechnol.* **2010**, *10*, 7747–7751. [CrossRef]
47. Zheng, X.; Ke, X.; Yu, P.; Wang, D.Q.; Pan, S.Y.; Yang, J.J.; Ding, C.M.; Xiao, S.M.; Luo, J.; Li, J.S. A facile strategy to construct silk fibroin based GTR membranes with appropriate mechanical performance and enhanced osteogenic capacity. *J. Mater. Chem. B* **2020**, *8*, 10407–10415. [CrossRef]
48. Zhang, Q.; Lv, S.; Lu, J.F.; Jiang, S.T.; Lin, L. Characterization of polycaprolactone/collagen fibrous scaffolds by electrospinning and their bioactivity. *Int. J. Biol. Macromol.* **2015**, *76*, 94–101. [CrossRef]
49. Liu, H.; Liu, W.J.; Luo, B.H.; Wen, W.; Liu, M.X.; Wang, X.Y.; Zhou, C.R. Electrospun composite nanofiber membrane of poly(l-lactide) and surface grafted chitin whiskers: Fabrication, mechanical properties and cytocompatibility. *Carbohydr. Polym.* **2016**, *147*, 216–225. [CrossRef]
50. Zarei, M.; Samimi, A.; Khorram, M.; Abdi, M.M.; Golestaneh, S.I. Fabrication and characterization of conductive polypyrrole/chitosan/collagen electrospun nanofiber scaffold for tissue engineering application. *Int. J. Biol. Macromol.* **2021**, *168*, 175–186. [CrossRef]
51. Bian, T.R.; Zhang, H.; Xing, H.Y. Preparation and biological properties of collagen/nano-hydroxyapatite composite nanofibers based on ordered nano-hydroxyapatite ceramic fibers. *Colloids Surf. A Physicochem. Eng. Asp.* **2020**, *602*, 124802. [CrossRef]
52. Li, L.Y.; Zhao, Y.Q.; He, Y.; Chi, C.F.; Wang, B. Physicochemical and antioxidant properties of acid- and pepsin-soluble collagens from the scales of miiuy croaker (*Miichthys miiuy*). *Mar. Drugs* **2018**, *16*, 394. [CrossRef] [PubMed]

53. Chen, J.D.; Li, L.; Yi, R.Z.; Gao, R.; He, J.L. Release kinetics of tilapia scale collagen I peptides during tryptic hydrolysis. *Food Hydrocoll.* **2018**, *77*, 931–936. [CrossRef]
54. Jiang, L.; Jiang, Y.C.; Stiadle, J.; Wang, X.F.; Wang, L.X.; Li, Q.; Shen, C.Y.; Thibeault, S.L.; Turng, L.S. Electrospun nanofibrous thermoplastic polyurethane/poly(Glycerol sebacate) hybrid scaffolds for vocal fold tissue engineering applications. *Mater. Sci. Eng. C* **2019**, *94*, 740–749. [CrossRef]
55. Cong, K.; He, J.Y.; Yang, R.J. Using twin screw extrusion reaction (TSER) to produce thermoplastic polyurethane (TPU): Tunable, stoichiometric and eco-friendly. *Polym. Adv. Technol.* **2021**, *32*, 3495–3504. [CrossRef]
56. Krishnakumar, G.S.; Gostynska, N.; Dapporto, M.; Campodoni, E.; Montesi, M.; Panseri, S.; Tampieri, A.; Kon, E.; Marcacci, M.; Sprio, S.; et al. Evaluation of different crosslinking agents on hybrid biomimetic collagen-hydroxyapatite composites for regenerative medicine. *Int. J. Biol. Macromol.* **2018**, *106*, 739–748. [CrossRef]
57. Lalia, B.S.; Janajreh, I.; Hashaikeh, R. A facile approach to fabricate superhydrophobic membranes with low contact angle hysteresis. *J. Membr. Sci.* **2017**, *539*, 144–151. [CrossRef]
58. Zhu, Z.G.; Wang, W.; Qi, D.P.; Luo, Y.F.; Liu, Y.R.; Xu, Y.; Cui, F.Y.; Wang, C.; Chen, X.D. Calcinable polymer membrane with revivability for efficient oily-water remediation. *Adv. Mater.* **2018**, *30*, 1801870. [CrossRef]
59. Yuan, M.Q.; Dai, F.F.; Li, D.; Fan, Y.Q.; Xiang, W.; Tao, F.H.; Cheng, Y.X.; Deng, H.B. Lysozyme/collagen multilayers layer-by-layer deposited nanofibers with enhanced biocompatibility and antibacterial activity. *Mater. Sci. Eng. C* **2020**, *112*, 110868. [CrossRef]

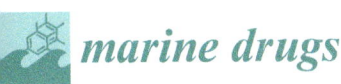

Article

# A Novel Gelatinase from Marine *Flocculibacter collagenilyticus* SM1988: Characterization and Potential Application in Collagen Oligopeptide-Rich Hydrolysate Preparation

Jian Li [1,2], Jun-Hui Cheng [2], Zhao-Jie Teng [2], Xia Zhang [3], Xiu-Lan Chen [2], Mei-Ling Sun [4], Jing-Ping Wang [2], Yu-Zhong Zhang [4], Jun-Mei Ding [5,*], Xin-Min Tian [1,*] and Xi-Ying Zhang [2,*]

1. Xinjiang Key Laboratory of Biological Resources and Genetic Engineering, College of Life Science and Technology, Xinjiang University, Urumqi 830046, China; fighter1216217564@163.com
2. State Key Laboratory of Microbial Technology, Marine Biotechnology Research Center, Institute of Marine Science and Technology, Shandong University, Qingdao 250100, China; 201820299@mail.sdu.edu.cn (J.-H.C.); tengpaper@163.com (Z.-J.T.); cxl0423@sdu.edu.cn (X.-L.C.); jp1120714999@163.com (J.-P.W.)
3. Department of Molecular Biology, Qingdao Vland Biotech Inc., Qingdao 266102, China; zhangx@vlandgroup.com
4. College of Marine Life Sciences, and Frontiers Science Center for Deep Ocean Multispheres and Earth System, Ocean University of China, Qingdao 266003, China; sunml1990@yeah.net (M.-L.S.); zhangyz@sdu.edu.cn (Y.-Z.Z.)
5. Engineering Research Center of Sustainable Development and Utilization of Biomass Energy, Ministry of Education, Yunnan Normal University, Kunming 650500, China
* Correspondence: djm3417@163.com (J.-M.D.); tianxm06@lzu.edu.cn (X.-M.T.); zhangxiying@sdu.edu.cn (X.-Y.Z.)

**Citation:** Li, J.; Cheng, J.-H.; Teng, Z.-J.; Zhang, X.; Chen, X.-L.; Sun, M.-L.; Wang, J.-P.; Zhang, Y.-Z.; Ding, J.-M.; Tian, X.-M.; et al. A Novel Gelatinase from Marine *Flocculibacter collagenilyticus* SM1988: Characterization and Potential Application in Collagen Oligopeptide-Rich Hydrolysate Preparation. *Mar. Drugs* 2022, 20, 48. https://doi.org/10.3390/md20010048

Academic Editor: Sik Yoon

Received: 6 December 2021
Accepted: 30 December 2021
Published: 3 January 2022

**Publisher's Note:** MDPI stays neutral with regard to jurisdictional claims in published maps and institutional affiliations.

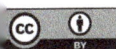

**Copyright:** © 2022 by the authors. Licensee MDPI, Basel, Switzerland. This article is an open access article distributed under the terms and conditions of the Creative Commons Attribution (CC BY) license (https://creativecommons.org/licenses/by/4.0/).

**Abstract:** Although the S8 family in the MEROPS database contains many peptidases, only a few S8 peptidases have been applied in the preparation of bioactive oligopeptides. Bovine bone collagen is a good source for preparing collagen oligopeptides, but has been so far rarely applied in collagen peptide preparation. Here, we characterized a novel S8 gelatinase, Aa2_1884, from marine bacterium *Flocculibacter collagenilyticus* SM1988$^T$, and evaluated its potential application in the preparation of collagen oligopeptides from bovine bone collagen. Aa2_1884 is a multimodular S8 peptidase with a distinct domain architecture from other reported peptidases. The recombinant Aa2_1884 over-expressed in *Escherichia coli* showed high activity toward gelatin and denatured collagens, but no activity toward natural collagens, indicating that Aa2_1884 is a gelatinase. To evaluate the potential of Aa2_1884 in the preparation of collagen oligopeptides from bovine bone collagen, three enzymatic hydrolysis parameters, hydrolysis temperature, hydrolysis time and enzyme-substrate ratio (E/S), were optimized by single factor experiments, and the optimal hydrolysis conditions were determined to be reaction at 60 °C for 3 h with an E/S of 400 U/g. Under these conditions, the hydrolysis efficiency of bovine bone collagen by Aa2_1884 reached 95.3%. The resultant hydrolysate contained 97.8% peptides, in which peptides with a molecular weight lower than 1000 Da and 500 Da accounted for 55.1% and 39.5%, respectively, indicating that the hydrolysate was rich in oligopeptides. These results indicate that Aa2_1884 likely has a promising potential application in the preparation of collagen oligopeptide-rich hydrolysate from bovine bone collagen, which may provide a feasible way for the high-value utilization of bovine bone collagen.

**Keywords:** peptidase; the MEROPS S8 family; bovine bone collagen; oligopeptides; hydrolysate

## 1. Introduction

Bioactive oligopeptides are referred to peptides that consist of 2–20 amino acids, which have various bioactivities [1]. In addition to being efficient amino acid sources, bioactive oligopeptides have been reported to possess many physiological functions and attractive physic properties in pharmacy (e.g., anticancer, antimicrobial, antihypertensive and anti-inflammatory activities, anticoagulant, and immunomodulatory), foods (gelling activity and emulsifying property), cosmetic (antioxidant and water holding capacity), and other functional products (foaming ability and hydrophobicity) [2–5]. In recent years, collagen oligopeptides attract more and more attention due to their various bioactive properties, such as angiotensin I converting enzyme (ACE) inhibitory activity, antioxidant activity, immunomodulatory and antimicrobial activities [6–9], and beneficial effects on human health, including improving skin health, muscle strength, and bone density [10–12], and reducing obesity, joint pain, and blood pressure [13–15]. Collagen oligopeptides have been widely applied in food, cosmetics, healthcare, and pharmaceutical industries [16–18].

Enzymatic hydrolysis is now the common method to prepare collagen bioactive peptides from collagen-rich animal tissues, such as skin, bones, tendons, and ligaments. Nowadays, the common enzymes for preparing collagen bioactive peptides are proteases from plants, animals, and bacteria, such as serine proteases alcalase of the MEROPS S8 family and trypsin and α-chymotrypsin of the MEROPS S1 family, aspartic protease pepsin of the MEROPS A1 family, cysteine protease papain of the MEROPS C1 family, and metalloprotease thermolysin of the MEROPS M4 family [6,19–22]. The S8 family is the second largest family of serine proteases after the S1 family [23]. In the S8 family, many members have activity on gelatin, the denatured form of collagen, and some are collagenolytic proteases, such as the thermostable protease from *Geobacillus collagenovorans* MO-1 [24], MCP-01 from *Pseudoalteromonas* sp. SM9913 [25], myroicolsin from *Myroides profundi* D25 [26], and P57 from *Photobacterium* sp. A5-7 [27]. Due to their activity on natural or denatured collagen, these S8 peptidases may have potentials in collagen oligopeptide preparation. However, only a few S8 peptidases have been used in preparing collagen oligopeptides, or their potentials have been evaluated. In addition to alcalase that are from *Bacillus* and have been used in collagen oligopeptide preparation [28], MCP-01 has also been shown to have a potential in preparing collagen bioactive peptides from codfish skin [7]. It is still necessary to identify more S8 peptidases suitable for preparing collagen bioactive peptides.

Recently, we isolated and identified a novel marine bacterium *Flocculibacter collagenilyticus* SM1988$^T$ (hereafter SM1988) that has a high collagenase production [29]. According to the genome and secretome analyses of this strain, Aa2_1884 was the most abundant of the 6 secreted S8 proteases and was predicted to be a potential collagenase [29]. The aim of this study was to characterize Aa2_1884 and to evaluate its potential in preparing collagen bioactive peptides. In this study, Aa2_1884 was expressed in *Escherichia coli* and biochemically characterized. The potential of Aa2_1884 in preparing collagen oligopeptides from bovine bone collagen was further evaluated. The results indicate that Aa2_1884 is a novel multimodular gelatinase with a good potential in preparing collagen oligopeptide from bovine bone collagen.

## 2. Results and Discussion

### 2.1. Aa2_1884 Is a Novel Multimodular Peptidase of the S8 Family

The amino acid sequence of protein Aa2_1884 (WP_199608745.1) deduced from the genome of strain SM1988 is composed of 1135 amino acid residues, containing a signal peptide with a length of 34 amino acid residues at the N terminus based on the SignalP 5.0 prediction. Aa2_1884 is annotated as an S8 family serine peptidase by BLASTP through the non-redundant protein database. InterProScan analysis indicated that, in addition to the predicted signal peptide, Aa2_1884 has five conserved domains (Figure 1), including an inhibitor I9 domain (Tyr72-Thr175, IPR010259), a peptidase S8 domain (Gly209-Lys661, IPR000209), a protease associated (PA) domain (Ser466-Leu545, IPR003137), a fibronectin type-III (FN3) domain (Leu711-Arg790, IPR041469), and a domain of unknown function (DUF11) (Lys817-Val863, IPR001434). The inhibitor I9 domain likely functions as a molecular chaperone to assist the protein folding of Aa2_1884 [30,31]. The peptidase S8 domain is the catalytic domain, containing the characteristic catalytic triad of the S8 family, namely

Asp218, His287, and Ser622 (Figure 2). The PA domain is an inserted domain in the peptidase S8 domain, which has been shown to play a role in collagen binding in some S8 proteases [27,32]. FN3 domain has been found in several proteases [33,34], whose function in proteases, however, has not been revealed. DUF11 domain is also present in peptidase brachyurin-T of the S1 family from *Caldilinea aerophile* based on InterProScan prediction (Figure 1). However, its function in peptidases such as brachyurin-T and Aa2_1884 needs further study.

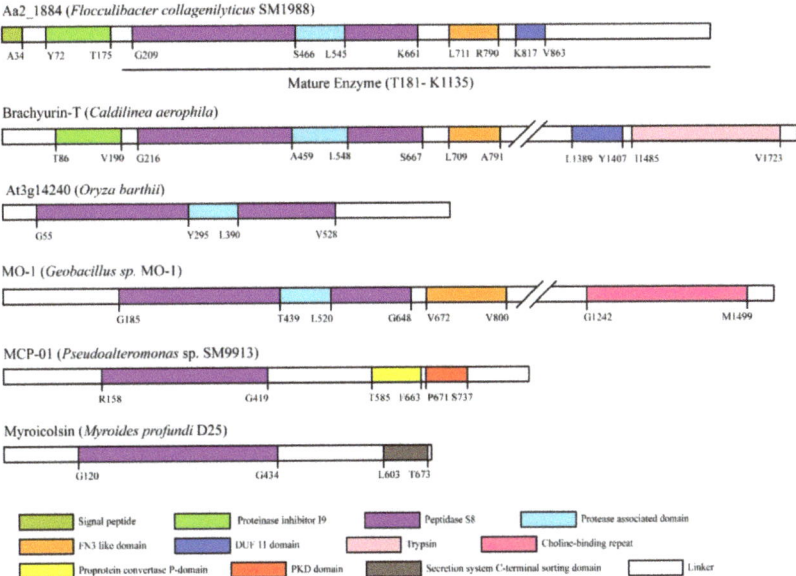

Figure 1. Domain architectures of Aa2_1884 and similar proteases predicted by InterPro. Marked numbers show the corresponding position of predicted domains in the amino acid sequences of the proteases.

Among the characterized peptidases, Aa2_1884 shares the highest sequence identity (44.05%) with brachyurin-T of the S1 family [35]. It is also most close to brachyurin-T in the phylogenetic tree (Figure 3). However, the domain architectures of these two enzymes are different. Compared to brachyurin-T, Aa2_1884 lacks the C-terminal Trypsin domain (Figure 1). Among all the characterized peptidases, none were found to have the same domain architecture as Aa2_1884 (Figure 1). These data suggest that Aa2_1884 is a novel multimodular protease of the S8 family. In addition, as shown in Figure 2, sequence alignment indicated that Aa2_1884 contains several motifs that are conserved in reported S8 collagenases, which suggests that Aa2_1884 may have collagenolytic activity.

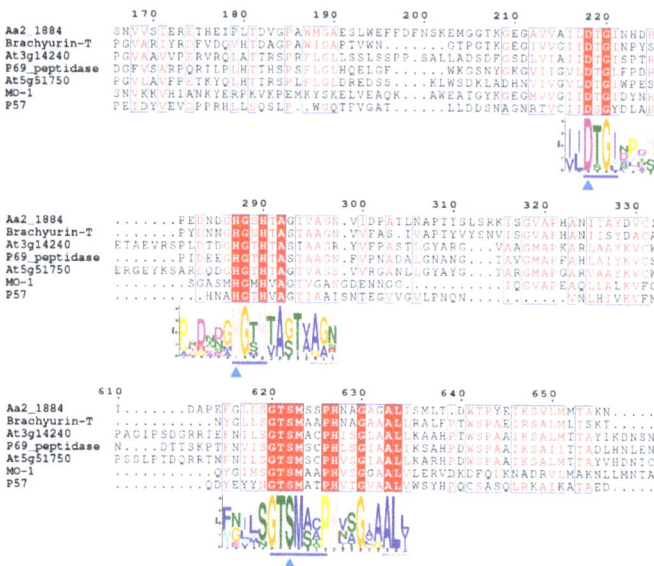

**Figure 2.** Sequence alignment of Aa2_1884 with similar proteases and reported S8 collagenases using the ClustalW program. Similar amino acid residues are boxed and shown in red, conserved amino acid residues are shown with red background. Amino acid residues constituting the catalytic triad of the MEROPS S8 family are marked with blue triangles, and motifs containing these residues are marked with blue underlines. Aa2_1884 (WP_199608745) is from *Flocculibacter collagenilyticus* SM1988, brachyurin-T (YP_005442656) from *Caldilinea aerophile*, At3g14240 (MER0006049) from *Oryza barthii*, P69 peptidase (XP_002275452) from *Vitis vinifera*, At5g51750 (XP_009789180) from *Nicotiana sylvestris*, MO-1 (BAF30978) from *Geobacillus* sp. MO-1, and P57 (KT923662) protease from *Photobacterium* sp. A5-7.

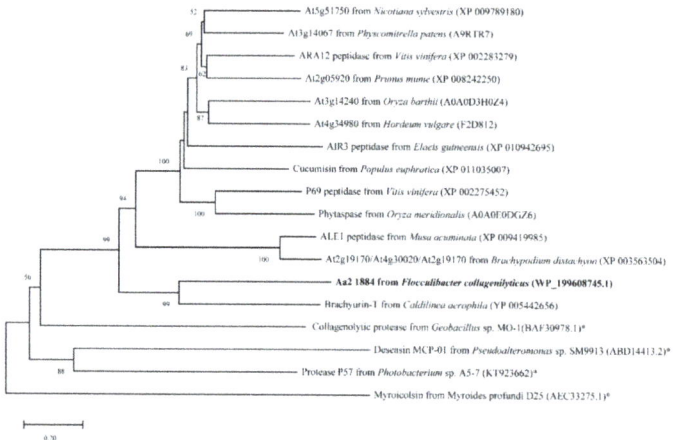

**Figure 3.** Neighbor-joining (NJ) phylogenetic tree based on amino acid sequences of Aa2_1884 and similar proteases. The tree was constructed with MEGA X. Bootstrap values (>50%) based on 1000 replicates were presented at nodes. Bar, 0.20. The reported S8 collagenases are indicated by asterisks.

## 2.2. Aa2_1884 Is a Gelatinase with High Activity toward Denatured Collagens

To characterize Aa2_1884, the gene of Aa2_1884 was over-expressed in *Escherichia coli* BL21 (DE3) with the vector pET-22b (+) containing a C-terminal His tag. The recombinant Aa2_1884 protein was purified by affinity chromatography on a His Bind Ni chelating column and gel filtration chromatography on a Sephadex G200 column. Sodium dodecyl sulfate polyacrylamide gel electrophoresis (SDS-PAGE) analysis showed that the purified Aa2_1884 had an apparent molecular weight of approximately 100,000 Da (Figure 4a). The N-terminal sequence of the purified Aa2_1884 was determined to T181-D-V-G-P-A186 by N-terminal sequencing. Thus, on the basis of its N-terminal sequence and molecular weight, mature Aa2_1884 should contain 955 amino acid residues from Thr181 to Lys1135 (Figure 1). The signal peptide and the inhibitor I9 domain are cleaved off during maturation.

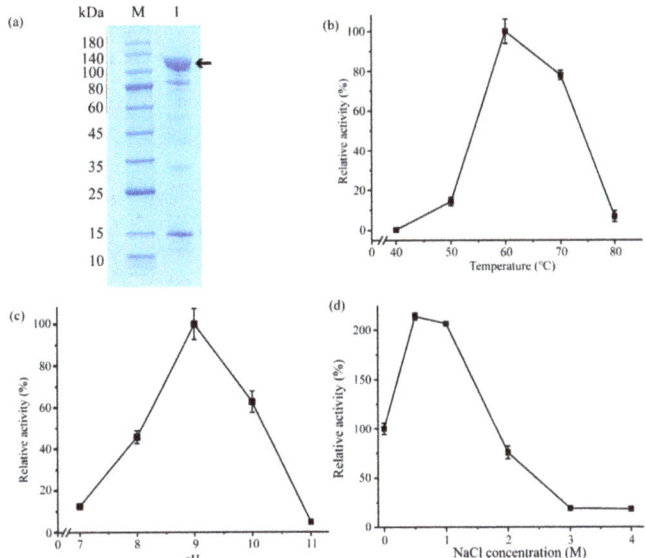

**Figure 4.** Purification and characterization of Aa2_1884: (**a**) SDS-PAGE analysis of purified Aa2_1884. Lane M, protein mass markers. Lane 1, purified Aa2_1884. The protein band of Aa2_1884 is indicated by an arrow; (**b**) Effect of temperature on the activity of Aa2_1884. The experiment was performed in Tris-HCl buffer (50 mM, pH 9.0) at 40–80 °C, and the enzyme activity at 60 °C was taken as 100%; (**c**) Effect of pH on the activity of Aa2_1884. The enzyme activity was measured at 60 °C with 40 mM Britton–Robinson buffers ranged from pH 7 to pH 11. The enzyme activity at pH 9.0 was taken as 100%; (**d**) Effect of NaCl concentration on the activity of Aa2_1884. The activity was measured at 60 °C in Tris-HCl buffer (50 mM, pH 9.0) containing different concentrations of NaCl from 0 to 4 M. The enzyme activity in the Tris-HCl buffer with 0 M NaCl was taken as 100%. In (**b**–**d**), bovine bone collagen was used as the substrate in the experiments. The graphs show data from triplicate experiments (mean ± SD).

Sequence alignment implied that Aa2_1884 may have collagenolytic activity. Indeed, Aa2_1884 had noticeable activity towards bovine bone collagen at temperatures of 50–70 °C, with an optimal temperature at 60 °C. However, it had almost no activity towards bovine bone collagen at 40 °C (Figure 4b). At 60 °C, Aa2_1884 also had activity towards bovine tendon collagen, gelatin, and casein, but no activity toward elastin-orcein (Table 1). As collagen is denatured at temperatures more than 40 °C, these results indicate that Aa2_1884 can hydrolyze denatured collagen, but not natural collagen. Therefore, Aa2_1884 is a gelatinase, rather than a collagenase. With bovine bone collagen as the substrate, Aa2_1884 showed the highest activity at pH 9.0 (Figure 4c), indicating that it is an alkaline protease.

In the buffer containing different NaCl (0–4 M), Aa2_1884 showed the highest activity at 0.5–1 M NaCl (Figure 4d). These characteristics reflect the adaptation of Aa2_1884 to the marine salty and alkaline environment.

Table 1. The substrate specificity of Aa2_1884 [$].

| Substrate | Enzymatic Activity (U/mL) |
|---|---|
| Bovine bone collagen | 801.15 ± 46.45 |
| Bovine tendon collagen | 761.27 ± 43.41 |
| Gelatin | 834.00 ± 61.39 |
| Casein | 51.75 ± 1.85 |
| Elastin-orcein | – |

[$] The activities of Aa2_1884 towards different substrates were measured in Tris-HCl (50 mM, pH 9.0) at 60 °C. The data represent the mean ± SD of three experimental repeats.

We also analyzed the effects of metal ions and protease inhibitors on the activity of Aa2_1884. As shown in Table 2, $Ca^{2+}$, $Ba^{2+}$, $Sr^{2+}$, and $Mg^{2+}$ significantly increased the activity of Aa2_1884 towards bovine bone collagen, $Zn^{2+}$ and $Fe^{2+}$ severely inhibited its activity, and $Ni^{2+}$, $Co^{2+}$, and $Mn^{2+}$ completely inhibited its activity (Table 2). Surprisingly, none of the four tested inhibitors, phenylmethylsulfonyl fluoride (PMSF), ethylenediamine tetraacetic acid (EDTA), ethylene glycol tetraacetic acid (EGTA), or o-phenanthroline (o-P), had inhibitory effect on the activity of Aa2_1884 (Figure 5), which is an unusual phenomenon for an S8 peptidase. Among these inhibitors, PSMF is a classical inhibitor to serine proteases, however, there are also some exceptions. Kexin has been reported to be resistant to PMSF [36]. Kexin is a typical S8 peptidase produced by *Saccharomyces cerevisiae*, which contains 814 amino acid residues. Different from Aa2_1884, Kexin contains only a P-proprotein domain in addition to the Peptidase S8 domain [37]. It still remains elusive why kexin is resistant to PMSF. Thus, the underlying mechanisms of kexin and Aa2_1884 to resist PMSF need further investigation.

Table 2. Effects of metal ions on the activity of Aa2_1884 [a].

| Metal Ion | Relative Activity (%) | | Metal Ion | Relative Activity (%) | |
|---|---|---|---|---|---|
| | 2 mM | 4 mM | | 2 mM | 4 mM |
| Control | 100 | 100 | $K^+$ | 108.62 ± 8.24 | 116.60 ± 4.18 |
| $Ca^{2+}$ | 263.67 ± 7.06 | 251.90 ± 10.14 | $Sn^{2+}$ | 97.01 ± 0.12 | 100.32 ± 4.40 |
| $Ba^{2+}$ | 250.54 ± 11.34 | 276.80 ± 10.14 | $Zn^{2+}$ | 56.50 ± 2.99 | 40.69 ± 1.33 |
| $Sr^{2+}$ | 245.91 ± 6.45 | 210.87 ± 29.18 | $Fe^{2+}$ | 43.73 ± 4.78 | 5.05 ± 2.04 |
| $Mg^{2+}$ | 217.58 ± 7.25 | 217.25 ± 32.74 | $Ni^{2+}$ | – [b] | – |
| $Li^+$ | 111.41 ± 4.40 | 116.60 ± 4.18 | $Co^{2+}$ | – | – |
| $Cu^{2+}$ | 100.32 ± 2.96 | 122.83 ± 2.43 | $Mn^{2+}$ | – | – |

[a] The activity of Aa2_1884 was measured in Tris-HCl (50 mM, pH 9.0) at 60 °C with bovine bone collagen as the substrate. The activity (657.37 U/mL) without any metal ion was used as a control (100%). The data represent the mean ± SD of three experimental repeats. [b] "–" means that enzyme activity was not detectable.

The S8 family, the second largest family of serine peptidases, contains more than 200 peptidases in the MEROPS database (https://www.ebi.ac.uk/merops/cgi-bin/famsum?family=S8, accessed on 6 December 2021). In this family, only a small number have collagenolytic activity, but many have gelatinolytic activity. Different from those with collagenolytic activity, Aa2_1884 has no activity towards native collagen. On the other hand, although Aa2_1884 has gelatinolytic activity, it has a distinct domain architecture and is resistant to PMSF, compared to those with gelatinolytic activity in the S8 family. Therefore, Aa2_1884 is a new gelatinase of the S8 family. The S8 family includes diverse peptidases produced by bacteria, archaea, and eukaryotes from various environments, and most are secreted endopeptidases. Therefore, both the temperature and pH optima of the S8 peptidases are in a wide range due to the adaptation of the peptidases to their respective environments [38]. For example, assays of subtilisins from *Bacillus* species are typically performed at pH 8.2–8.6 and 25 °C [39]. The pH optima of the S8 peptidases from archaea are usually in the range of 7.5–10.7, and their temperature optima are in a wide range of 55–115 °C [40]. The pH optima of the S8 collagenases from bacteria are within the range of 7.1–9.3, and their temperature optima are usually 50–60 °C [24,26,41,42]. The optimal temperature and pH of Aa2_1884 are 60 °C and pH 9.0, which fall in the optimal temperature and pH ranges of the S8 peptidases.

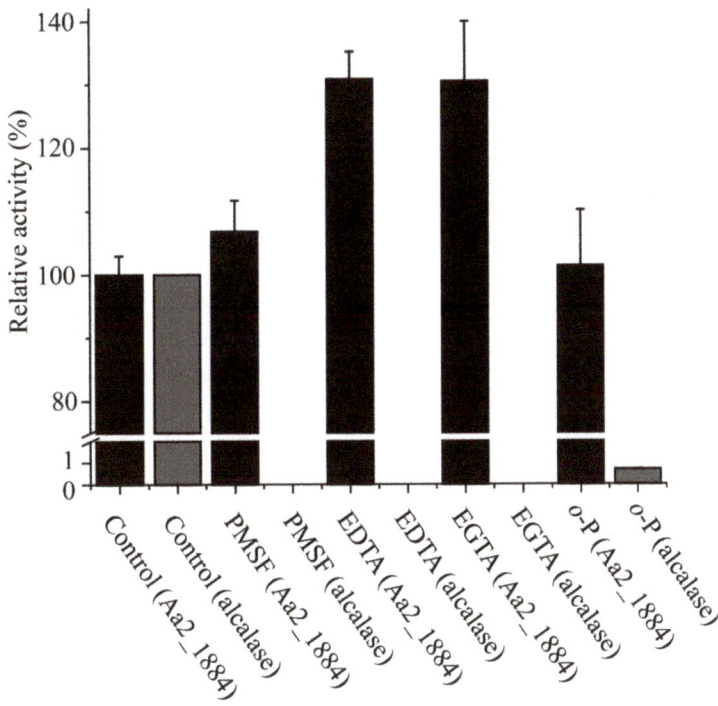

**Figure 5.** Effects of protease inhibitors on the activity of Aa2_1884. Aa2_1884 and the control enzyme alcalase were incubated at 4 °C for 1 h in 50 mM Tris-HCl (pH 9.0) containing 2 mM of each inhibitor, PMSF, EDTA, EGTA, or o-P. After incubation, the residual activity toward bovine bone collagen was measured at 60 °C, pH 9.0. The activity of Aa2_1884 without any inhibitor was taken as 100%. The graphs show data from triplicate experiments (mean ± SD).

### 2.3. Aa2_1884 Shows High Hydrolytic Efficiency on Bovine Bone Collagen

As Aa2_1884 had high activity towards bovine bone collagen at 60 °C (Figure 4b), it may have a potential in preparing collagen bioactive peptides from bovine bone collagen. Thus, attempts were made to prepare peptides from bovine bone collagen with Aa2_1884 as a tool. To determine the optimal hydrolysis conditions, three enzymatic hydrolysis parameters were optimized by single factor experiments, including hydrolysis temperature, hydrolysis time and enzyme-substrate ratio (E/S). On the basis of the residual amount of collagen, the appropriate hydrolysis temperature and time of Aa2_1884 were determined to be 55–65 °C (Figure 6a) and ≥3 h (Figure 6b), respectively. When the E/S was more than 400 U/g, no more obvious decrease in the amount of residual collagen was detected (Figure 6c). Hence, considering the hydrolysis efficiency and economic benefit, the optimal conditions of Aa2_1884 for the hydrolysis of bovine bone collagen on the laboratory scale were determined to be reaction at 60 °C for 3 h with an E/S ratio of 400 U/g. Under these hydrolysis conditions, the maximum hydrolytic efficiency of bovine bone collagen reached 95.3 ± 0.3%, indicating that Aa2_1884 is a good enzyme for the hydrolysis of bovine bone collagen. We then prepared bovine bone collagen hydrolysate with Aa2_1884 under the determined hydrolysis conditions.

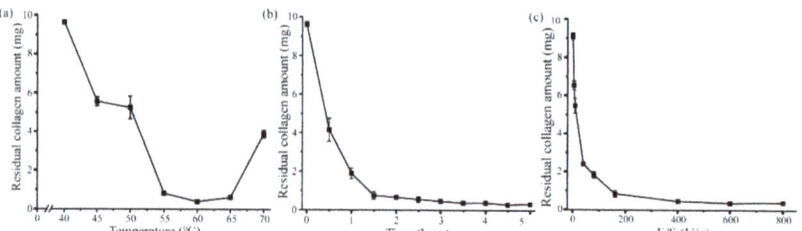

**Figure 6.** Effects of temperature, time and E/S on the hydrolysis efficiency of bovine bone collagen: (a) Effect of hydrolysis temperature determined at the hydrolysis time of 3 h and the hydrolysis E/S of 400 U/g; (b) Effect of hydrolysis time determined at the hydrolysis temperature of 60 °C and the hydrolysis E/S of 400 U/g; (c) Effect of hydrolysis E/S determined at the hydrolysis temperature of 60 °C and the hydrolysis time of 3 h. The graphs show data from triplicate experiments (mean ± SD).

*2.4. The Collagen Hydrolysate Prepared with Aa2_1884 Is Rich in Collagen Oligopeptides*

To evaluate the quality of the prepared hydrolysate, we analyzed the contents of amino acids and peptides, amino acid composition, and molecular weight distribution of peptides in the hydrolysate. According to the ninhydrin method, there were 2.2 ± 0.1% free amino acids and 97.8 ± 0.1% peptides in the hydrolysate. Analysis of the composition of free amino acids in the hydrolysate by automatic amino acid analyzer also showed that there was only a small amount of free amino acids in the hydrolysate (Table 3). Thus, the hydrolysate is rich in peptides. In the hydrolysate, glycine is the most abundant (17.2%), followed by proline (10.1%). In addition, there were 1.0% hydroxylysine and 8.2% hydroxyproline in the peptides in the hydrolysate (Table 3). As hydroxylysine and hydroxyproline are two unique amino acids in collagen, our results indicated that the hydrolysate is rich in collagen peptides. The molecular weight distribution of peptides in the hydrolysate was analyzed by high performance liquid chromatography (HPLC) (Figure 7). The results showed that peptides with a molecular weight lower than 3000 Da, 1000 Da, and 500 Da accounted for approximately 71.6 ± 0.2%, 55.1 ± 0.2%, and 39.5 ± 0.2%, respectively (Table 4), indicating that the hydrolysate is rich in collagen oligopeptides.

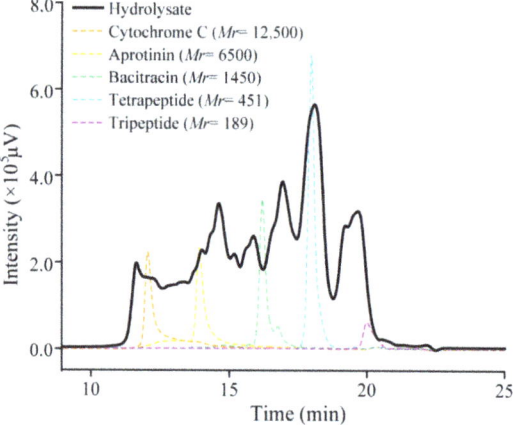

**Figure 7.** Size exclusion chromatography analysis of the molecular weight distribution of peptides in the hydrolysate. The hydrolysate dissolved in deionized water was analyzed by HPLC with a TSK gel G2000 SWXL column.

**Table 3.** Composition and content of free and total amino acids in the hydrolysate [a].

| Amino Acid | Total Amino Acids (g/100 g) | Free Amino Acids (g/100 g) |
|---|---|---|
| Ala | 6.87 ± 0.05 | 0.07 ± 0.02 |
| Arg | 7.16 ± 0.06 | |
| Asp | 3.39 ± 0.03 | 0.10 ± 0.02 |
| Cit | 0.07 ± 0.03 | |
| Cys | 0.56 ± 0.04 | 0.12 ± 0.01 |
| Glu | 4.04 ± 0.03 | |
| Gly | 17.21 ± 0.12 | 0.02 ± 0.01 |
| His | 0.67 ± 0.02 | |
| Ile | 1.54 ± 0.04 | 0.07 ± 0.01 |
| Leu | 2.73 ± 0.06 | 0.04 ± 0.01 |
| Lys | 3.23 ± 0.05 | |
| Met | 0.75 ± 0.06 | 0.10 ± 0.01 |
| Orn | 0.17 ± 0.01 | |
| Phe | 1.83 ± 0.11 | |
| Pro | 10.10 ± 0.08 | |
| Ser | 3.03 ± 0.03 | 0.15 ± 0.04 |
| Thr | 2.47 ± 0.03 | |
| Trp [b] | – | |
| Tyr | 0.79 ± 0.10 | 0.09 ± 0.07 |
| Val | 2.10 ± 0.02 | 0.14 ± 0.01 |
| Hylys | 1.04 ± 0.05 | 0.19 ± 0.05 |
| Hypro | 8.18 ± 0.11 | |

[a] Composition and content of free and total amino acids in the hydrolysate were analyzed by using an amino acid analyzer. The data represent the mean ± SD of three experimental repeats; [b] Trp was not detectable because it was destroyed in the process of acid hydrolysis.

**Table 4.** Molecular weight distribution of peptides in the hydrolysate [a].

| Molecular-Weight Range (Da) | Hydrolysate (%) |
|---|---|
| >10,000 | 9.68 ± 0.13 |
| 5000–10,000 | 6.25 ± 0.02 |
| 3000–5000 | 12.46 ± 0.11 |
| 1000–3000 | 16.49 ± 0.09 |
| 500–1000 | 15.60 ± 0.07 |
| <500 | 39.50 ± 0.20 |

[a] The content of each range of peptides in the hydrolysate were calculated based on the percentage of the area of corresponding molecular weight range in the total chromatograph area of the hydrolysate in the HPLC chromatogram.

### 2.5. Antioxidant Activity of Bovine Bone Collagen Hydrolysate

The antioxidant activity of the hydrolysate was further evaluated by measuring its free radical scavenging activity towards 1,1-diphenyl-2-picryl-hydrazyl radical (DPPH•) with hyaluronic acid (HA) as a control. The scavenging ratio of the hydrolysate to DPPH• increased with the hydrolysate concentration, which reached 32.8 ± 1.1% at the concentration of 10 mg/mL (Figure 8). In addition, as shown in Figure 8, the DPPH• scavenging ratio of the hydrolysate was obviously higher than that of HA, especially at high concentrations. A comparison of the DPPH• scavenging ratio of the hydrolysate with those of some reported collagen hydrolysates are shown in Table 5. The differences in the DPPH• scavenging ratios among the hydrolysates are likely attributed to the differences in the collagen sources, the preparation methods, and the enzymes used.

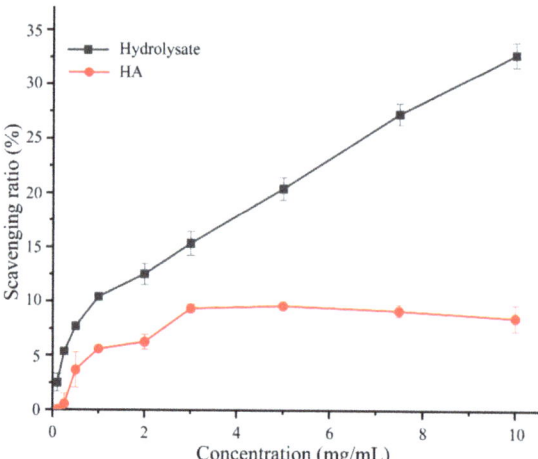

**Figure 8.** Antioxidant activity towards DPPH• of the hydrolysate and hyaluronic acid (HA).

**Table 5.** Antioxidant activity towards DPPH• of collagen hydrolysates prepared from different collagen sources by different methods.

| Antioxidant Activity | Hydrolysate Concentration (mg/mL) | Enzyme | Method | Collagen Source | Reference |
|---|---|---|---|---|---|
| 32.8% [a] | 10 | Aa2_1884 (S8) | Enzymolysis | Bovine bone | This study |
| 40.7% [a] | 30 | A69 (M4) | Enzymolysis | Bovine bone | [43] |
| 341.91% [a] | 10 | MCP-01 (S8) | Enzymolysis | Fish skin | [7] |
| 50% [a] | 8.38 | | SWH [b] | Fish bone | [44] |
| 50% [a] | 7.58 | | SWH | Fish skin | [44] |
| 50% [a] | 5.81 | Pepsin | Enzymolysis | Fish skin | [45] |
| 50% [a] | 1.57 | Pepsin | Enzymolysis and fraction isolation | Fish skin | [46] |

[a] DPPH• scavenging ratio, [b] SWH, subcritical water hydrolysis.

As oligopeptides from various proteins have been demonstrated as beneficial compounds for skin protection or against diseases such as hypertension, hypercholesterolemia, and atherosclerosis, oligopeptides have been widely prepared from a variety of proteins, including proteins from various plant fruits and seeds, and proteins from skins and meats of various marine and terrestrial animals [4,47,48]. Protein hydrolysates containing oligopeptides have been prepared with both commercial and non-commercial proteases. For example, a loach protein hydrolysate prepared with papain contained approximately 30% oligopeptides with a molecular weight lower than 500 Da, and exhibited good hydroxyl radical scavenging and antioxidant activities [49]. A salmon skin hydrolysate prepared with alcalase and papain contained approximately 90% oligopeptides with a molecular weight lower than 1000 Da, and showed the ACE inhibitory effect from different fractions collected by reversed-phase HPLC [19]. A 1301 Da peptide from the cod fish skin hydrolysate prepared with pepsin, trypsin, and α-chymotrypsin exhibited potent ACE inhibitory and antioxidant activities [20]. A shrimp hydrolysate prepared with the crude enzyme from *Bacillus* sp. SM98011 contained approximately 41% oligopeptides with molecular mass lower than 3000 Da, and exhibited good hydroxyl radical scavenger and antioxidant activities [50]. A codfish skin hydrolysate prepared with the collagenolytic protease MCP-01 from *Pseudoalteromonas* sp. SM9913 contained 60% oligopeptides with a molecular weight lower than 1000 Da, and exhibited good hydroxyl radical scavenging activity and promoted an effect on cell viability of human dermal fibroblasts [7]. A bovine bone collagen hydrolysate prepared with the thermolysin-like protease A69 from *Anoxybacillus caldiproteolyticus* 1A02591 contained 21.1% oligopeptides with a molecular weight lower than 1000 Da, and exhibited good moisture-retention ability and antioxidant activity [43]. The hydrolysate prepared from Bigeye tuna skin collagen contained peptides with molecular weights of 300–425 Da and had DPPH• scavenging activity [51]. It has been demonstrated that di-/tripeptides can be absorbed in their intact forms in human intestine without further hydrolysis [5]. Thus, protein hydrolysates containing more oligo-peptides with a molecular weight of <1000 Da or even <500 Da are preferred in cosmetics, functional food, and nutraceuticals [52].

Collagen used in collagen oligopeptides preparation have been extracted from the bones and skins of various animals, such as fish skins and bones [7,44,53], and goat skin [54]. Bovine bone is a by-product of beef processing industry and its annual production is huge due to the large number of global slaughtered cattle. Bovine bone is rich in collagen and therefore, is a cheap and good source for collagen preparation. However, bovine bone collagen has rarely been used in collagen oligopeptide preparation to our knowledge. In this study, we used Aa2_1884 to prepare collagen oligopeptides from bovine bone collagen. Aa2_1884 showed a high hydrolysis efficiency (95%) on bovine bone collagen and the resultant hydrolysate contained a high proportion of collagen oligopeptides, 55.1% peptides with a molecular weight lower than 1000 Da, and 39.5% peptides with a molecular weight lower than 500 Da. These data suggest that Aa2_1884 has a promising potential in preparing collagen oligopeptides from bovine bone collagen, which may provide a feasible way for the high-value utilization of bovine bone collagen.

## 3. Materials and Methods

### 3.1. Materials

Bovine tendon collagen was purchased from Worthington (Lakewood, NJ, USA), and bovine bone collagen from Kinry Biotech Co., Ltd. (Jinan, China). Casein (from bovine milk), gelatin (from cold water fish skin), elastin-orcein, EGTA, o-P, aprotinin, and cytochrome C were purchased from Sigma (St. Louis, MO, USA). Alcalase was purchased from Vazyme Biotech Co., Ltd. (Nanjing, China). PMSF was purchased from BBI (Shanghai, China). EDTA was purchased from HUSHI (Shanghai, China). Bacitracin was purchased from Aladdin (Shanghai, China). Tripeptide GGG and tetrapeptide GGYR were synthesized by Qiangyao Biotechnology Co., Ltd. (Shanghai, China). DPPH• was purchased from Tokyo Chemical Industry (Tokyo, Japan). HA was purchased from Shandong Freda Bioeng Co., Ltd. (Jinan, China). Other chemicals were of analytical grade and commercially available.

### 3.2. Sequence Analysis

The domains of Aa2_1884 (WP_199608745) from *Flocculibacter collagenilyticus* SM1988 (CP05988) and of the other proteases shown in Figure 1 were predicted by InterPro (https://www.ebi.ac.uk/interpro/; 6 December 2021) [55]. The signal peptide of Aa2_1884 was predicted by the SignalP 5.0 server (https://services.healthtech.dtu.dk/service.php?SignalP-5.0; 6 December 2021) [56]. For sequence alignment, previously reported MCP-01 (ABD14413) from *Pseudoalteromonas* sp. SM9913, the collagenolytic protease (BAF30978) from *Geobacillus* sp. MO-1, myroicolsin (AEC33275) from *Myroides profundi* D25, and P57 (KT923662) from *Photobacterium* sp. A5-7 were selected to align with Aa2_1884 by ClustalW with bootstrap of 1000 [57]. The sequence alignment was displayed using ESPript 3.0 [58]. The conserved sites were predicted by MEME (https://meme-suite.org/meme/; 6 December 2021) [59]. The phylogenetic tree was constructed via MEGA X [60].

### 3.3. Protein Expression and Purification

The genome DNA of strain SM1988 was extracted with bacterial genomic DNA isolation kit (BioTeke, Beijing, China) according to the manufacturer's instructions. The gene sequence of Aa2_1884 was amplified by PCR using the genome DNA of strain SM1988 with primers 1884-F (5′-AAGAAGGAGATATACATATGATGAAAATAGAACATAGT-3′) and 1884-R (5′-TGGTGGTGGTGGTGCTCGAGTTTATTGTCACACGTGGTT-3′). The primers were synthesized by Tsingke Biotechnology Co., Ltd. (Qingdao, China). The PCR product was then cloned into vector pET-22b (+) (Vazyme) with a C-terminal His tag. The constructed plasmid carrying the gene sequence of Aa2_1884 was verified by sequencing and then transformed into Fe2 BL21 (DE3). Recombinant *E. coli* cells were cultured in Lysogeny broth (LB) medium with 100 µg/mL ampicillin at 37 °C, 180 rpm to an $OD_{600}$ of 0.8–1.0. Then, 0.2 mM isopropyl β-D-1-thiogalactopyranoside (IPTG) was added, and the cells were further incubated at 15 °C, 120 rpm for 5 days [26]. After incubation, cells were lysed by a high-pressure cracker and centrifuged at 4656× *g*, 4 °C for 1 h, and the supernatant was collected. The recombinant Aa2_1884 protein was extracted from the supernatant by an His binding Ni chelating column, and then purified on a Sephadex G200 gel filtration column (GE, Boston, MA, USA) using fast protein liquid chromatography (FPLC) on AKTA purifier (GE, Boston, MA, USA) [61]. The purified Aa2_1884 was analyzed by 12.5% SDS-PAGE. Protein concentration was determined by a BCA protein assay kit (Thermo, Waltham, MA, USA) with bovine serum albumin (BSA) as the standard according to the manufacturer's instructions.

*3.4. Enzyme Assay*

The activities of Aa2_1884 toward bovine bone collagen, bovine tendon collagen, and gelatin at 60 °C were measured by the method provided by Worthington Biochemical Co. (Lakewood, NJ, USA) [26]. For collagen, a mixture of 5 mg substrate and 1 mL enzyme solution was incubated at 60 °C in Tris-HCl buffer for 0.5 h with continuous stirring. For gelatin, 100 µL enzyme solution was incubated with 100 µL of 2% (*w/v*) gelatin at 60 °C for 10 min. The reaction was stopped by the addition of 10 µL of 1.25 M trichloroacetic acid. The released amino acids were quantified using the colorimetric ninhydrin method [62] with L-leucine as the standard. One unit of enzyme activity was defined as the amount of enzyme that released 1 nmol of L-leucine per hour from collagen or gelatin [26]. The caseinolytic activity was determined at 60 °C using the method described by He et al. [63]. A reaction mixture containing 100 µL enzyme solution and 100 µL of 2% (*w/v*) casein was incubated at 60 °C for 10 min, and then the reaction was terminated by 200 µL trichloroacetic acid (0.4 M). The mixture was centrifuged at 17,935× *g* for 10 min, and 100 µL of the supernatant was incubated with 500 µL of sodium carbonate solution (0.4 M) and 100 µL of the Folin-phenol reagent at 40 °C for 20 min. After the reaction, the $OD_{660}$ of the mixture was measured. One unit of enzyme activity was defined as the amount of enzyme that liberated 1 mg tyrosine per minute [63]. The elastolytic activity at 60 °C was determined using the method described by Chen [64]. A mixture of 250 µL enzyme solution and 5 mg elastin-orcein was incubated at 60 °C for 1 h. After the reaction, the residual elastin-orcein was removed by centrifugation. The $OD_{590}$ of the supernatant was recorded. One unit of enzyme activity was defined as the amount of enzyme that caused an increase of 0.01 in $OD_{590}$ per minute [64].

*3.5. Enzyme Characterization*

The optimal temperature was determined by measuring the activity of Aa2_1884 toward bovine bone collagen in Tris-HCl buffer (50 mM, pH 9.0) at 40, 50, 60, 70, and 80 °C. The optimal pH was determined by measuring the activity of Aa2_1884 toward bovine bone collagen at 60 °C in 40 mM Britton–Robinson buffers from pH 7.0 to pH 11.0. The effect of NaCl concentration on the activity of Aa2_1884 was determined by measuring the activity of Aa2_1884 toward bovine bone collagen in Tris-HCl buffer (50 mM, pH 9.0) containing NaCl of different concentrations (0–4 M) at 60 °C. To evaluate the effect of metal ions ($Li^+$, $K^+$, $Ca^{2+}$, $Mg^{2+}$, $Cu^{2+}$, $Ni^{2+}$, $Mn^{2+}$, $Ba^{2+}$, $Fe^{2+}$, $Zn^{2+}$, $Co^{2+}$, $Sn^{2+}$, $Sr^{2+}$) on the enzymatic activity, Aa2_1884 was incubated in Tris-HCl buffer (50 mM, pH 9.0) containing each metal ion (2 mM or 4 mM) at 4 °C for 1 h, and the enzymatic activity toward bovine bone collagen was then measured at 60 °C. For the inhibitory experiment, Aa2_1884 and alcalase were incubated at 4 °C for 1 h with 2 mM of an inhibitor, PMSF, EDTA, EGTA, or *o*-P. After incubation, the residue activity toward bovine bone collagen was measured at 60 °C and pH 9.0.

## 3.6. Optimization of the Enzymatic Hydrolysis Parameters

Three parameters, hydrolysis temperature, hydrolysis time, and E/S, which influence the efficiency of the enzymatic hydrolysis, were optimized via single-factor experiments, in which enzymatic hydrolysis of 10 mg bovine bone collagen in 1 mL 50 mM Tris-HCl (pH 9.0) was performed at 180 rpm in a shaking bath. Each parameter was determined under the optimum conditions of the other two parameters. To determine the hydrolysis temperature, the enzymatic hydrolysis was performed at different hydrolysis temperature (40, 45, 50, 55, 60, 65, 70 °C). To determine the hydrolysis time, the enzymatic hydrolysis was performed for different time (0.5, 1, 1.5, 2, 2.5, 3, 3.5, 4, 4.5, 5 h). To determine the E/S, the enzymatic hydrolysis was performed with different E/S (0, 4, 8, 40, 80, 160, 400, 600, 800 U/g collagen). After the hydrolysis, the reaction system was heated at 90 °C for 15 min to terminate the reaction, and then centrifuged at 4 °C for 20 min. The precipitate was freeze-dried and weighted, which was taken as the residual amount of collagen.

## 3.7. Preparation and Evaluation of Collagen Hydrolysate

To prepare peptides from bovine bone collagen, 10 mg bovine bone collagen was hydrolyzed under the determined parameters (at 60 °C for 3 h with an E/S ratio of 400 U/g). After hydrolysis, the reaction system was heated at 90 °C for 15 min and then centrifuged at 4 °C for 20 min. The supernatant was collected, freeze-dried, and weighted, which was the prepared hydrolysate.

Ten milligrams of the hydrolysate were dissolved in 1 mL deionized water. With L-leucine as the standard, the content of free amino acids in the hydrolysate solution was determined by the ninhydrin method [62]. The content of peptides in the hydrolysate was calculated by subtracting the content of free amino acids from that of the hydrolysate in the solution [43]. The compositions of free and total amino acids of the hydrolysate were analyzed by using an amino acid analyzer HITACHI 835 (Tokyo, Japan). The molecular mass distribution of peptides in the hydrolysates were analyzed by the method described by [7]. Briefly, the hydrolysate was dissolved with deionized water, and then analyzed by HPLC (LC-20AD, SHIMADZU, Tokyo, Japan) equipped with a TSK gel G2000 SWXL column (300 × 7.8 mm; range, <150,000 Da; void volume, 5.7 mL; Tosoh, Japan) that was eluted with the buffer containing 45% acetonitrile and 1% trifluoroacetic acid in deionized water at a flow rate of 0.5 mL/min HPLC under 220 nm monitoring. The calibration standards for molecular mass were tripeptide Gly-Gly-Gly (GGG, $M_r$ 189), tetrapeptide Gly-Gly-Tyr-Arg (GGYR, $M_r$ 451), bacitracin ($M_r$ 1422), aprotinin ($M_r$ 6511), and cytochrome C ($M_r$ 12400). Based on the calibration standards, the chromatogram of the hydrolysate was separated into several fractions (<500 Da, 500–1000 Da, 1000–3000 Da, 3000–5000 Da, 5000–10,000 Da, and >10,000 Da), and the content of each fraction was determined by its relative peak area.

## 3.8. Analysis of the Antioxidant Activity of the Collagen Hydrolysate

The antioxidant activity of the prepared hydrolysate was analyzed by measuring its free radical scavenging activity towards 1,1-diphenyl-2-picryl-hydrazyl radical (DPPH•) according to the method described by Sun [65]. HA was used as a positive control due to its widespread application in scavenging free radical. To determine the DPPH• scavenging activity, 1 mL hydrolysate samples in incremental concentrations (0.1, 0.25, 0.5, 1, 2, 3, 5, 7.5, 10 mg/mL) were reacted with 2 mL of 100 μM DPPH• (dissolved in ethanol solution) for 40 min at room temperature (25 °C) in dark, and then the absorbance of the reaction solution was detected at 525 nm. DPPH solution was replaced with ethanol solution to obtain the result of background of sample, and the hydrolysate sample was replaced with water to obtain the result of blank control.

The free radical scavenging activity (D) was calculated as follows:

$$D(\%) = [1 - (A_i - A_j)/A_0] * 100 \tag{1}$$

where $A_i$ was the absorbance of the sample, $A_j$ was the background absorbance of the sample, and $A_0$ was the absorbance of the blank control.

## 4. Conclusions

As only a few peptidases of the S8 family so far have been applied in the preparation of bioactive oligopeptides, there is still a need to develop more S8 serine peptidases with potentials in bioactive oligopeptide preparation. In this study, the peptidase Aa2_1884 from marine bacterium *Flocculibacter collagenilyticus* SM1988$^T$ was demonstrated to be a novel multimodular gelatinase of the S8 family, which has high activity towards gelatin and denatured collagens. Moreover, under the optimized enzymolysis conditions, Aa2_1884 has a high hydrolysis efficiency (95%) on bovine bone collagen. The prepared hydrolysate is rich in collagen oligopeptides and has antioxidant activity. The results in this study suggest that Aa2_1884 has a promising potential application in preparing collagen oligopeptides from bovine bone collagen. The collagen hydrolysate prepared with Aa2_1884 may have good bioactivities due to its high oligopeptide content as well as good antioxidant activity, which awaits further investigation.

**Author Contributions:** Conceptualization, X.-L.C. and Y.-Z.Z.; investigation, J.L. and J.-M.D.; methodology, J.L., J.-H.C., M.-L.S., J.-P.W. and X.Z.; software, Z.-J.T.; project administration, X.-L.C. and X.-Y.Z.; resources, X.-L.C. and X.-Y.Z.; supervision, X.-M.T. and X.-Y.Z.; writing—original draft preparation, J.L. and Z.-J.T.; writing—review and editing, X.-L.C. and X.-Y.Z. All authors have read and agreed to the published version of the manuscript.

**Funding:** This work was funded by the National Science Foundation of China (grant numbers U2006205, U1706207, 31670038 and 31971535, awarded to X.-L.C., Y.-Z.Z., X.-L.C. and Y.-Z.Z., respectively), the National Key R&D Program of China (2018YFC0310704 awarded to X.-L.C.), the Major Scientific and Technological Innovation Project (MSTIP) of Shandong Province (2019JZZY010817 awarded to Y.-Z.Z.), Taishan Scholars Program of Shandong Province (tspd20181203, awarded to Y.-Z.Z.), and Scientific Research Think Tank of Biological Manufacturing Industry in Qingdao (QDSWZK202002 awarded to Y.-Z.Z.).

**Data Availability Statement:** The amino acid sequence of Aa2_1884 has been submitted to NCBI database under the accession number WP_199608745, It can be found here: https://www.ncbi.nlm.nih.gov/protein/WP_199608745 (accessed on 6 December 2021).

**Acknowledgments:** The authors sincerely appreciate Jiaojiao Tian (Ocean University of China) for her assistance in the amino acid analyses. We also thank Jingyao Qu, Jing Zhu, and Zhifeng Li from State Key Laboratory of Microbial Technology, Shandong University, China for their help and guidance in LC-MS.

**Conflicts of Interest:** The authors declare no conflict of interest.

## References

1. Zamyatnin, A.A. Structural-functional diversity of the natural oligopeptides. *Prog. Biophys. Mol. Biol.* **2018**, *133*, 1–8. [CrossRef]
2. Suarez-Jimenez, G.M.; Burgos-Hernandez, A.; Ezquerra-Brauer, J.M. Bioactive peptides and depsipeptides with anticancer potential: Sources from marine animals. *Mar. Drugs* **2012**, *10*, 963–986. [CrossRef] [PubMed]
3. Nasri, R.; Nasri, M. Marine-derived bioactive peptides as new anticoagulant agents: A review. *Curr. Protein Pept. Sci.* **2013**, *14*, 199–204. [CrossRef]
4. Bhat, Z.F.; Kumar, S.; Bhat, H.F. Bioactive peptides of animal origin: A review. *J. Food Sci. Technol.* **2015**, *52*, 5377–5392. [CrossRef]
5. Shen, W.; Matsui, T. Current knowledge of intestinal absorption of bioactive peptides. *Food Funct.* **2017**, *8*, 4306–4314. [CrossRef] [PubMed]
6. Ngo-Son, A.; Katekaew, S. Purification and characterization of angiotensin converting enzyme-inhibitory derived from crocodile blood hydrolysates. *Food Sci. Technol.* **2019**, *39*, 818–823. [CrossRef]
7. Chen, X.L.; Peng, M.; Li, J.; Tang, B.L.; Shao, X.; Zhao, F.; Liu, C.; Zhang, X.Y.; Li, P.Y.; Shi, M.; et al. Preparation and functional evaluation of collagen oligopeptide-rich hydrolysate from fish skin with the serine collagenolytic protease from *Pseudoalteromonas* sp. SM9913. *Sci. Rep.* **2017**, *7*, 15716. [CrossRef] [PubMed]
8. Chalamaiah, M.; Yu, W.; Wu, J. Immunomodulatory and anticancer protein hydrolysates (peptides) from food proteins: A review. *Food Chem.* **2018**, *245*, 205–222. [CrossRef]

9. Salampessy, J.; Phillips, M.; Seneweera, S.; Kailasapathy, K. Release of antimicrobial peptides through bromelain hydrolysis of leatherjacket (*Meuchenia* sp.) insoluble proteins. *Food Chem.* 2010, *120*, 556–560. [CrossRef]
10. Kim, D.U.; Chung, H.C.; Choi, J.; Sakai, Y.; Lee, B.Y. Oral Intake of Low-Molecular-Weight Collagen Peptide Improves Hydration, Elasticity, and Wrinkling in Human Skin: A Randomized, Double-Blind, Placebo-Controlled Study. *Nutrients* 2018, *10*, 826. [CrossRef]
11. Liu, J.; Wang, J.; Guo, Y. Effect of Collagen Peptide, Alone and in Combination with Calcium Citrate, on Bone Loss in Tail-Suspended Rats. *Molecules* 2020, *25*, 782. [CrossRef] [PubMed]
12. Zdzieblik, D.; Oesser, S.; Baumstark, M.W.; Gollhofer, A.; König, D. Collagen peptide supplementation in combination with resistance training improves body composition and increases muscle strength in elderly sarcopenic men: A randomised controlled trial. *Br. J. Nutr.* 2015, *114*, 1237–1245. [CrossRef] [PubMed]
13. Qiao, L.; Li, B.; Chen, Y.; Li, L.; Chen, X.; Wang, L.; Lu, F.; Luo, G.; Li, G.; Zhang, Y. Discovery of Anti-Hypertensive Oligopeptides from Adlay Based on In Silico Proteolysis and Virtual Screening. *Int. J. Mol. Sci.* 2016, *17*, 2099. [CrossRef] [PubMed]
14. Lee, E.J.; Hur, J.; Ham, S.A.; Jo, Y.; Lee, S.; Choi, M.J.; Seo, H.G. Fish collagen peptide inhibits the adipogenic differentiation of preadipocytes and ameliorates obesity in high fat diet-fed mice. *Int. J. Biol. Macromol.* 2017, *104*, 281–286. [CrossRef]
15. Zdzieblik, D.; Oesser, S.; Gollhofer, A.; König, D. Improvement of activity-related knee joint discomfort following supplementation of specific collagen peptides. *Appl. Physiol. Nutr. Metab.* 2017, *42*, 588–595. [CrossRef] [PubMed]
16. Bello, A.E.; Oesser, S. Collagen hydrolysate for the treatment of osteoarthritis and other joint disorders: A review of the literature. *Curr. Med. Res. Opin.* 2006, *22*, 2221–2232. [CrossRef]
17. Kang, M.C.; Yumnam, S.; Kim, S.Y. Oral Intake of Collagen Peptide Attenuates Ultraviolet B Irradiation-Induced Skin Dehydration In Vivo by Regulating Hyaluronic Acid Synthesis. *Int. J. Mol. Sci.* 2018, *19*, 3551. [CrossRef]
18. Korhonen, H.; Pihlanto, A. Food-derived bioactive peptides—Opportunities for designing future foods. *Curr. Pharm. Des.* 2003, *9*, 1297–1308. [CrossRef]
19. Gu, R.-Z.; Li, C.-Y.; Liu, W.-Y.; Yi, W.-X.; Cai, M.-Y. Angiotensin I-converting enzyme inhibitory activity of low-molecular-weight peptides from Atlantic salmon (*Salmo salar* L.) skin. *Food Res. Int.* 2011, *44*, 1536–1540. [CrossRef]
20. Himaya, S.W.A.; Ngo, D.-H.; Ryu, B.; Kim, S.-K. An active peptide purified from gastrointestinal enzyme hydrolysate of Pacific cod skin gelatin attenuates angiotensin-1 converting enzyme (ACE) activity and cellular oxidative stress. *Food Chem.* 2012, *132*, 1872–1882. [CrossRef]
21. Li, Z.-R.; Wang, B.; Chi, C.-f.; Zhang, Q.-H.; Gong, Y.-d.; Tang, J.-J.; Luo, H.-y.; Ding, G.-f. Isolation and characterization of acid soluble collagens and pepsin soluble collagens from the skin and bone of Spanish mackerel (*Scomberomorous niphonius*). *Food Hydrocoll.* 2013, *31*, 103–113. [CrossRef]
22. Adekoya, O.A.; Sylte, I. The thermolysin family (M4) of enzymes: Therapeutic and biotechnological potential. *Chem. Biol. Drug Des.* 2009, *73*, 7–16. [CrossRef]
23. Rawlings, N. Introduction: Serine Peptidases and Their Clans. In *Handbook of Proteolytic Enzymes*, 2nd ed.; Academic Press: San Diego, CA, USA, 2004.
24. Okamoto, M.; Yonejima, Y.; Tsujimoto, Y.; Suzuki, Y.; Watanabe, K. A thermostable collagenolytic protease with a very large molecular mass produced by thermophilic *Bacillus* sp. strain MO-1. *Appl. Microbiol. Biotechnol.* 2001, *57*, 103–108. [CrossRef]
25. Chen, X.L.; Xie, B.B.; Lu, J.T.; He, H.L.; Zhang, Y. A novel type of subtilase from the psychrotolerant bacterium *Pseudoalteromonas* sp. SM9913: Catalytic and structural properties of deseasin MCP-01. *Microbiology* 2007, *153*, 2116–2125. [CrossRef] [PubMed]
26. Ran, L.Y.; Su, H.N.; Zhou, M.Y.; Wang, L.; Chen, X.L.; Xie, B.B.; Song, X.Y.; Shi, M.; Qin, Q.L.; Pang, X.; et al. Characterization of a novel subtilisin-like protease myroicolsin from deep sea bacterium *Myroides profundi* D25 and molecular insight into its collagenolytic mechanism. *J. Biol. Chem.* 2014, *289*, 6041–6053. [CrossRef] [PubMed]
27. Li, H.J.; Tang, B.L.; Shao, X.; Liu, B.X.; Zheng, X.Y.; Han, X.X.; Li, P.Y.; Zhang, X.Y.; Song, X.Y.; Chen, X.L. Characterization of a New S8 serine Protease from Marine Sedimentary *Photobacterium* sp. A5-7 and the Function of Its Protease-Associated Domain. *Front. Microbiol.* 2016, *7*, 2016. [CrossRef] [PubMed]
28. Abdul-Hamid, A.; Bakar, J.; Bee, G.H. Nutritional quality of spray dried protein hydrolysate from Black Tilapia (*Oreochromis mossambicus*). *Food Chem.* 2002, *78*, 69–74. [CrossRef]
29. Li, J.; Cheng, J.H.; Teng, Z.J.; Sun, Z.Z.; He, X.Y.; Wang, P.; Shi, M.; Song, X.Y.; Chen, X.L.; Zhang, Y.Z.; et al. Taxonomic and Enzymatic Characterization of *Flocculibacter collagenilyticus* gen. nov., sp. nov., a Novel Gammaproteobacterium With High Collagenase Production. *Front. Microbiol.* 2021, *12*, 621161. [CrossRef]
30. Li, Y.; Hu, Z.; Jordan, F.; Inouye, M. Functional Analysis of the Propeptide of Subtilisin E as an Intramolecular Chaperone for Protein Folding: Refolding And Inhibitory Abilities of Propeptide Mutants (*). *J. Biol. Chem.* 1995, *270*, 25127–25132. [CrossRef]
31. Kojima, S.; Minagawa, T.; Miura, K. The propeptide of subtilisin BPN' as a temporary inhibitor and effect of an amino acid replacement on its inhibitory activity. *FEBS Lett.* 1997, *411*, 128–132. [CrossRef]
32. Luo, X.; Hofmann, K. The protease-associated domain: A homology domain associated with multiple classes of proteases. *Trends Biochem. Sci.* 2001, *26*, 147–148. [CrossRef]
33. Kagawa, T.F.; O'Connell, M.R.; Mouat, P.; Paoli, M.M.; O'Toole, P.W.; Cooney, J.C. Model for substrate interactions in C5a peptidase from *Streptococcus pyogenes*: A 1.9 A crystal structure of the active form of ScpA. *J. Mol. Biol.* 2009, *386*, 754–772. [CrossRef]

34. Morrissey, J.H. Chapter 641—Coagulation Factor VIIa. In *Handbook of Proteolytic Enzymes*, 3rd ed.; Rawlings, N.D., Salvesen, G., Eds.; Academic Press: Cambridge, MA, USA, 2013; pp. 2905–2908.
35. Page, M.J.; Craik, C.S. Chapter 669—Brachyurins. In *Handbook of Proteolytic Enzymes*, 3rd ed.; Rawlings, N.D., Salvesen, G., Eds.; Academic Press: Cambridge, MA, USA, 2013; pp. 3049–3052.
36. Fuller, R.S.; Brake, A.; Thorner, J. Yeast prohormone processing enzyme (KEX2 gene product) is a $Ca^{2+}$-dependent serine protease. *Proc. Natl. Acad. Sci. USA* **1989**, *86*, 1434–1438. [CrossRef]
37. Zhou, A.; Martin, S.; Lipkind, G.; LaMendola, J.; Steiner, D.F. Regulatory roles of the P domain of the subtilisin-like prohormone convertases. *J. Biol. Chem.* **1998**, *273*, 11107–11114. [CrossRef] [PubMed]
38. Rawlings, N.D.; Barrett, A.J. Chapter 559—Introduction: Serine Peptidases and Their Clans. In *Handbook of Proteolytic Enzymes*, 3rd ed.; Rawlings, N.D., Salvesen, G., Eds.; Academic Press: Cambridge, MA, USA, 2013; pp. 2491–2523.
39. Graycar, T.P.; Bott, R.R.; Power, S.D.; Estell, D.A. Chapter 693—Subtilisins. In *Handbook of Proteolytic Enzymes*, 3rd ed.; Rawlings, N.D., Salvesen, G., Eds.; Academic Press: Cambridge, MA, USA, 2013; pp. 3148–3155.
40. Sacco, E.; Elena Regonesi, M.; Vanoni, M. Chapter 711—Archaean Serine Proteases. In *Handbook of Proteolytic Enzymes*, 3rd ed.; Rawlings, N.D., Salvesen, G., Eds.; Academic Press: Cambridge, MA, USA, 2013; pp. 3224–3233.
41. Uesugi, Y.; Arima, J.; Usuki, H.; Iwabuchi, M.; Hatanaka, T. Two bacterial collagenolytic serine proteases have different topological specificities. *Biochim. Biophys. Acta* **2008**, *1784*, 716–726. [CrossRef] [PubMed]
42. Tsuruoka, N.; Nakayama, T.; Ashida, M.; Hemmi, H.; Nakao, M.; Minakata, H.; Oyama, H.; Oda, K.; Nishino, T. Collagenolytic serine-carboxyl proteinase from Alicyclobacillus sendaiensis strain NTAP-1: Purification, characterization, gene cloning, and heterologous expression. *Appl. Environ. Microbiol.* **2003**, *69*, 162–169. [CrossRef] [PubMed]
43. Cheng, J.-H.; Zhang, X.-Y.; Wang, Z.; Zhang, X.; Liu, S.-C.; Song, X.-Y.; Zhang, Y.-Z.; Ding, J.-M.; Chen, X.-L.; Xu, F. Potential of Thermolysin-like Protease A69 in Preparation of Bovine Collagen Peptides with Moisture-Retention Ability and Antioxidative Activity. *Mar. Drugs* **2021**, *19*, 676. [CrossRef] [PubMed]
44. Asaduzzaman, A.K.M.; Getachew, A.T.; Cho, Y.-J.; Park, J.-S.; Haq, M.; Chun, B.-S. Characterization of pepsin-solubilised collagen recovered from mackerel (*Scomber japonicus*) bone and skin using subcritical water hydrolysis. *Int. J. Biol. Macromol.* **2020**, *148*, 1290–1297. [CrossRef]
45. Medina-Medrano, J.R.; Quiñones-Muñoz, T.A.; Arce-Ortíz, A.; Torruco-Uco, J.G.; Hernández-Martínez, R.; Lizardi-Jiménez, M.A.; Varela-Santos, E. Antioxidant Activity of Collagen Extracts Obtained from the Skin and Gills of *Oreochromis* sp. *J. Med. Food* **2019**, *22*, 722–728. [CrossRef]
46. Zhang, J.B.; Zhao, Y.Q.; Wang, Y.M.; Chi, C.F.; Wang, B. Eight Collagen Peptides from Hydrolysate Fraction of Spanish Mackerel Skins: Isolation, Identification, and In Vitro Antioxidant Activity Evaluation. *Mar. Drugs* **2019**, *17*, 224. [CrossRef]
47. Yu, C.; Xiong, Y.L.; Jie, C. Andoxidant and emulsifying properties of potato protein hydrolysate in soybean oil-in-water emulsions. *Food Chem.* **2010**, *120*, 101–108.
48. Jahanbani, R.; Ghaffari, S.M.; Salami, M.; Vahdati, K.; Sepehri, H.; Sarvestani, N.N.; Sheibani, N.; Moosavi-Movahedi, A.A. Antioxidant and Anticancer Activities of Walnut (*Juglans regia* L.) Protein Hydrolysates Using Different Proteases. *Plant. Food Hum. Nutr.* **2016**, *71*, 402–409. [CrossRef] [PubMed]
49. You, L.J. Effect of degree of hydrolysis on the antioxidant activity of loach (*Misgurnus anguillicaudatus*) protein hydrolysates. *Innov. Food Sci. Emerg.* **2009**, *10*, 235–240. [CrossRef]
50. He, H.; Chen, X.; Sun, C.; Zhang, Y.; Gao, P. Preparation and functional evaluation of oligopeptide-enriched hydrolysate from shrimp (*Acetes chinensis*) treated with crude protease from *Bacillus* sp. SM98011. *Bioresour. Technol.* **2006**, *97*, 385–390. [CrossRef] [PubMed]
51. Haq, M.; Ho, T.C.; Ahmed, R.; Getachew, A.T.; Cho, Y.-J.; Park, J.-S.; Chun, B.-S. Biofunctional properties of bacterial collagenolytic protease-extracted collagen hydrolysates obtained using catalysts-assisted subcritical water hydrolysis. *J. Ind. Eng. Chem.* **2020**, *81*, 332–339. [CrossRef]
52. Yamamoto, S.; Deguchi, K.; Onuma, M.; Numata, N.; Sakai, Y. Absorption and Urinary Excretion of Peptides after Collagen Tripeptide Ingestion in Humans. *Biol. Pharm. Bull.* **2016**, *39*, 428–434. [CrossRef] [PubMed]
53. Ahmed, R.; Haq, M.; Chun, B.-S. Characterization of marine derived collagen extracted from the by-products of bigeye tuna (*Thunnus obesus*). *Int. J. Biol. Macromol.* **2019**, *135*, 668–676. [CrossRef] [PubMed]
54. Pratiwi, A.; Hakim, T.R.; Abidin, M.Z.; Fitriyanto, N.A.; Jamhari, J.; Rusman, R.; Erwanto, Y. Angiotensin-converting enzyme inhibitor activity of peptides derived from Kacang goat skin collagen through thermolysin hydrolysis. *Vet. World* **2021**, *14*, 161–167. [CrossRef]
55. Blum, M.; Chang, H.Y.; Chuguransky, S.; Grego, T.; Kandasaamy, S.; Mitchell, A.; Nuka, G.; Paysan-Lafosse, T.; Qureshi, M.; Raj, S.; et al. The InterPro protein families and domains database: 20 years on. *Nucleic Acids Res.* **2021**, *49*, D344–D354. [CrossRef]
56. Almagro Armenteros, J.J.; Tsirigos, K.D.; Sønderby, C.K.; Petersen, T.N.; Winther, O.; Brunak, S.; von Heijne, G.; Nielsen, H. SignalP 5.0 improves signal peptide predictions using deep neural networks. *Nat. Biotechnol.* **2019**, *37*, 420–423. [CrossRef]
57. Thompson, J.D.; Higgins, D.G.; Gibson, T.J. CLUSTAL W: Improving the sensitivity of progressive multiple sequence alignment through sequence weighting, position-specific gap penalties and weight matrix choice. *Nucleic Acids Res.* **1994**, *22*, 4673–4680. [CrossRef]
58. Robert, X.; Gouet, P. Deciphering key features in protein structures with the new ENDscript server. *Nucleic Acids Res.* **2014**, *42*, W320–W324. [CrossRef]

59. Bailey, T.L.; Boden, M.; Buske, F.A.; Frith, M.; Grant, C.E.; Clementi, L.; Ren, J.; Li, W.W.; Noble, W.S. MEME SUITE: Tools for motif discovery and searching. *Nucleic Acids Res.* **2009**, *37*, W202–W208. [CrossRef]
60. Kumar, S.; Stecher, G.; Li, M.; Knyaz, C.; Tamura, K. MEGA X: Molecular Evolutionary Genetics Analysis across Computing Platforms. *Mol. Biol. Evol.* **2018**, *35*, 1547–1549. [CrossRef] [PubMed]
61. Zhao, G.Y.; Chen, X.L.; Zhao, H.L.; Xie, B.B.; Zhou, B.C.; Zhang, Y.Z. Hydrolysis of insoluble collagen by deseasin MCP-01 from deep-sea *Pseudoalteromonas* sp. SM9913: Collagenolytic characters, collagen-binding ability of C-terminal polycystic kidney disease domain, and implication for its novel role in deep-sea sedimentary particulate organic nitrogen degradation. *J. Biol. Chem.* **2008**, *283*, 36100–36107. [CrossRef] [PubMed]
62. Yemm, E.W.; Cocking, E.C.; Ricketts, R.E. The determination of amino-acids with ninhydrin. *Analyst* **1955**, *80*, 209–214. [CrossRef]
63. He, H.L.; Chen, X.L.; Li, J.W.; Zhang, Y.Z.; Gao, P.J. Taste improvement of refrigerated meat treated with cold-adapted Protease. *Food Chem.* **2004**, *84*, 307–311. [CrossRef]
64. Chen, X.L.; Xie, B.B.; Bian, F.; Zhao, G.Y.; Zhao, H.L.; He, H.L.; Zhou, B.C.; Zhang, Y.Z. Ecological function of myroilysin, a novel bacterial M12 metalloprotease with elastinolytic activity and a synergistic role in collagen hydrolysis, in biodegradation of deep-sea high-molecular-weight organic nitrogen. *Appl. Environ. Microbiol.* **2009**, *75*, 1838–1844. [CrossRef]
65. Sun, M.L.; Zhao, F.; Shi, M.; Zhang, X.Y.; Zhou, B.C.; Zhang, Y.Z.; Chen, X.L. Characterization and Biotechnological Potential Analysis of a New Exopolysaccharide from the Arctic Marine Bacterium *Polaribacter* sp. SM1127. *Sci. Rep.* **2015**, *5*, 18435. [CrossRef]

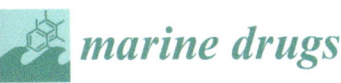

Article

# Growth Factor-Free Vascularization of Marine-Origin Collagen Sponges Using Cryopreserved Stromal Vascular Fractions from Human Adipose Tissue

Sara Freitas-Ribeiro [1,2], Gabriela S. Diogo [1,2], Catarina Oliveira [1,2], Albino Martins [1,2], Tiago H. Silva [1,2], Mariana Jarnalo [3,4], Ricardo Horta [3,4], Rui L. Reis [1,2] and Rogério P. Pirraco [1,2,*]

1. 3B's Research Group, I3Bs—Research Institute on Biomaterials, Biodegradables and Biomimetics, University of Minho, Headquarters of the European Institute of Excellence on Tissue Engineering and Regenerative Medicine, Barco, 4805-017 Guimarães, Portugal
2. ICVS/3B's—PT Government Associate Laboratory, Braga, 4710-057 Guimarães, Portugal
3. Department of Plastic and Reconstructive Surgery, and Burn Unity, Centro Hospitalar de São João, 4200-319 Porto, Portugal
4. Faculty of Medicine, University of Porto, 4200-319 Porto, Portugal
* Correspondence: rpirraco@i3bs.uminho.pt

**Abstract:** The successful integration of transplanted three-dimensional tissue engineering (TE) constructs depends greatly on their rapid vascularization. Therefore, it is essential to address this vascularization issue in the initial design of constructs for perfused tissues. Two of the most important variables in this regard are scaffold composition and cell sourcing. Collagens with marine origins overcome some issues associated with mammal-derived collagen while maintaining their advantages in terms of biocompatibility. Concurrently, the freshly isolated stromal vascular fraction (SVF) of adipose tissue has been proposed as an advantageous cell fraction for vascularization purposes due to its highly angiogenic properties, allowing extrinsic angiogenic growth factor-free vascularization strategies for TE applications. In this study, we aimed at understanding whether marine collagen 3D matrices could support cryopreserved human SVF in maintaining intrinsic angiogenic properties observed for fresh SVF. For this, cryopreserved human SVF was seeded on blue shark collagen sponges and cultured up to 7 days in a basal medium. The secretome profile of several angiogenesis-related factors was studied throughout culture times and correlated with the expression pattern of CD31 and CD146, which showed the formation of a prevascular network. Upon in ovo implantation, increased vessel recruitment was observed in prevascularized sponges when compared with sponges without SVF cells. Immunohistochemistry for CD31 demonstrated the improved integration of prevascularized sponges within chick chorioalantoic membrane (CAM) tissues, while in situ hybridization showed human cells lining blood vessels. These results demonstrate the potential of using cryopreserved SVF combined with marine collagen as a streamlined approach to improve the vascularization of TE constructs.

**Keywords:** stromal vascular fraction; vascularization; blue shark skin collagen; 3D constructs

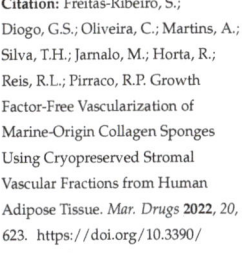

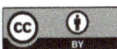

## 1. Introduction

Vascularization is a critical aspect of every tissue engineering (TE) approach for thick perfused tissues. A comprehensive network of capillaries is necessary to ensure, upon anastomosis with the host's circulation, the proper delivery of nutrients and oxygen to all cells of the engineered tissue, avoiding necrotic events and promoting integration with the surrounding tissue. TE approaches for thick tissues not specifically addressing vascularization rely, in an initial phase after implantation, on passive diffusion, which is limited to ~150 μm [1]. Although the hypoxic environment created by the lack of oxygen potentiates the host vessel's invasion towards the implanted construct, the rate of spontaneous vascular ingrowth is slow [2] and does not satisfy the metabolic needs of cells, leading to necrosis at the bulk of the graft. As a result, the successful use of TE constructs in the clinic is mainly limited to thin engineered constructs in which this rate of neovascularization from the host combined with diffusion is sufficient [3,4]. Therefore, most current strategies for engineering thick 3D constructs encompass a prevascularization step. Prevascularization uses endothelial cells (ECs) to form capillary-like networks before implantation, which will ideally anastomose with the circulation of the host tissue after implantation [5]. ECs are seeded alone or in combination with other supportive cell types and most frequently require supplementation with angiogenic growth factors [6,7]. However, the sourcing of ECs is an issue since macrovascular cells such as HUVECs are often used but are arguably not the most suited for capillary network formation [8]. Moreover, supplementation with extrinsic angiogenic growth factors fails to reproduce the growth factor kinetics involved in native vasculogenesis, which often leads to the formation of a non-mature network [9]. In this context, adipose tissue's stromal vascular fraction (SVF) may be extremely important due to its intrinsic angiogenic potential [10]. This fraction can be isolated after the enzymatic digestion of adipose tissue obtained from liposuction or abdominoplasties, which otherwise would be discarded. Several cell populations encompass the SVF, namely endothelial and hematopoietic cells, mesenchymal and endothelial progenitors, pericytes, fibroblasts, and preadipocytes [10–12]. As previously reported, the pericytes and endothelial progenitors present in this fraction have the potential to spontaneously assemble in capillary-like networks in vitro without the need for angiogenic growth factor supplementation, both in 2D [13] and 3D settings [14]. However, freshly isolated SVF is usually used for this purpose, which may be disadvantageous for widespread clinical applications. The use of preserved SVF is therefore underexplored and warrants further investigation. Another important factor for the vascularization of 3D TE constructs is the biomaterial used. The use of natural origin polymers with intrinsic biocompatible properties has revealed a promising approach [15]. [15] Of these polymers, collagen is the most broadly used, as it is the major structural component of the native extracellular matrix (ECM) in living tissues and provides several cues for directing cellular behavior. Among the latter, adhesive motifs are included, which are powerful regulators of cell responses, such as cell spreading or stem cell differentiation [16]. Although collagen from mammalian sources is mostly used to produce TE constructs [17–21], regulatory and religious issues [22] have boosted the search for other collagen sources. Marine collagen is one such source. This type of collagen can be isolated from a number of marine species. In particular, the skin and bones of fish, sea urchin waste, jellyfish, and starfish have high collagen contents [15] with similar properties to mammalian collagen type I [23]. Due to by-catch, the blue shark is one of the most caught shark species [24], and its by-products are highly available and, thus, desirable for collagen extraction [25,26]. We have previously developed blue shark skin collagen sponges with interconnected micro-porous structures that promote not only human adipose stem cells adhesion but also ECM production and cell proliferation and infiltration within scaffolds, indicating a great potential for vascularization purposes [27].

Considering all of the above, blue shark collagen sponges were used as 3D matrices to explore the capacity of cryopreserved SVF to spontaneously yield a prevascular network in vitro in the absence of extrinsic angiogenic growth factors. This was achieved by assessing the spontaneous formation of capillary-like structures in vitro and by evaluating vessel recruitment, constructing the integration of the prevascular network with the host tissue after in ovo implantation using a chick chorioalantoic membrane (CAM) model.

## 2. Results

### 2.1. Generation of Prevascularized Collagen Sponges in an Extrinsic Angiogenic Growth Factor Free Manner

We investigated the potential of cryopreserved SVF to create a prevascular network, in the absence of extrinsic angiogenic growth factors, after seeding in a blue shark collagen sponge (Figure 1A). Highly interconnected microporous sponges were produced by resorting to a cryogelation method, as previously described [27] (Figure 1B). SVF was isolated from human adipose subcutaneous tissue and cryopreserved in 10% DMSO in FBS for at least 7 days. SVF was then thawed and seeded on collagen sponges and cultured for 7 days without angiogenic growth factor supplementation, as previously described for fresh SVF [13] (Figure 1A). After that period, the expression pattern of endothelial marker CD31 and pericytes CD146 revealed the presence of endothelial cells together with pericytes organized in a complex and interconnected capillary-like network, confirming that SVF maintained its capacity to create a prevascular network without angiogenic growth factor supplementation even after cryopreservation (Figure 1C).

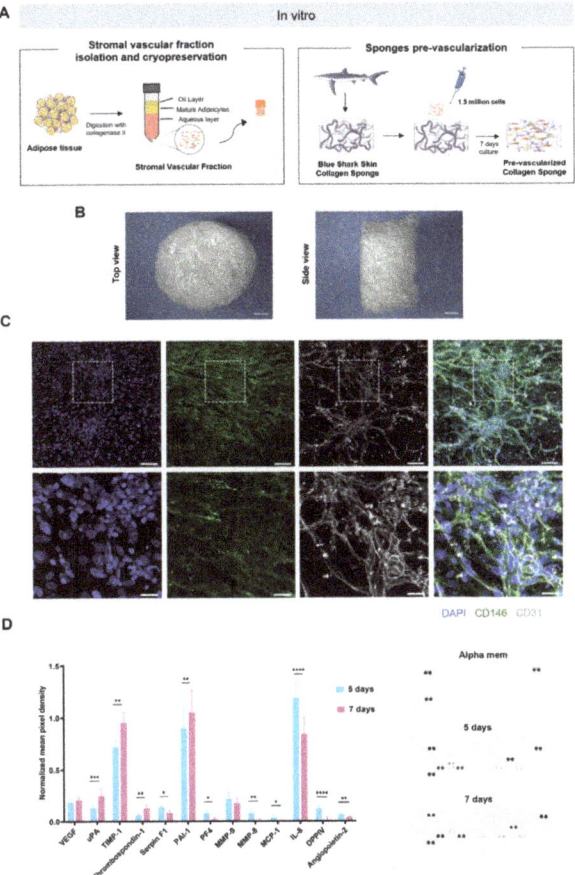

**Figure 1.** Generation of pre-vascularized collagen sponges. (**A**) In vitro experimental design. (**B**) Representative macroscopic images of shark skin collagen sponge's macroporosity after freeze drying. Scale bar: 1000 μm. (**C**) Representative immunocytochemistry images of the network-like organization of SVF-derived CD31-expressing cells (white) interconnected with pericytes CD146-expressing cells (green), within collagen sponges after 7 days of culture in the absence of extrinsic angiogenic growth factors. Cell nuclei were counterstained with DAPI (blue). Scale bar: 75 μm (**top**) and 25 μm (**bottom**). (**D**) Angiogenic secretome profile of SVF cells seeded in collagen sponges at different culture periods. Conditioned media were collected at days 5 and 7 for dot blot analysis of angiogenesis-related factors. Protein expression profiles were measured using mean intensity and normalized to the reference spots. Data are presented as mean ± std dev and were analyzed using a paired $t$-test (* $p < 0.0332$, ** $p < 0.0021$, *** $p < 0.0002$, and **** $p < 0.0001$).

## 2.2. Profiling of Angiogenesis-Related Proteins in Prevascularized Collagen Sponges Secretome

Given the confirmation of prevascular network formation, we sought to understand if and how the secretome profile changed throughout the culture time. To achieve this, a multiplex analysis of secretome targeting angiogenesis-related proteins was performed on secretome samples collected after 5 and 7 days of culture (Figure 1D). The selection of these timepoints was based on previous studies from our lab [13]. The secretion of important angiogenic modulators such as VEGF and MMP-9 remained unchanged from one time point to the other. However, an increase in the secretion of several factors specifically involved in ECM remodeling (uPA, PAI-1, and TIMP-1) was verified from day 5 to 7, while macrophage-related factors decreased over culture time (IL-8, MCP-1). Interestingly, no expression of angiogenic proteins other than the ones detected for the first timepoint was found for the later timepoint.

## 2.3. In Ovo Evaluation of Angiogenic Potential

Upon the in vitro confirmation of prevascular network formations, the in ovo angiogenic potential of the prevascularized collagen sponge was assessed by using a chick CAM assay (Figure 2A). After prevascularization, collagen sponges were implanted into the CAM of chicken eggs. A control group consisting of sponges without seeded cells was also implanted. For the evaluation and quantification of angiogenesis, the area around the implantation site was fixed, photographed, and finally excised and paraffin embedded. Results demonstrate host vessel recruitment in both the prevascularized and control sponges (Figure 2B). However, vessel quantification demonstrated a significantly higher number of recruited vessels for prevascularized sponges when comparing with sponges without SVF cells (Figure 2C), strongly suggesting a beneficial role of prevascularization with SVF in post-implantation vascularization. Concurrently, histological analysis after H&E staining clearly presented a higher CAM tissue ingrowth towards the bulk of prevascularized sponges in contrast with the control group with empty sponges where host tissue was very much limited to the outside of the sponge's structure (Figure 2D). Importantly, no significant immune reaction was visible for both groups. Together with the higher number of recruited vessels, these results strongly suggest a positive effect of prevascularization with SVF upon the integration of implanted collagen sponges with the CAM tissue. In situ hybridization results show that human origin cells from the SVF persist in the CAM tissue after 4 days of implantation (Figure 3A) and, importantly, incorporate new vessels, suggesting a net contribution to the higher vessel density determined above. The contribution of implanted SVF cells to neo-vessel formation was further confirmed after immunohistochemistry for human CD31, which clearly demonstrates CD31-positive cells lining blood vessel walls in the interface between CAM tissues and collagen sponges (Figure 3B).

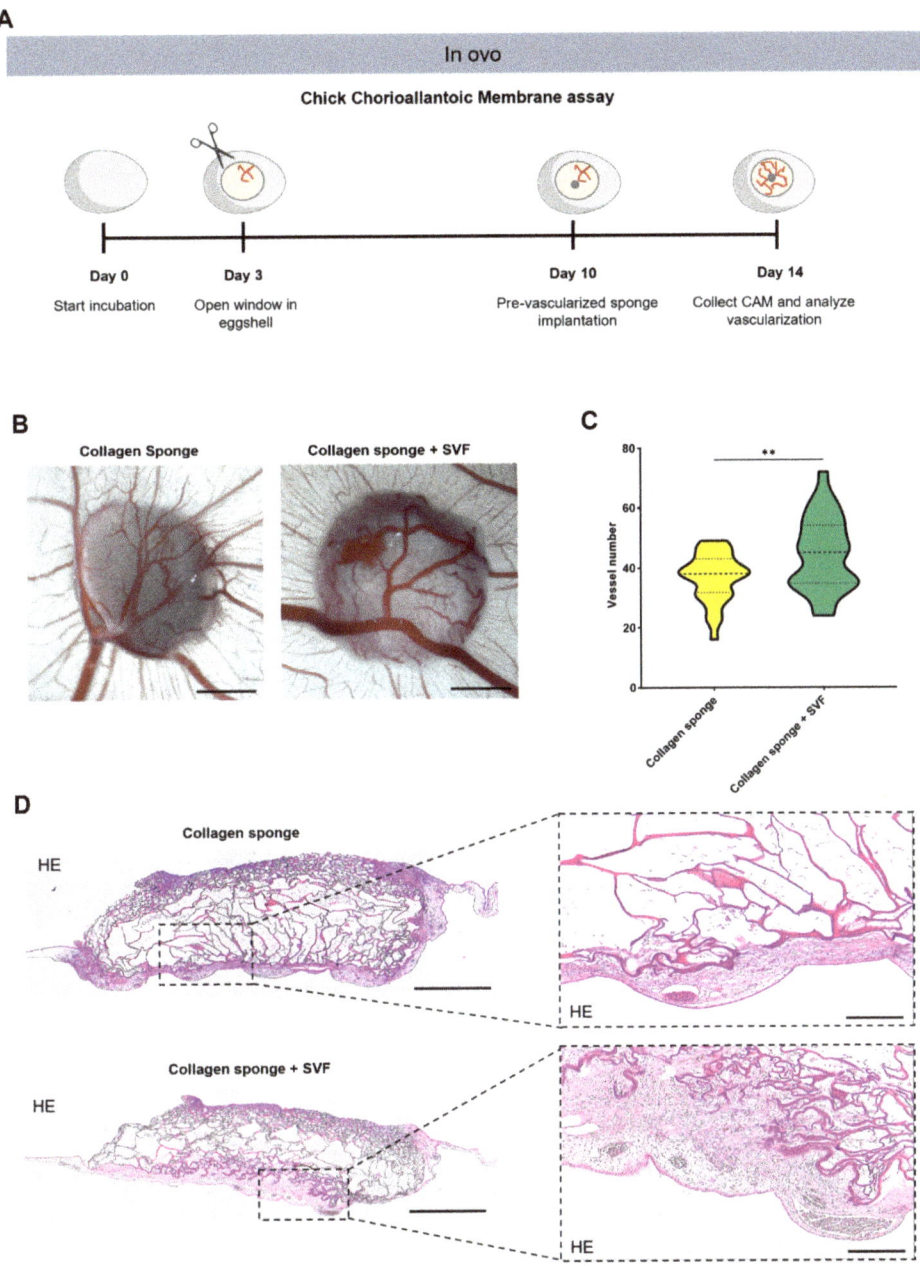

**Figure 2.** In ovo angiogenic potential upon implantation in Chick Chorioallantoic Membrane (CAM). (**A**) In vivo experimental design. (**B**) Representative micrographs of recruited vessels after 4 days of implantation of collagen sponges with and without SVF. Scale bar: 2000 μm. (**C**) Quantification of recruited vessels after 4 days of implantation of collagen sponge with and without SVF. Data are presented as violin plot illustrating the kernel density distribution frequency of recruited vessels and analyzed using an unpaired $t$-test (** $p < 0.0021$). (**D**) Representative micrographs of hematoxylin and eosin staining in collagen sponges with and without SVF. Scale bar: 500 μm (**left**) and 50 μm (**right**).

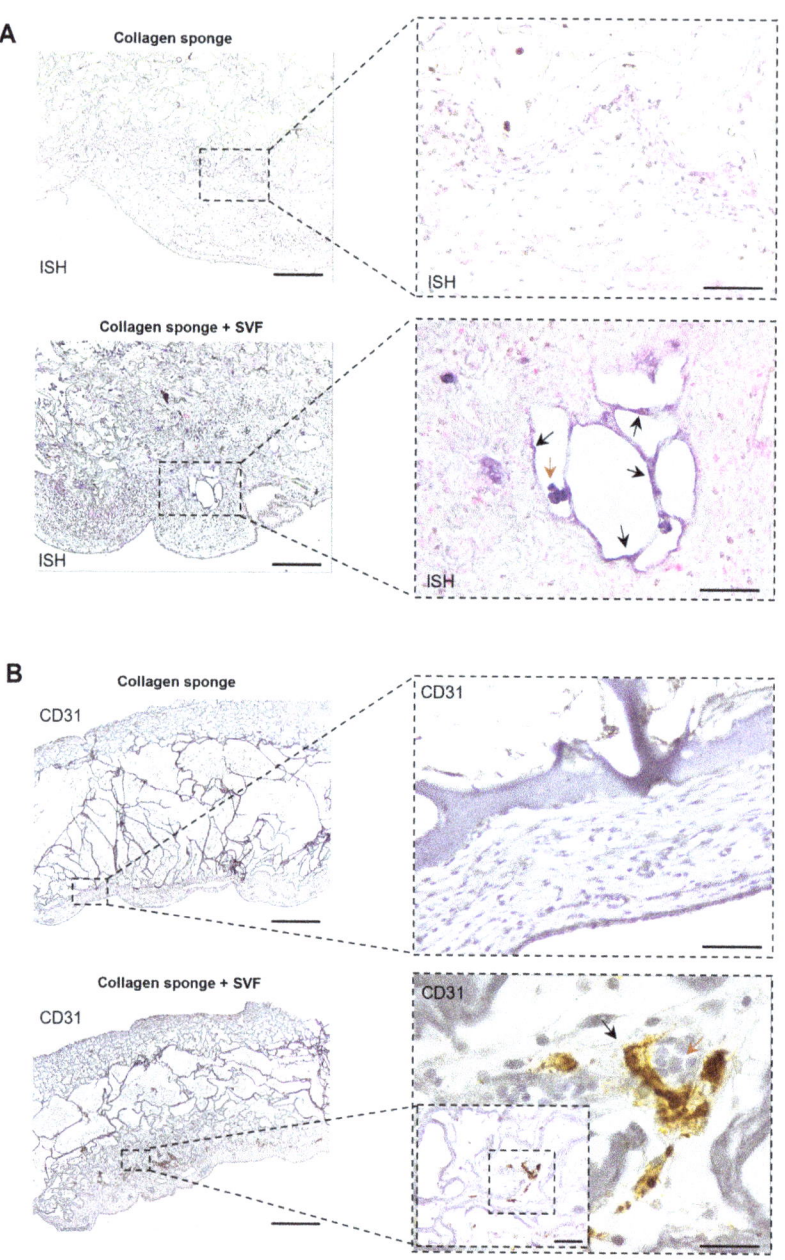

**Figure 3.** In ovo angiogenic potential upon implantation in Chick Chorioallantoic Membrane (CAM). (**A**) Representative images of the in situ hybridization performed with a DNA probe that stains human cellular nuclei (blue, arrows) in contrast with chicken nuclei (pink). The implanted cells infiltrated the host tissue and vasculature as highlighted by black arrows. Chicken erythrocytes identified by orange arrows. Scale bars: 200 µm (**left**) and 50 µm (**right**). (**B**) Representative immunohistochemistry images of the collagen sponge after 4 days of implantation showing human CD31-positive cells (brown). Human CD31 expression patterns demonstrated the integration of the pre-vascular network in the CAM, as highlighted by black arrows. Chicken erythrocytes identified by orange arrows. Scale bars: 500 µm (**left**) and 20 µm (**right**) and 50 µm (**inset right**).

## 3. Discussion

The fast and efficient establishment of blood perfusion in engineered constructs after transplantation represents one of the major challenges for the incorporation of TE products into the clinical practice. Some early vascularization approaches focused on vascular ingrowth stimulation in tissue constructs by optimizing scaffolds' material properties [28] or by incorporating growth factor delivery systems [29,30]. Both strategies proved to be inefficient, however, since vascular ingrowth is a slow process [2]. To overcome this, TERM strategies started to incorporate the in vitro creation of a prevascular network. ECs are seeded in scaffolds and supplemented with angiogenic growth factors that induce a vasculogenic-like process, ultimately forming a prevascular network [31]. However, the native vasculogenic process requires different growth factors produced by different cell types that interact with target receptors in a coordinated manner to ultimately yield a mature vascular network [9]. This is why early prevascularization strategies using only ECs, typically HUVECs, were often found to yield non-mature prevascular that is prone to regression after some period of time [32]. However, to recapitulate, the in vitro complexity of native vasculogenesis is a formidable challenge, both technically and in terms of costs due to the diverse cell types and different culture media and growth factors required. These facts urge the development of a streamlined and more cost-effective strategy to promote the vascularization of constructs.

In recent years, the SVF of adipose tissue became a focus of attention mainly due to its intrinsic angiogenic potential. However, studies demonstrating the angiogenic potential of SVF commonly use freshly isolated samples, which may limit its clinical applicability to specialized centers. The development of cell-banking strategies for SVF while maintaining its angiogenic potential would boost its clinical potential. The development of cell-banking strategies for SVF while maintaining its angiogenic potential would boost its clinical potential. Some studies describe the use of cryopreserved SVF for the production of vascularized adipose tissue, showing its ability to create capillary-like structures after preservation [33]. However, such studies use supplementation with angiogenic growth factors to induce capillary-like structure formation, which introduces a significant degree of complexity to the system. A previous study from our laboratory has shown that fresh SVF can spontaneously produce capillary-like structures as early as 5 days of culture, without the addition of angiogenic growth factors, representing a cost reduction and a more organic vasculogenic process since it is orchestrated by the cells themselves [13]. In this sense, we explored if cryopreserved SVF, in the absence of extrinsic angiogenic growth factors, retained this ability to spontaneously create a prevascular network in 3D conditions. SVF consists of a heterogeneous population of cells with an intrinsic capacity to secrete several angiogenic-associated growth factors, creating the perfect angiogenic microenvironment capable of promoting the formation of in vitro capillary-like networks in the absence of extrinsic angiogenic growth factors [13].

Vasculogenesis and angiogenesis are complex processes involving the coordinated action of several families of growth factors such as the vascular endothelial growth factor (VEGF), platelet-derived growth factor (PDGF), tissue inhibitor of metalloproteinases (TIMP), fibroblast growth factor (FGF), angiopoietin (ANG), interleukins (ILs), and matrix metalloproteinases (MMPs). All these players contribute not only ro capillary formation but, critically, to their stabilization and maturation [13]. In the 3D SVF cultures reported herein, we verified the protein expression of several angiogenic modulators over the culture time. Factors involved in ECM remodeling, namely urokinase (uPA), plasminogen activator inhibitor (PAI-1), and TIMP-1, increased from day 5 to day 7. Plasminogen activators such as (uPA) are key mediators of the ECM degradation process by converting inactive plasminogen to active plasmin, and it is in turn capable of degrading specific matrix constituents and of activating matrix-degrading metalloproteases such as MMP-9 [34]. Concurrently, it has been demonstrated that the increased production of uPA by microvascular ECs in response to angiogenic stimuli is accompanied by an increase in the production of the PAI-1 [35], which is in line with what we observed. This is most likely related with the need of a proteolytic balance that allows ECM degradation for cell migration but in a controlled fashion to keep the three-dimensional matrix intact, into which ECs form capillary-like networks [36]. The secretion of MMPs inhibitors is also influenced by this synergistic effect. Increased TIMP-1 expression is important for vessel stabilization by limiting matrix degradation and allowing matrix depositions that could explain its increase over culture times [37]. The decrease in IL-8 and MCP-1 expression also suggests that the angiogenic process is more directed to capillaries stabilization and maturation. In an initial phase of angiogenesis, MCP-1 recruits macrophages [38] that in turn secrete a variety of angiogenic-related factors such as thrombospondin-1 and IL-8 [39]. The latter is in fact essential for EC proliferation and migration [40,41], allowing capillary formation and elongation. The role of MCP-1 in angiogenesis promotion is not exclusively for macrophage recruitment. It up-regulates VEGF expression [42], increases vascular permeability [43], and is involved in pericytes recruitment [44]. The incorporation of pericytes initiates the stabilization and maturation of new vessels [45]. They are capable of modulating the ECM remodeling capacity of ECs by inducing the upregulation of PAI-1 in ECs and, in this way, limiting its migration and branching [46]. We verified the presence and incorporation of pericytes in the pre-vascular nerwork after 7 days, together with an increase over culture time of the levels of thrombospondin-1 and a decrease in levels of IL-8 and MCP-1 and stagnation in VEGF release. This strongly suggests a move towards the stage of capillary stabilization and maturation. This is further reinforced by decreased levels of ANG-2, involved in angiogenesis initiation [47]. The synergy between all cells present in the SVF and the secretion of all of these factors ultimately led to the formation of a prevascular network, as demonstrated by CD31's expression pattern, and it is anchored by perivascular cells identified by the expression of CD146 and the lack of expression of CD31. Although the present study did not directly compare the angiogenic capacity of cryo-preserved and fresh SVF, our results are in agreement with what was reported by Costa et al. for fresh SVF. That study showed the spontaneous formation of a network of capillaries, with increased secretions of several angiogenic modulators from 5 to 8 days of culture. All of this, of course, occurred in the absence of extrinsic angiogenic factors [13]. Collagen scaffolds also provided structural and mechanical support and permitted significant capillary formation within its structure in vitro. The ability of collagen, as a three-dimensional matrix, to support the adherence and proliferation of endothelial cells in vitro has been observed for several years [48]. While mammalian collagen is the standard, new collagen sources have emerged. The skin and bones of several marine organisms are abundant in collagen, presenting very similar characteristics to that of mammalian origin. Blue shark skin collagen demonstrated a comparable chondrogenic differentiation of human adipose stem cells compared to the commercial alternative comprising bovine collagen [27]. In the case of a direct comparison between collagen from marine tilapia skin and bovine skin collagen, both showed a similar performance in a wound-healing scenario, allowing fibroblasts infiltration, vascularization, reduced inflammation, and collagen deposition [49]. In fact, the existing differences are only noticeable in proline and hydroxyproline contents [27]. The lower content of this amino acids in comparison with mammalian collagen, affects the denaturation temperature and, consequently, its thermal stability, resulting in a faster degradation of scaffolds [50]. Despite presenting a faster degradation rate due to its lower denaturation temperature, the use of crosslinkers allowed the stabilization of sponges. The large pores created (averaging 250–300 μm) [27] with highly interconnective microporosities positively influenced endothelial cell migration, rearrangement, and vessel density. Microporosity is considered critical for the new vessel's size and number [51,52]. High pore interconnectivity results in significantly higher blood vessel density in vitro and increased blood vessel density and average invasion depth after implantation [53]. These architectural features present in the sponges used in this study allowed for the cell migration, proliferation, and organization of vascular networks, validating marine-derived collagen as a suitable raw material for TE of vascularized tissues. This alternative source of collagen for TE products not only surpasses disease-transmission concerns, such as bovine spongiform encephalopathy (BSE) [22], but also religious constraints, making it suitable for broader applications. Furthermore, new applications of marine by-products are of extreme importance, especially those that are environmentally friendly [54]. Its isolation represents low costs, creating value from products that are considered wasteful for the fish transformation industry.

To assess the in ovo functionality of the created prevascular network, a CAM assay was performed. The membrane of chick embryo provides a non-innervated and rapidly growing vascular bed, which can serve as a blood supply for engineered tissues and, therefore, be a useful model for testing prevascularization strategies [55]. In particular, its use has been reported in approaches ranging from cell sheets [56] to spheroids [57]. Herein, prevascularized collagen sponges were implanted onto the CAM and collected after 4 days. Empty sponges were implanted as controls. Both prevascularized and empty sponges were able to recruit blood vessels from the host in the implant region. Nonetheless, this effect was significantly improved for prevascularized constructs, suggesting that the presence of SVF can accelerate graft's vascularization in ovo. Furthermore, the rapid infiltration of the implanted construct by host cells, without visible inflammatory response, revealed a superior integration with CAM when SVF cells were present. It is known that the cell complexity present in SVF can have an effect on neovascularization in ischemic tissues [58,59]. By injecting SVF in a hind limb ischemic mouse model, previous studies demonstrated that SVF cells not only improved blood flow [58,59] but were also able to integrate blood vessel linings [58]. It is thought that this improvement is mainly mediated by angiogenic cytokines secreted from implanted cells [60]. Since the latter two studies were conducted by injecting cells, the residence time for implanted cells at the injured site was probably reduced; thus, the release of angiogenic stimulators is limited in time. While the encapsulation of SVF can improve residency times, the creation of a 3D prevascular network prior to implantation [61] may further accelerate the vascularization of the graft in vivo through a rapid connection to recipient blood vessels [61,62]. In fact, the maturation of the created prevascular network also influences the angiogenic potential. Cerino et al. demonstrated that faster inosculation and the enhanced survival of transplanted cells in full-thickness rat wounds is associated to pericytes, for which its number was significantly higher in more mature constructs [62]. In the present study, it was clearly demonstrated that implanted human cells, namely CD31-positive cells, were able to integrate newly formed blood vessels at the interface between the CAM and implanted sponges. While this was not specifically tested, no evidence of prevascular network inosculation with the host's circulation was found. Nevertheless, ISH and CD31 results, together with the demonstrated increase in vessel recruitment from the host, show that cryopreserved SVF had a positive effect on vascularization after implantation, underscoring the potential of this fraction for TE applications.

## 4. Materials and Methods

### 4.1. Collagen Acid Extraction

Collagen was extracted from blue shark (Prionace glauca) skin at Instituto de Investigaciones Marinas (CSCI, Vigo, Spain), according to a previously described protocol [27]. Blue shark skin was stirred with 0.1M NaOH in a cold room (3–5 °C) for 24 h to remove non-collagenous proteins and pigments. After a centrifugation step, the remaining pellet was washed with distilled water and incubated overnight with 0.5 M acetic acid under agitation to start the acid extraction process. The obtained extract was centrifuged at 10 °C, and the supernatant dialyzed against distilled water for 2 days in a cold room (3–5 °C). Finally, the obtained collagen extract was freeze-dried.

### 4.2. Collagen Sponge Fabrication

The production of highly interconnective microporous collagen sponges was performed as previously described [27]. Briefly, the previously extracted collagen was solubilized at 1% (w/v) concentration in a 10 mM hydrochloric acid (HCl, Sigma-Aldrich, St. Louis, MO, USA) solution. Cryogelation and crosslinking reactions were carried out at

−20 °C for 4 h by the addition of 1-[3-(dimethylamino) propyl]-3-ethylcarbodiimide hydrochloride (EDC) (Mw: 191,70 g.mol$^{-1}$, Sigma-Aldrich, St. Louis, MO, USA) at 60 mM of final concentration. To remove the residual crosslinker, cryogels were rinsed with distilled water before freeze drying.

### 4.3. Isolation and Cryopreservation of Human Adipose-Derived SVF Cells

Human subcutaneous adipose tissues were obtained from surgical procedures performed at Hospital de S. João (Porto), after obtaining the patient's written informed consent, and within the scope of a collaboration protocol approved by the ethical committees of both institutions for this work (Comissão de Ética do Hospital de S. João/University of Minho: 217/19; CEICVS 008/2019). SVF was obtained as previously described [13]. Briefly, adipose tissue was digested with a collagenase type II (Sigma Aldrich, St. Louis, MO, USA) solution of 0.05% (w/v), for 45 min at 37 °C under agitation. After centrifugation, the obtained SVF was incubated with red blood lysis buffer and centrifuged, and the supernatant was resuspended in Minimum Essential Medium alpha-modification (α-MEM) (Life Technologies, Carlsbad, CA, USA) supplemented with 10% fetal bovine serum (FBS) and 1% antibiotic/antimycotic. Cell nuclei were stained using a solution of 3% (v/v) acetic acid (VWR, Lutterworth, UK) and 0.05 wt % methylene blue (Sigma Aldrich, St. Louis, MO, USA) in water to count nucleated cells. Finally, cells were cryopreserved in 10% (v/v) dimethyl sulfoxide (DMSO) in FBS with a controlled freeze rate of 1 °C/min for at least 7 days.

### 4.4. Cell Seeding

After thawing, a pool of five different donors was made. SVF was seeded on collagen sponges by dispensing 25 µL on top of the dried sponges and another 25 µL at the bottom of a 50 µL cell suspension comprising $1.5 \times 10^6$ cells. Constructs were incubated for 1 h at 37 °C, 5% $CO_2$, to allow maximum cell entrapment within the structures, and then fresh medium was added to a total volume of 1 mL. Constructs were cultured for 7 days in α-MEM to allow the formation of capillary-like structures.

### 4.5. Immunocytochemistry

After in vitro culture, constructs were fixed in a 10% (v/v) buffered formalin solution. A 3% (w/v) BSA was used to block non-specific binding, and cells were incubated overnight at 4 °C with primary antibody mouse anti-human CD31 (M0823) (1:30) (Dako, Cambridge, UK) and rabbit anti-human CD146 (ABCAAB75769) (1:50) (VWR, Lutterworth, UK). After repeated washes in PBS, secondary antibody Alexa Fluor 594 donkey anti-mouse (1:500) and AlexaFluor 488 donkey anti-rabbit (Molecular probes, Eugene, OR, USA) were incubated with cells for 4 h at room temperature. After washing with PBS, cell nuclei were counterstained with DAPI. The presence of capillary-like structures was verified in a confocal laser scanning microscope (SP8 Leica Microsystems CMS GmbH, Wetzlar, Germany).

### 4.6. Secretome Analysis

In order to analyze the expression profile of angiogenesis-related proteins during the prevascularization process, conditioned media were collected and centrifuged to remove cell debris after 5 and 7 days of culture. A control with basal media was also set up. Secreted proteins were analyzed using a Proteome Profiler human angiogenesis array (R&D Systems; Minneapolis, MN, USA) in accordance with manufacturer guidelines. Briefly, conditioned media were incubated with an assay-specific detection antibody cocktail for 1 h at room temperature. After a membrane blocking step, samples containing antibody cocktail were added to the respective membrane and incubated overnight at 4 °C under shaking. Membranes were then washed with 1× wash buffer, incubated with streptavidin-HRP for 30 min, and washed again. Membranes were incubated with Chemi Reagent Mix for 1 min, and spots detected by using chemiluminescence in an Odyssey Fc Imaging System

(LI-COR, Lincoln, NE, USA) and densitometry were quantified using Image studio 5.2 software (LI-COR, Lincoln, NE, USA)

*4.7. In ovo Implantation*

A CAM assay was performed as previously described [57,63]. White fertilized chicken eggs were incubated at 37 °C in a temperature incubator (Termaks KB8000, Bergen, Norway) for 3 days. After this, a window was opened into the shell to evaluate embryo viability. Prevascularized sponges ($n = 12$) were implanted on the CAM at day 10 of embryonic development, and the eggs returned to the incubator at 37 °C. Control groups with empty materials ($n = 12$) and without the material ($n = 12$) were also set up. After 4 days of implantation, embryos were sacrificed with 4 % (v/v) paraformaldehyde and subsequent incubation at −80 °C for 10 min. Then, the implanted materials with adjacent portions of CAM were cut and fixed with 4% (v/v) paraformaldehyde. Ex ovo images were captured using a Stemi 2000-C stereo microscope (Zeiss, Oberkochen, Germany).

*4.8. New Vessel Quantification*

The obtained ex ovo images were processed using ImageJ 1.52a (National Institutes of Health, Bethesda, MD, USA). Images were cropped to a defined area of 500 × 500 pixels, considering the implanted construct in the center of the image. The number of new/recruited vessels growing radially towards the constructed area was quantified by manual counting, in a blind fashion, by three independent operators.

*4.9. Histological Analysis*

After formalin fixation, CAM explants were processed in a MICRON STP120-2 spin tissue processor (MICRON, Walldorf, Germany), embedded in paraffin (Thermo Scientific, Waltham, MA, USA), and serially sectioned into 4 µm-thick sections.

*4.10. Hematoxylin and Eosin Staining*

Hematoxylin and eosin (H&E) staining was performed in CAM sections. Briefly, sections were deparaffinized with xylene, rehydrated in graded ethanol series and stained with hematoxylin and eosin in an MICROM HMS740 automatic stainer (MICROM, Walldorf, Germany). Afterwards, sections were dehydrated and mounted with resinous mounting medium Entellan® (Merck, Darmstadt, Germany). Histological sections were analyzed under a Leica DM750 microscope (Leica, Wetzlar, Germany).

*4.11. Immunohistochemistry*

CAM sections were deparaffinized and rehydrated in an MICROM HMS740 automatic stainer (MICROM, Walldorf, Germany). Immunohistochemical analysis was performed using a streptavidin–biotin peroxidase complex system. Briefly, after rehydration, slides were subjected to heat-induced antigen-retrieval with 10 mM citrate buffer at pH = 6 for 2 min at 98 °C. The slides were washed with PBS and then incubated with 3% hydrogen peroxide for 10 min to inactivate endogenous peroxidases. Another washing step was performed, and nonspecific binding was blocked with a 2.5% (v/v) horse serum (Vector Labs, Newark, CA, USA) for 30 min, before overnight incubation at 4 °C with mouse anti-human CD31 (1:30) (Dako, Cambridge, UK). Sections were washed with 0.1% tween in PBS and incubated with a secondary biotinylated antibody (Vector Labs, Newark, CA, USA) for 20 min. After thoroughly washed with 0.1% tween in PBS, samples were incubated with streptavidin-HRP (Vector Labs, Newark, CA, USA) for 20 min, followed by 3,3′diaminobenzidine (DAB) incubation (Vector Labs, Newark, CA, USA). Finally, all sections were counterstained with Mayer's hematoxylin, dehydrated and mounted with resinous mounting medium Entellan®(Merck, Darmstadt, Germany).

*4.12. In Situ Hybridization*

The presence of human cells within the implantation area was assessed using a human-specific DNA probe, according to the respective detection system BIO-AP REMBRANDT®Universal DISH & Detection kit (PanPath, Budel, The Netherlands). Briefly, after deparaffinization, proteolytic digestion was performed using a pepsin-HCL solution for 30 min at 37 °C, followed by dehydration in graded ethanol series. Sections were air-dried, and 1 drop of the probe was applied and covered with a coverslip. Samples were incubated at 95 °C for 5 min for DNA denaturation and then for 16 h at 37 °C in a moisturized environment for hybridization to occur. Samples were then washed in Tris-buffered saline (TBS) and incubated for 10 min with the stringency wash buffer. After rinsing with TBS, the detection was performed, and color was permitted to develop for 5 min at 37 °C in the dark. Samples were washed with water, counterstained with nuclear fast red, and observed under a Leica DM750 microscope (Leica, Wetzlar, Germany).

## 5. Conclusions

This study demonstrates that cryopreservation did not affect the capacity of SVF to spontaneously create an in vitro prevascular network in the absence of angiogenic growth factor supplementation in 3D conditions. Moreover, the angiogenic potential of SVF was further demonstrated after the in ovo implantation of prevascularized sponges resulting in improved vessel recruitment and improved construct integration within the CAM tissue. All together, these results demonstrate that the use of cryopreserved SVF, combined with marine-derived collagen, allows a simplified and cost-efficient method for assistance in the vascularization of TE constructs.

**Author Contributions:** Conceptualization, S.F.-R. and R.P.P.; formal analysis, S.F.-R. and R.P.P.; funding acquisition, R.P.P.; investigation, S.F.-R., G.S.D., C.O., A.M. and T.H.S.; methodology, S.F.-R., A.M., T.H.S. and R.P.P.; resources, M.J. and R.H.; supervision, R.P.P. and R.L.R.; validation, R.P.P.; writing—original draft, S.F.-R.; writing—review and editing, S.F.-R. and R.P.P. All authors have read and agreed to the published version of the manuscript.

**Funding:** This research has received funding from the European Research Council (ERC) under the European Union's Horizon 2020 research and innovation programme (Grant agreement No. 805411); Portuguese Foundation for Science and Technology under doctoral fellowship PD/BD/135252/2017 and individual grant IF/00347/2015; European Regional Development Fund, through INTERREG España-Portugal 2014-2020 under BLUEBIOLAB (0474_BLUEBIOLAB_1_E) project, through Atlantic Area Programme under BLUEHUMAN (EAPA_151/2016) project and through NORTE2020/PT2020 Programme under ATLANTIDA (Norte-01-0145-FEDER-000040) project.

**Institutional Review Board Statement:** The study was conducted in accordance with the Declaration of Helsinki and approved by the Ethics Committee of Hospital de S. João/University of Minho (217/19; CEICVS 008/2019).

**Data Availability Statement:** Not applicable.

**Acknowledgments:** We thank Cármen G. Sotelo (IIM-CSI, Vigo, Spain) for the kind offer of blue shark skin collagen.

**Conflicts of Interest:** The authors declare no conflict of interest.

## References

1. Rouwkema, J.; Koopman, B.F.; van Blitterswijk, C.; Dhert, W.; Malda, J. Supply of Nutrients to Cells in Engineered Tissues. *Biotechnol. Genet. Eng. Rev.* **2009**, *26*, 163–178. [CrossRef] [PubMed]
2. Clark, E.R.; Clark, E.L. Microscopic observations on the growth of blood capillaries in the living mammal. *Am. J. Anat.* **1939**, *64*, 251–301. [CrossRef]
3. Nishida, K.; Yamato, M.; Hayashida, Y.; Watanabe, K.; Yamamoto, K.; Adachi, E.; Nagai, S.; Kikuchi, A.; Maeda, N.; Watanabe, H.; et al. Corneal Reconstruction with Tissue-Engineered Cell Sheets Composed of Autologous Oral Mucosal Epithelium. *N. Engl. J. Med.* **2004**, *351*, 1187–1196. [CrossRef]

4. Miyagawa, S.; Sawa, Y.; Sakakida, S.; Taketani, S.; Kondoh, H.; Memon, I.A.; Imanishi, Y.; Shimizu, T.; Okano, T.; Matsuda, H. Tissue Cardiomyoplasty Using Bioengineered Contractile Cardiomyocyte Sheets to Repair Damaged Myocardium: Their Integration with Recipient Myocardium. *Transplantation* **2005**, *80*, 1586–1595. [CrossRef]
5. Shafiee, S.; Shariatzadeh, S.; Zafari, A.; Majd, A.; Niknejad, H. Recent Advances on Cell-Based Co-Culture Strategies for Prevascularization in Tissue Engineering. *Front. Bioeng. Biotechnol.* **2021**, *9*, 1155. [CrossRef] [PubMed]
6. Kniebs, C.; Kreimendahl, F.; Köpf, M.; Fischer, H.; Jockenhoevel, S.; Thiebes, A.L. Influence of Different Cell Types and Sources on Pre-Vascularisation in Fibrin and Agarose–Collagen Gels. *Organogenesis* **2020**, *16*, 14–26. [CrossRef]
7. Qian, Z.; Sharma, D.; Jia, W.; Radke, D.; Kamp, T.; Zhao, F. Engineering stem cell cardiac patch with microvascular features representative of native myocardium. *Theranostics* **2019**, *9*, 2143–2157. [CrossRef]
8. Jackson, C.; Nguyen, M. Human microvascular endothelial cells differ from macrovascular endothelial cells in their expression of matrix metalloproteinases. *Int. J. Biochem. Cell Biol.* **1997**, *29*, 1167–1177. [CrossRef]
9. Sacharidou, A.; Stratman, A.N.; Davis, G.E. Molecular Mechanisms Controlling Vascular Lumen Formation in Three-Dimensional Extracellular Matrices. *Cells Tissues Organs* **2012**, *195*, 122–143. [CrossRef]
10. Sun, Y.; Chen, S.; Zhang, X.; Pei, M. Significance of Cellular Cross-Talk in Stromal Vascular Fraction of Adipose Tissue in Neovascularization. *Arter. Thromb. Vasc. Biol.* **2019**, *39*, 1034–1044. [CrossRef]
11. Bourin, P.; Bunnell, B.A.; Casteilla, L.; Dominici, M.; Katz, A.J.; March, K.L.; Redl, H.; Rubin, J.P.; Yoshimura, K.; Gimble, J.M. Stromal cells from the adipose tissue-derived stromal vascular fraction and culture expanded adipose tissue-derived stromal/stem cells: A joint statement of the International Federation for Adipose Therapeutics and Science (IFATS) and the International Society for Cellular Therapy (ISCT). *Cytotherapy* **2013**, *15*, 641–648. [CrossRef] [PubMed]
12. Ramakrishnan, V.M.; Boyd, N.L. The Adipose Stromal Vascular Fraction as a Complex Cellular Source for Tissue Engineering Applications. *Tissue Eng. Part B Rev.* **2018**, *24*, 289–299. [CrossRef] [PubMed]
13. Costa, M.; Cerqueira, M.T.; Santos, T.C.; Sampaio-Marques, B.; Ludovico, P.; Marques, A.P.; Pirraco, R.P.; Reis, R.L. Cell sheet engineering using the stromal vascular fraction of adipose tissue as a vascularization strategy. *Acta Biomater.* **2017**, *55*, 131–143. [CrossRef] [PubMed]
14. Mytsyk, M.; Cerino, G.; Reid, G.; Sole, L.; Eckstein, F.; Santer, D.; Marsano, A. Long-Term Severe In Vitro Hypoxia Exposure Enhances the Vascularization Potential of Human Adipose Tissue-Derived Stromal Vascular Fraction Cell Engineered Tissues. *Int. J. Mol. Sci.* **2021**, *22*, 7920. [CrossRef]
15. Coppola, D.; Oliviero, M.; Vitale, G.A.; Lauritano, C.; D'Ambra, I.; Iannace, S.; De Pascale, D. Marine Collagen from Alternative and Sustainable Sources: Extraction, Processing and Applications. *Mar. Drugs* **2020**, *18*, 214. [CrossRef]
16. Heino, J. The collagen family members as cell adhesion proteins. *BioEssays* **2007**, *29*, 1001–1010. [CrossRef]
17. Marino, D.; Luginbühl, J.; Scola, S.; Meuli, M.; Reichmann, E. Bioengineering Dermo-Epidermal Skin Grafts with Blood and Lymphatic Capillaries. *Sci. Transl. Med.* **2014**, *6*, 221ra14. [CrossRef]
18. Nilforoushzadeh, M.A.; Sisakht, M.M.; Amirkhani, M.A.; Seifalian, A.M.; Banafshe, H.R.; Verdi, J.; Nouradini, M. Engineered skin graft with stromal vascular fraction cells encapsulated in fibrin–collagen hydrogel: A clinical study for diabetic wound healing. *J. Tissue Eng. Regen. Med.* **2020**, *14*, 424–440. [CrossRef]
19. Lugo-Cintrón, K.M.; Ayuso, J.M.; White, B.R.; Harari, P.M.; Ponik, S.M.; Beebe, D.J.; Gong, M.M.; Virumbrales-Muñoz, M. Matrix density drives 3D organotypic lymphatic vessel activation in a microfluidic model of the breast tumor microenvironment. *Lab Chip* **2020**, *20*, 1586–1600. [CrossRef]
20. McCoy, M.G.; Seo, B.R.; Choi, S.; Fischbach, C. Collagen I hydrogel microstructure and composition conjointly regulate vascular network formation. *Acta Biomater.* **2016**, *44*, 200–208. [CrossRef]
21. Montaño, I.; Schiestl, C.; Schneider, J.; Pontiggia, L.; Luginbühl, J.; Biedermann, T.; Böttcher-Haberzeth, S.; Braziulis, E.; Meuli, M.; Reichmann, E. Formation of Human Capillaries In Vitro: The Engineering of Prevascularized Matrices. *Tissue Eng. Part A* **2010**, *16*, 269–282. [CrossRef] [PubMed]
22. European Medicines Agency. Note for guidance on minimising the risk of transmitting animal spongiform encephalopathy agents via human and veterinary medicinal products (EMA/410/01 rev.3). *Off. J. Eur. Union* **2011**, *73*, 1–18.
23. Sotelo, C.G.; Comesaña, M.B.; Ariza, P.R.; Pérez-Martín, R.I. Characterization of Collagen from Different Discarded Fish Species of the West Coast of the Iberian Peninsula. *J. Aquat. Food Prod. Technol.* **2015**, *25*, 388–399. [CrossRef]
24. Fowler, G.M.; Campana, S.E. Commercial by-catch rates of blue shark (prionace glauca) from longline fisheries in the Canadian Atlantic. *Collect. Vol. Sci. Pap. ICCAT* **2009**, *64*, 1650–1667.
25. Elango, J.; Lee, J.W.; Wang, S.; Henrotin, Y.; De Val, J.E.M.S.; Regenstein, J.M.; Lim, S.Y.; Bao, B.; Wu, W. Evaluation of Differentiated Bone Cells Proliferation by Blue Shark Skin Collagen via Biochemical for Bone Tissue Engineering. *Mar. Drugs* **2018**, *16*, 350. [CrossRef]
26. Nomura, Y.; Yamano, M.; Hayakawa, C.; Ishii, Y.; Shirai, K. Structural Property and in Vitro Self-assembly of Shark Type I Collagen. *Biosci. Biotechnol. Biochem.* **1997**, *61*, 1919–1923. [CrossRef]
27. Diogo, G.S.; Carneiro, F.; Freitas-Ribeiro, S.; Sotelo, C.G.; Pérez-Martín, R.I.; Pirraco, R.P.; Reis, R.L.; Silva, T.H. Prionace glauca skin collagen bioengineered constructs as a promising approach to trigger cartilage regeneration. *Mater. Sci. Eng. C* **2020**, *120*, 111587. [CrossRef]
28. Joshi, V.S.; Lei, N.Y.; Walthers, C.M.; Wu, B.; Dunn, J.C. Macroporosity enhances vascularization of electrospun scaffolds. *J. Surg. Res.* **2013**, *183*, 18–26. [CrossRef]

29. Perets, A.; Baruch, Y.; Weisbuch, F.; Shoshany, G.; Neufeld, G.; Cohen, S. Enhancing the vascularization of three-dimensional porous alginate scaffolds by incorporating controlled release basic fibroblast growth factor microspheres. *J. Biomed. Mater. Res.* **2003**, *65A*, 489–497. [CrossRef]
30. Oliviero, O.; Ventre, M.; Netti, P. Functional porous hydrogels to study angiogenesis under the effect of controlled release of vascular endothelial growth factor. *Acta Biomater.* **2012**, *8*, 3294–3301. [CrossRef]
31. Sharma, D.; Ross, D.; Wang, G.; Jia, W.; Kirkpatrick, S.J.; Zhao, F. Upgrading prevascularization in tissue engineering: A review of strategies for promoting highly organized microvascular network formation. *Acta Biomater.* **2019**, *95*, 112–130. [CrossRef] [PubMed]
32. Liao, H.; He, H.; Chen, Y.; Zeng, F.; Huang, J.; Wu, L.; Chen, Y. Effects of long-term serial cell passaging on cell spreading, migration, and cell-surface ultrastructures of cultured vascular endothelial cells. *Cytotechnology* **2014**, *66*, 229–238. [CrossRef] [PubMed]
33. Wittmann, K.; Dietl, S.; Ludwig, N.; Berberich, O.; Hoefner, C.; Storck, K.; Blunk, T.; Bauer-Kreisel, P. Engineering Vascularized Adipose Tissue Using the Stromal-Vascular Fraction and Fibrin Hydrogels. *Tissue Eng. Part A* **2015**, *21*, 1343–1353. [CrossRef]
34. Collen, D. The Plasminogen (Fibrinolytic) System. *Thromb. Haemost.* **1999**, *82*, 259–270. [CrossRef]
35. Pepper, M.S.; Sappino, A.P.; Montesano, R.; Orci, L.; Vassalli, J.-D. Plasminogen activator inhibitor-1 is induced in migrating endothelial cells. *J. Cell. Physiol.* **1992**, *153*, 129–139. [CrossRef] [PubMed]
36. Pepper, M.; Montesano, R. Proteolytic balance and capillary morphogenesis. *Cell Differ. Dev.* **1990**, *32*, 319–327. [CrossRef]
37. Kraling, B.; Wiederschain, D.; Boehm, T.; Rehn, M.; Mulliken, J.; Moses, M. The role of matrix metalloproteinase activity in the maturation of human capillary endothelial cells in vitro. *J. Cell Sci.* **1999**, *112*, 1599–1609. [CrossRef] [PubMed]
38. Charo, I.F.; Taubman, M.B. Chemokines in the Pathogenesis of Vascular Disease. *Circ. Res.* **2004**, *95*, 858–866. [CrossRef]
39. Jaffe, E.; Ruggiero, J.; Falcone, D. Monocytes and macrophages synthesize and secrete thrombospondin. *Blood* **1985**, *65*, 79–84. [CrossRef]
40. Koch, A.E.; Polverini, P.J.; Kunkel, S.L.; Harlow, L.A.; DiPietro, L.A.; Elner, V.M.; Elner, S.G.; Strieter, R.M. Interleukin-8 as a macrophage-derived mediator of angiogenesis. *Science* **1992**, *258*, 1798–1801. [CrossRef]
41. Li, A.; Dubey, S.; Varney, M.L.; Dave, B.J.; Singh, R.K. IL-8 Directly Enhanced Endothelial Cell Survival, Proliferation, and Matrix Metalloproteinases Production and Regulated Angiogenesis. *J. Immunol.* **2003**, *170*, 3369–3376. [CrossRef] [PubMed]
42. Hong, K.H.; Ryu, J.; Han, K.H. Monocyte chemoattractant protein-1–induced angiogenesis is mediated by vascular endothelial growth factor-A. *Blood* **2005**, *105*, 1405–1407. [CrossRef] [PubMed]
43. Yamada, M.; Kim, S.; Egashira, K.; Takeya, M.; Ikeda, T.; Mimura, O.; Iwao, H. Molecular Mechanism and Role of Endothelial Monocyte Chemoattractant Protein-1 Induction by Vascular Endothelial Growth Factor. *Arter. Thromb. Vasc. Biol.* **2003**, *23*, 1996–2001. [CrossRef] [PubMed]
44. Ma, J.; Wang, Q.; Fei, T.; Han, J.-D.J.; Chen, Y.-G. MCP-1 mediates TGF-β–induced angiogenesis by stimulating vascular smooth muscle cell migration. *Blood* **2006**, *109*, 987–994. [CrossRef] [PubMed]
45. Mendes, L.F.F.; Pirraco, R.P.; Szymczyk, W.; Frias, A.M.; Santos, T.C.; Reis, R.L.; Marques, A.P. Perivascular-Like Cells Contribute to the Stability of the Vascular Network of Osteogenic Tissue Formed from Cell Sheet-Based Constructs. *PLoS ONE* **2012**, *7*, e41051. [CrossRef] [PubMed]
46. McIlroy, M.; O'Rourke, M.; McKeown, S.R.; Hirst, D.G.; Robson, T. Pericytes influence endothelial cell growth characteristics: Role of plasminogen activator inhibitor type 1 (PAI-1). *Cardiovasc. Res.* **2006**, *69*, 207–217. [CrossRef]
47. Lobov, I.B.; Brooks, P.C.; Lang, R.A. Angiopoietin-2 displays VEGF-dependent modulation of capillary structure and endothelial cell survival in vivo. *Proc. Natl. Acad. Sci. USA* **2002**, *99*, 11205–11210. [CrossRef]
48. Montesano, R.; Orci, L.; Vassalli, P. In vitro rapid organization of endothelial cells into capillary-like networks is promoted by collagen matrices. *J. Cell Biol.* **1983**, *97*, 1648–1652. [CrossRef]
49. Chen, J.; Gao, K.; Liu, S.; Wang, S.; Elango, J.; Bao, B.; Dong, J.; Liu, N.; Wu, W. Fish Collagen Surgical Compress Repairing Characteristics on Wound Healing Process In Vivo. *Mar. Drugs* **2019**, *17*, 33. [CrossRef]
50. Gauza-Włodarczyk, M.; Kubisz, L.; Mielcarek, S.; Włodarczyk, D. Comparison of thermal properties of fish collagen and bovine collagen in the temperature range 298–670 K. *Mater. Sci. Eng. C* **2017**, *80*, 468–471. [CrossRef]
51. Bai, F.; Wang, Z.; Lu, J.; Liu, J.; Chen, G.; Lv, R.; Wang, J.; Lin, K.; Zhang, J.; Huang, X. The Correlation Between the Internal Structure and Vascularization of Controllable Porous Bioceramic Materials In Vivo: A Quantitative Study. *Tissue Eng. Part A* **2010**, *16*, 3791–3803. [CrossRef] [PubMed]
52. Somo, S.I.; Akar, B.; Bayrak, E.S.; Larson, J.C.; Appel, A.A.; Mehdizadeh, H.; Cinar, A.; Brey, E.M. Pore Interconnectivity Influences Growth Factor-Mediated Vascularization in Sphere-Templated Hydrogels. *Tissue Eng. Part C Methods* **2015**, *21*, 773–785. [CrossRef] [PubMed]
53. Mehdizadeh, H.; Sumo, S.; Bayrak, E.S.; Brey, E.M.; Cinar, A. Three-dimensional modeling of angiogenesis in porous biomaterial scaffolds. *Biomaterials* **2013**, *34*, 2875–2887. [CrossRef] [PubMed]
54. Kirkfeldt, T.S.; Santos, C.F. A Review of Sustainability Concepts in Marine Spatial Planning and the Potential to Supporting the UN Sustainable Development Goal 14. *Front. Mar. Sci.* **2021**, *8*, 1244. [CrossRef]
55. Moreno-Jiménez, I.; Kanczler, J.M.; Hulsart-Billstrom, G.; Inglis, S.; Oreffo, R.O. The Chorioallantoic Membrane Assay for Biomaterial Testing in Tissue Engineering: A Short-Term In Vivo Preclinical Model. *Tissue Eng. Part C Methods* **2017**, *23*, 938–952. [CrossRef] [PubMed]

56. Silva, A.S.; Santos, L.F.; Mendes, M.C.; Mano, J.F. Multi-layer pre-vascularized magnetic cell sheets for bone regeneration. *Biomaterials* **2020**, *231*, 119664. [CrossRef]
57. Feijão, T.; Neves, M.I.; Sousa, A.; Torres, A.L.; Bidarra, S.J.; Orge, I.D.; Carvalho, D.T.; Barrias, C.C. Engineering injectable vascularized tissues from the bottom-up: Dynamics of in-gel extra-spheroid dermal tissue assembly. *Biomaterials* **2021**, *279*, 121222. [CrossRef]
58. Sumi, M.; Sata, M.; Toya, N.; Yanaga, K.; Ohki, T.; Nagai, R. Transplantation of adipose stromal cells, but not mature adipocytes, augments ischemia-induced angiogenesis. *Life Sci.* **2007**, *80*, 559–565. [CrossRef]
59. Koh, Y.J.; Koh, B.I.; Kim, H.; Joo, H.J.; Jin, H.K.; Jeon, J.; Choi, C.; Lee, D.H.; Chung, J.H.; Cho, C.-H.; et al. Stromal Vascular Fraction From Adipose Tissue Forms Profound Vascular Network Through the Dynamic Reassembly of Blood Endothelial Cells. *Arter. Thromb. Vasc. Biol.* **2011**, *31*, 1141–1150. [CrossRef]
60. Nakagami, H.; Maeda, K.; Morishita, R.; Iguchi, S.; Nishikawa, T.; Takami, Y.; Kikuchi, Y.; Saito, Y.; Tamai, K.; Ogihara, T.; et al. Novel Autologous Cell Therapy in Ischemic Limb Disease Through Growth Factor Secretion by Cultured Adipose Tissue–Derived Stromal Cells. *Arter. Thromb. Vasc. Biol.* **2005**, *25*, 2542–2547. [CrossRef]
61. Klar, A.S.; Güven, S.; Zimoch, J.; Zapiórkowska, N.A.; Zapiórkowska, T.; Böttcher-Haberzeth, S.; Meuli-Simmen, C.; Martin, I.; Scherberich, A.; Reichmann, E.; et al. Characterization of vasculogenic potential of human adipose-derived endothelial cells in a three-dimensional vascularized skin substitute. *Pediatr. Surg. Int.* **2016**, *32*, 17–27. [CrossRef] [PubMed]
62. Cerino, G.; Gaudiello, E.; Muraro, M.G.; Eckstein, F.; Martin, I.; Scherberich, A.; Marsano, A. Engineering of an angiogenic niche by perfusion culture of adipose-derived stromal vascular fraction cells. *Sci. Rep.* **2017**, *7*, 14252. [CrossRef] [PubMed]
63. Oliveira, C.; Granja, S.; Neves, N.; Reis, R.L.; Baltazar, F.; Silva, T.H.; Martins, A. Fucoidan from Fucus vesiculosus inhibits new blood vessel formation and breast tumor growth in vivo. *Carbohydr. Polym.* **2019**, *223*, 115034. [CrossRef] [PubMed]

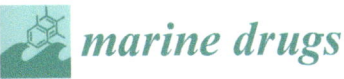

Article

# A Collagen Basketweave from the Giant Squid Mantle as a Robust Scaffold for Tissue Engineering

Anastasia Frolova [1,*], Nadezhda Aksenova [2,3], Ivan Novikov [4], Aitsana Maslakova [5], Elvira Gafarova [1], Yuri Efremov [1,2], Polina Bikmulina [1], Vadim Elagin [6], Elena Istranova [2], Alexandr Kurkov [2], Anatoly Shekhter [2], Svetlana Kotova [2,3], Elena Zagaynova [7] and Peter Timashev [1,2,3,8]

1. World-Class Research Center "Digital Biodesign and Personalized Healthcare", Sechenov First Moscow State Medical University (Sechenov University), 8-2 Trubetskaya Street, 119991 Moscow, Russia; gafarova_e_r@staff.sechenov.ru (E.G.); efremov_yu_m@staff.sechenov.ru (Y.E.); bikmulina_p_yu@staff.sechenov.ru (P.B.); timashev_p_s@staff.sechenov.ru (P.T.)
2. Institute for Regenerative Medicine, Sechenov First Moscow State Medical University (Sechenov University), 8-2 Trubetskaya Street, 119991 Moscow, Russia; aksenova_n_a@staff.sechenov.ru (N.A.); istranova_e_v@staff.sechenov.ru (E.I.); kurkov_a_v@staff.sechenov.ru (A.K.); shekhter_a_b@staff.sechenov.ru (A.S.); kotova_s_l@staff.sechenov.ru (S.K.)
3. N.N. Semenov Federal Research Center for Chemical Physics, RAS, 4 Kosygin Street, 119991 Moscow, Russia
4. Research Institute of Eye Diseases, 11 Rossolimo Street, 119021 Moscow, Russia; i.novikov@niigb.ru
5. Faculty of Biology, Department of Human and Animal Physiology, M.V. Lomonosov Moscow State University, 1-12 Leninskie Gory, 119991 Moscow, Russia; aitsana.dokrunova@gmail.com
6. Institute of Experimental Oncology and Biomedical Technologies, Privolzhsky Research Medical University, Minin and Pozharsky Square 10/1, 603950 Nizhny Novgorod, Russia; elagin.vadim@gmail.com
7. Institute of Experimental Oncology and Biomedical Technologies, National Research Lobachevsky State University of Nizhny Novgorod, Prospekt Gagarina (Gagarin Avenue) 23, 603950 Nizhny Novgorod, Russia; ezagaynova@gmail.com
8. Chemistry Department, M.V. Lomonosov Moscow State University, 1 Leninskiy Gory, 119991 Moscow, Russia
* Correspondence: frolova_a_a_2@staff.sechenov.ru

**Abstract:** The growing applications of tissue engineering technologies warrant the search and development of biocompatible materials with an appropriate strength and elastic moduli. Here, we have extensively studied a collagenous membrane (GSCM) separated from the mantle of the Giant squid Dosidicus Gigas in order to test its potential applicability in regenerative medicine. To establish the composition and structure of the studied material, we analyzed the GSCM by a variety of techniques, including amino acid analysis, SDS-PAGE, and FTIR. It has been shown that collagen is a main component of the GSCM. The morphology study by different microscopic techniques from nano- to microscale revealed a peculiar packing of collagen fibers forming laminae oriented at 60–90 degrees in respect to each other, which, in turn, formed layers with the thickness of several microns (a basketweave motif). The macro- and micromechanical studies showed high values of the Young's modulus and tensile strength. No significant cytotoxicity of the studied material was found by the cytotoxicity assay. Thus, the GSCM consists of a reinforced collagen network, has high mechanical characteristics, and is non-toxic, which makes it a good candidate for the creation of a scaffold material for tissue engineering.

**Keywords:** biomechanical properties; collagen membrane; AFM; SEM; tensile test; giant squid; Dosidicus Gigas; jumbo squid; outer tunic; tissue engineering

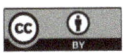

## 1. Introduction

The basic objective of tissue engineering consists of obtaining such a scaffold material that would promote complete or at least partial regeneration of internal organs, skin, vascular, bone, cartilage, and other tissues. For a construct to successfully engraft in the body, its parameters ought to be similar to those of the region in which the construct will function. The construct's biocompatibility, biodegradability, as well as mechanical properties determine its potential to substitute the corresponding live tissue in the body.

The interest to collagen-based materials is stipulated by the fact that collagen is biocompatible with the recipients' tissues, can biodegrade, is non-toxic, non-carcinogenic and non-immunogenic, and combines many characteristics of synthetic polymers (strength, stiffness, ability to form various supramolecular structures, etc.).

Currently, a plethora of pharmaceutical preparations and medical devices have been created using collagen as a base [1].

Collagen is one of basic natural materials which have application in tissue engineering [2–6]. In many types of connective tissue, it is a fibrillar protein and the main component responsible for the tissue integrity, shape, elasticity, and strength.

Connective tissue is present in all the organs and tissues in the body and comprises ~60–90% of their weight. Such collagenous structures as tendons [7,8] and ligaments [9] have a certain structural hierarchy of collagen to withstand intensive mechanical loads (extension and compression). The common idea about them has been that tendons and ligaments are structurally similar, if not identical [10]. Ligaments [10–12] and tendons [7,10,13] consist of tightly packed parallel collagen fibers. Ligaments differ from tendons by the predominance of elastic fibers; therefore, they are characterized by a lower strength but higher flexibility as compared to tendons. The distinctions between them stem from the connections they create; ligaments connect a bone with another bone, and tendons connect a muscle with a bone. A number of studies are dedicated to the restoration of tendon ruptures using different materials [14,15].

The skin is also an interesting and sophisticated collagen-based organ [16]. The skin structure resembles a net consisting of differently oriented collagen fibers [17–19]. One of the basic functions of the skin is to protect internal organs and tissues from mechanical injuries. Skin as a material exhibits a viscoelastic behavior, and its mechanical response to a stress involves both a viscous component related to energy dissipation and an elastic component related to energy storage [20,21]. Collagen fibers comprise 75% of the skin tissue dry weight [22], and it is those fibers that are responsible for the skin strength. The skin's mechanical properties are important for a number of applications, including surgery, dermatology, forensic medicine, etc. [23]. The problem of skin replacement and search of the appropriate materials has long been discussed (see, for example, a review [24]).

The anulus fibrosus, an outer fibrous ring of the intervertebral disc, is yet another example of a collagen-based tissue that undergoes mechanical stresses of various directions and has a corresponding collagen packing [25,26].

The knowledge of the mechanical characteristics of tissues and organs, and the conditions in which they must function, help to create or select a material that would be appropriate for their complete or partial replacement [27,28]. The basic mechanical properties include the strength, stiffness, viscosity, elasticity, plasticity, brittleness, etc.

Table 1 presents examples of tissues with a certain collagen packing related to their mechanical properties and materials for tissue engineered constructs meant to replace such tissues.

**Table 1.** Mechanical properties of some collagen-based tissues and materials for tissue engineered constructs.

| Tissue/Material | Treatment | Tensile Test Data | | References |
|---|---|---|---|---|
| | | Ultimate Tensile Strength, UTS (MPa) | Young's Modulus (MPa) | |
| Human Skin | | 27.2 ± 9.3 MPa | 98.9 ± 97 MPa | [23,29] |
| Reconstructed anterior cruciate ligament (ACL) rabbit model | Glutaraldehyde cross-linked prostheses | 26 MPa | | [30] |
| Reconstructed anterior cruciate ligament (ACL) rabbit model | Carbodiimide cross-linked prostheses | 12 MPa | | [30] |
| Reconstructed anterior cruciate ligament (ACL) rabbit model | Sham-operated controls | 49 ± 20 MPa | | [30] |
| Human patellar tendon | | 60–100 MPa | 300–400 MPa | [31] |
| Human native rotator cuff tendon | | 11.5 ± 5 MPa | 50–170 MPa | [32] |
| TSPC seeded knitted silk–collagen sponge scaffold for functional shoulder repair rabbit model | TSPC seeded | Control group 5.9 ± 1 MPa; TCPC group 8.3 ± 1.5 MPa | Control group 44.3 ± 12.1 MPa; TCPC group 67.8 ± 14.6 MPa | [33] |
| Human Achilles tendon | | 40 ± 8 MPa | 1600 ± 200 MPa | [34] |
| Rabbit Achilles tendon | | 4.5 MPa | 45 MPa | [14] |
| Human fibrocartilage | | 10 MPa | | [26] |
| Human compact bone | | 0.03 MPa | 15,000 MPa (Depending on type and size of the bones) | [35] |
| Human vaginal tissue | | 0.82–2.62 MPa | | [36] |
| Human cornea | | 3.81 ± 0.4 MPa | | [37] |
| DBP, decellularized bovine pericardium | | Along 23 MPa Across 20 MPa | Along 120 MPa Across 50 MPa | [38] |
| Normal human skin (NHS) | | 2.8 MPa | | [39] |
| ASC from bovine hide scaffolds by electrospinning | | 0.4 MPa | | [39] |
| Un-crosslinked collagen film from bovine tendon | | 10 ± 0.5 MPa | | [40] |
| Un-crosslinked collagen film from (Coll type I) | | 37.7 ± 4.5 MPa | 1100 ± 100 MPa | [41] |
| Collagen films from rat tail (Coll type I) | | 100 MPa | 27 MPa | [42] |
| Chitosan-AS collagen biofilms from mantle *D. gigas* | | 33.5 ± 4 MPa | | [43] |
| Collagen fiber films from cattle skin | | Dry 17.25 ± 0.07 MPa Wet 2.61 ± 0.05 MPa | | [44] |
| Fresh (non-treated) pulmonary heart valves pigs | | 0.5 ± 0.2 MPa | | [45] |

In the view of creating tissue engineered constructs with predefined mechanical properties, the mantle of squids attracts special attention, since these animals, living in the deep under great pressure, must have a robust musculature and outer coating to protect their internal organs. The morphological features of the squids' mantle affect the mechanisms of their locomotion [46].

Among many species of cephalopods, the Giant squid (Humboldt squid) represents the most important object of fishing, which covers 30% of the world fishing volume and about 4% of the entire world market of squids [47]. It is the biggest of the known mollusks. This species of large predatory squids lives in the eastern Pacific region, along the Peru coast at depths of 200 to 700 m. Its mantle can reach almost two meters in length, while its lifespan is only about 2 years, since the squid dies upon spawning [48].

A number of publications have appeared recently on the use of marine collagen, obtained, for example, from fish scales [49], mantle, fins, and tentacles of squids [50], and even sea cucumbers [51]. Uriarte-Montoya et al. (2010) described a film for application in the food and medical industries, prepared from collagen extracted from the mantle of the Giant squid of the *Dosidicus gigas* species [43]. Adamowicz et al. (2021) conducted a study on the use of the decellularized mantle of *Loligo vulgaris* squid in tissue engineering as a material for the urethra reconstruction [52]. Collagen-based materials prepared from the mantle of the Giant squid might also become a prospective carrier in tissue engineering, however, no studies on this idea have been reported so far.

Oliveira et al. (2021) discuss the application directions and advantages of marine collagen, as well as the need for the research in this area, aiming at strengthening this biopolymer's position on the world's collagen market [53]. Physically, biochemically, and spectroscopically, marine collagen is identical to mammalian collagen [54,55].

Application of mollusks for collagen production has other advantages, including safety from Creutzfeldt–Jakob disease, which is associated with collagen obtained from cattle, and no ethical or religious barriers.

In this study, our objective was to assess the possibility of using a material obtained from the mantle of the Giant squid, *Dosidicus gigas*, for the tasks of regenerative medicine, based on the data on its chemical composition, structural analysis, biomechanical properties, and cytotoxicity. The studied material represented a collagenous membrane prepared from the squid's outer tunic (hereafter, Giant Squid Collagenous Membrane, GSCM).

## 2. Results

*2.1. Collagen Is a Basic Component of the GSCM*

2.1.1. Amino Acid Analysis

According to the amino acid analysis, the content of hydroxyproline (Hyp) in the GSCM was 86.3 residues, proline (Pro)—91.3 residues per 1000 residues (Table 2). The Hyp percentage in the studied specimen was 10.13 weight %.

The specimen also contained a large amount (330 per 1000 residues) of glycine (Gly). The weight percentage of Gly was 22.18%. This finding is related to the fact that a molecule of collagen consists of a triple helix formed by three polypeptide helical strands, and each helical chain is formed by three-residue-long repeats, with glycine as one of the three residues. Thus, the primary structure of collagen is characterized by a large content of glycine. The high content of glutamic acid (Glu) in the specimen is explained by the presence of proline (Pro) since Pro is synthesized from glutamic acid.

Table 2. Amino acid composition of the D. gigas CM.

| Name of Amino Acids | Abbreviation | Letter Code | Molecular Mass, g/mol | Residues per 1000 Residues | w% * |
|---|---|---|---|---|---|
| Alanine | Ala | A | 89.094 | 86.2 | 6.87 |
| Arginine | Arg | R | 174.203 | 56.4 | 8.79 |
| Aspartic acid | Asp | D | 133.104 | 62.9 | 7.49 |
| Cysteine | Cys | C | 121.154 | 3.5 | 0.74 |
| Glutamic acid | Glu | E | 147.131 | 86.4 | 11.38 |
| Glycine | Gly | G | 75.067 | 330.0 | 22.18 |
| Histidine | His | H | 155.156 | 7.7 | 1.07 |
| Hydroxyproline | Hyp | O | 131.131 | 86.3 | 10.13 |
| Hydroxylysine | Hyl | | 162.187 | 10.3 | 1.5 |
| Isoleucine | Ile | I | 131.175 | 13.9 | 1.64 |
| Leucine | Leu | L | 131.175 | 29.5 | 3.47 |
| Lysine | Lys | K | 146.189 | 14.0 | 1.83 |
| Methionine | Met | M | 149.208 | 10.4 | 1.39 |
| Phenylalanine | Phe | F | 165.192 | 11.1 | 1.64 |
| Proline | Pro | P | 115.132 | 91.3 | 9.4 |
| Serine | Ser | S | 105.093 | 41.1 | 3.86 |
| Threonine | Thr | T | 119.119 | 27.9 | 2.97 |
| Tyrosine | Tyr | Y | 181.191 | 6.4 | 1.04 |
| Valine | Val | V | 117.148 | 24.9 | 2.61 |
| Total | | | | 1000 | |
| | Hyp/Hyl | | | 8.4 | |

* Percentage of amino acids to the mass of the test sample.

### 2.1.2. SDS-PAGE

The SDS-PAGE analysis showed four main bands in the studied GSCM (Figure 1). Two bands had the molecular weights of 133.3 and 151.6 kDa, and they were assigned to two α-chains of collagen, α1 and α2. The two high-molecular components, with the weights of 295.7 kDa and 300 kDa, were identified as a β-chain consisting of two α-chains and a γ-chain consisting of three α-chains, respectively.

## 2.2. Hydration and Thermal Properties of the GSCM

### 2.2.1. FTIR Spectroscopy

The IR spectrum of the GSCM (blue curve in Figure 2) shows bands at 876, 918, 939, 972, 1030, 1060, 1080, and 1119 cm$^{-1}$, which are characteristic of carbohydrate moieties (CO stretching and COC stretching); an Amide III band at 1236 cm$^{-1}$ (associated with CN stretching and NH deformation); bands positioned at 1336 and 1451 cm$^{-1}$, attributable to methylene vibrations ($CH_2$ deformation and $CH_3$ deformation); N–H in-plane bend and the C–N stretching vibrations at 1540 cm$^{-1}$ (Amid II). The polypeptide backbone CO stretching vibration is found in the range of 1600–1700 cm$^{-1}$: bands at 1740 cm$^{-1}$ due to carbonyl vibrations, and the one 1630 cm$^{-1}$ due to Amide I. The spectrum shows bands at 2878 and 2927 cm$^{-1}$ assigned to aliphatic chains (CH stretching and $CH_3$ stretching) an Amide B band at 3073 cm$^{-1}$ (NH stretching), and a broad band at 3500–3300 cm$^{-1}$ related to Amide A (NH stretching) and OH vibrations [56–60].

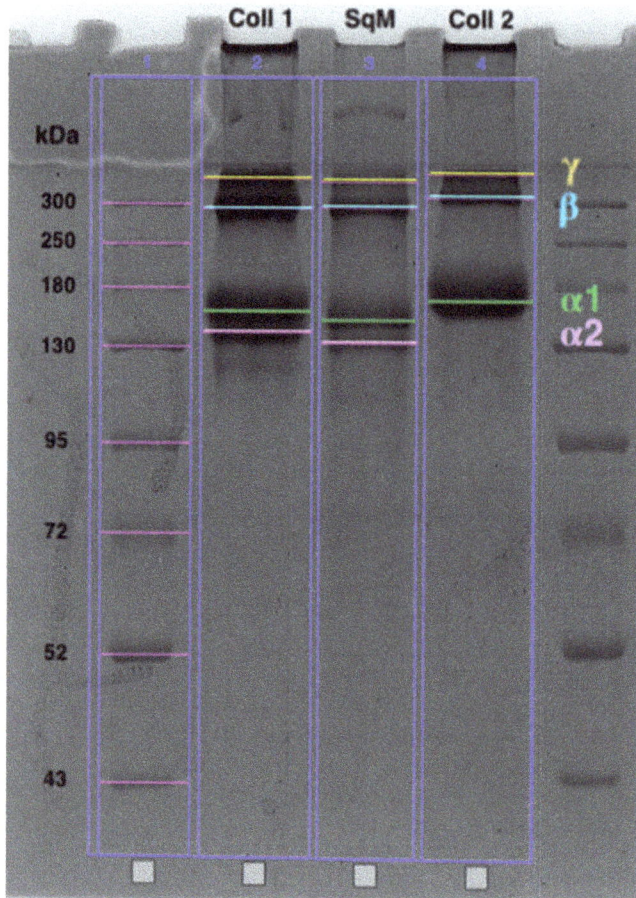

**Figure 1.** Evaluation of the GSCM collagen chains' electrophoretic mobility in 8% PAAG under the denaturing and reducing conditions. Collagen Type I (Coll 1) and Type II (Coll 2) were used as collagen standards. SqM—collagen extracted from the GSCM. The high range protein ladder bands are shown in kDa.

For comparison, the FTIR spectra of collagens Type I and Type II were examined [61]. The spectra of both samples are presented in Figure 2, and the band positions are presented in Table S1. FTIR confirmed a similar triple helical structure with the secondary α-chain structure for all three samples [56]. The IR spectra of the GSCM and collagen type II differed slightly in regard to the bands at 1740, 2800–2930, and 3620–3690 cm$^{-1}$ (associated with OH stretching and H-bonding). From the general view of the spectra, one can assume that the GSCM belongs to collagen Type II, but the increased intensity of bands at 2930 and 1740 cm$^{-1}$ indicates that it rather belongs to a mixture of collagens Type I and Type II. These results confirm the results of SDS-PAGE (see Section 2.1, Figure 1).

The position of the Amide I band in the GSCM spectrum is in agreement with the literature data on the Amide I band in the spectra of oligopeptides containing Gly, Pro, and Ala in various combinations, as well as the spectra of polyproline [60]. This is consistent with the results of the study of the amino acid composition, demonstrating that the main amino acids of the GSCM are Gly, Pro, Hyp, and Glu (see Section 2.1, Table 2).

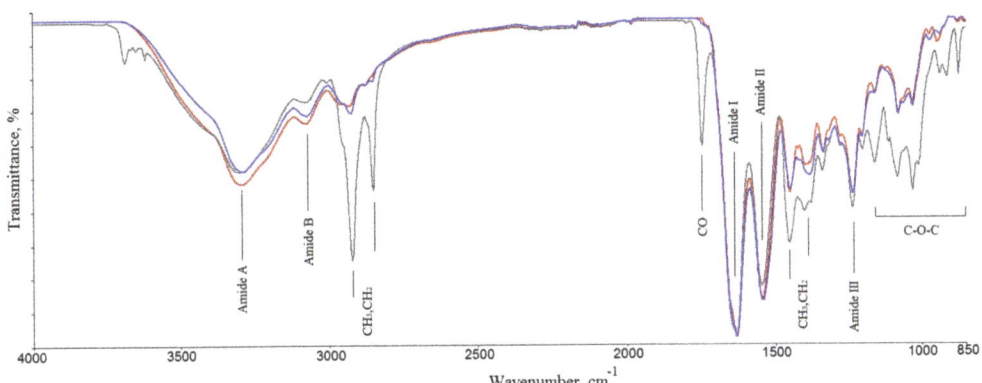

**Figure 2.** FT-IR spectra of the GSCM is the blue curve; collagen Type I is the gray curve; collagen Type II is the red curve.

### 2.2.2. TGA/DSC Studies

A typical weight loss vs. temperature curve (a thermogravimetric, TG curve), as well as a DSC curve, for the GSCM are displayed in Figure 3. In TG curves, there were two temperatures at which the onset of the thermal degradation occurred. The DSC curves showed two endothermic peaks. The broad endothermic peak in DSC curves in the temperature range of 50–170 °C is associated with thermal dehydration [62–64]. This process was accompanied by a ~10% weight loss (the TG curve). The broad and multimodal endothermic peak in the temperature range of 220–330 °C is assigned to the collagen matrix thermal denaturation and destruction. The latter process was accompanied by a ~65% weight loss (TG curves). According to [64], for dehydrated collagen type I, the endothermic peak of denaturation was observed at Tdn = 225 °C. It can be assumed that, below the temperature of Tdn ~225–235 °C, the interchain hydrogen bonds rupture, dehydrated collagens unfold, and amorphous polymers form. The second stage of destruction was observed at Tdst > 235 °C. In general, the GSCM TG and DSC curves were similar to those for collagenous materials [62,64].

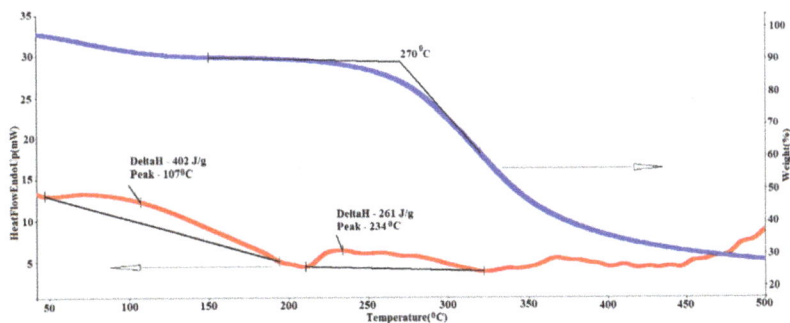

**Figure 3.** TG (blue) and DSC (red) curves for the GSCM.

### 2.2.3. Shrinkage Temperature

The shrinkage temperature of the GSCM was experimentally found at 58 °C. The swelling degree was measured as 102% in distilled water and as 176% in PBS. The much higher degree of swelling in the PBS medium is due to the fact that ions present in the saline facilitate hydration of collagen fibers.

### 2.3. Morphological Properties of the GSCM

#### 2.3.1. Histological Studies

The histological studies of the GSCM cross-sections showed that the material had a layered structure that consisted of 8–12 tightly packed "laminae" with the total thickness of ~50–70 µm (Figure 4(A1,B1,C1,D1)). The thickness of each lamina was ~5–7 µm. When stained with hematoxylin and eosin, the material of laminae had uniform eosinophilic staining (Figure 4(A1)). However, the picrosirius red stain (Figure 4(B1)), especially, when using phase contrast (Figure 4(C1)) and polarized light microscopy (Figure 4(D1)) showed that in some regions the material had a fibrillar structure due to poorly visible small collagen fibers oriented along the laminae. In the polarized light microscopy images, these fibers produced a bright glow in the material, testifying the birefringence (anisotropy) specific for oriented fibers in collagen.

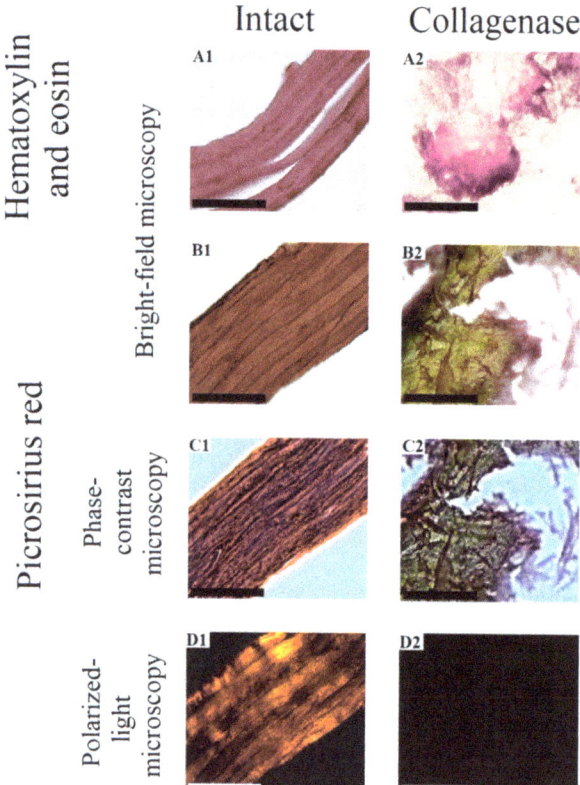

**Figure 4.** Morphological and optical characteristics of the GSCM before and after the collagenase treatment. (**A1**) As seen at a cross-section, the GSCM consists of parallel uniform pink (eosinophilic) layers—"laminae"; (**A2**) lysis of the material with homogenization, loss of crisp contours, and appearing purple (basophilic) regions; (**B1**) predominantly red staining of laminae with regions of poorly visible fine-fibred structure; (**B2**) loss of the red and appearance of yellow (picrinophilic) staining in most parts of the material with single loose and multidirectional red collagen fibers; (**C1**) a somewhat more visible fibrillar structure of the material than that in (**B1**); (**C2**) scattered collagen fibers among the picrinophilic material are more visible than they are in (**B2**); (**D1**) laminae produce a bright yellow-green, yellow-orange, and orange-red glow due to the collagen fibers within their structure; (**D2**) no material glow was noted; ×1000 (Scale bar = 50 µm).

### 2.3.2. Scanning Electronic Microscopy Studies (SEM)

The SEM studies revealed that the GSCM surface had a multilayered basketweave structure, with laminae laid at different angles, which resembled a reinforcing mesh. The angle between the laminae was ~60–90° (Figure 5a,b).

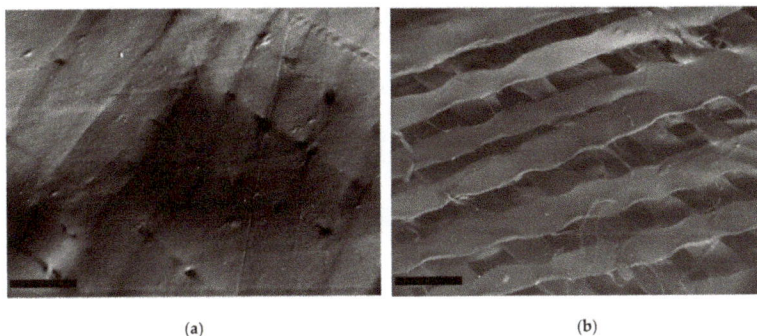

**Figure 5.** SEM-BSE images of the GSCM surface. (**a**) Native surface, and (**b**) a region inside a fracture zone of the material (Scale bar = 100 μm).

The reinforcing layers consisting of laminae have a definite mutual layer-by-layer orientation. Each layer represents a set of parallel laminae with the width of 38–50 μm and thickness of 4.0–4.5 μm. In turn, each lamina consists of tightly packed parallel collagen fibers longitudinally packed along the whole lamina length (Figure 6a,b). Besides, there is a thin layer that covers the upper reinforcing layer with laminae (Figure 6c). This surface is extremely stable chemically (it was not damaged by the sample preparation procedure) and is formed by a randomly crossed motif of collagen fibers and fibrils.

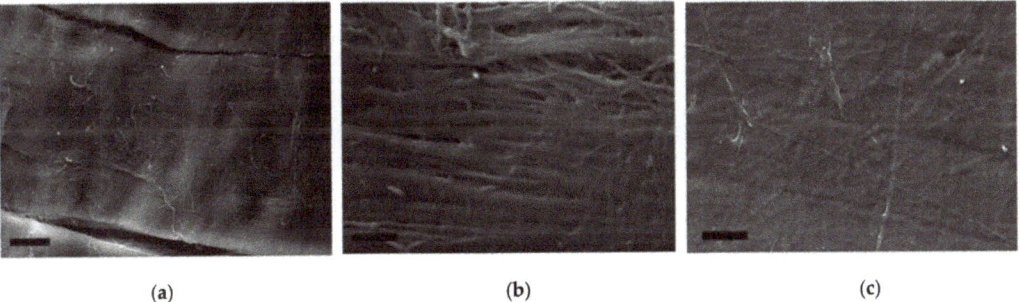

**Figure 6.** Microtopography of the dried GSCM (SEM-SE). (**a**) the surface of a lamina comprising the reinforcing layer (Scale bar = 10 μm), (**b**) the enlarged fragment of the lamina surface (Scale bar = 1 μm), and (**c**) the layer covering the GSCM reinforcing layers (Scale bar = 20 μm).

We also studied the GSCM cross-section using SEM, which showed the layered structure, in agreement with the histological data. The SEM images (Figure 7a,b) demonstrate that laminae change their angle in each layer, thus making a basketweave multilayered collagen structure.

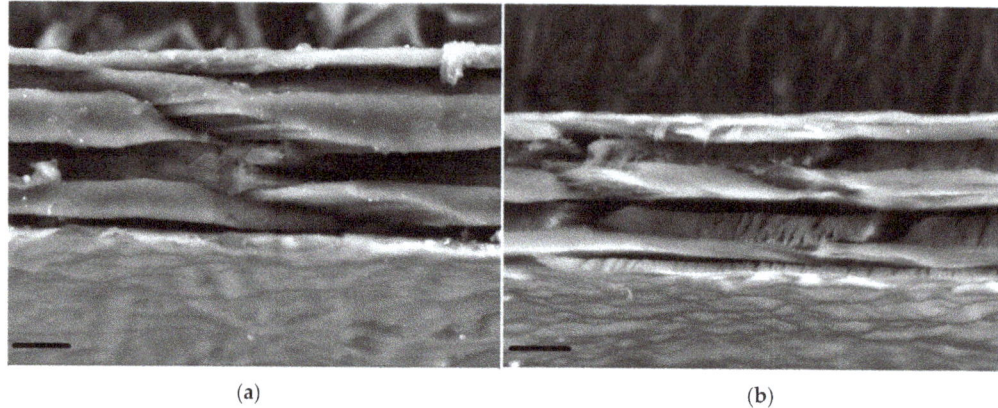

**Figure 7.** A SEM-BSE image of the GSCM cross-section. (a,b) Two different regions (Scale bar = 10 μm).

2.3.3. Laser Scanning Microscopy (LSM) (Second Harmonics Generation Signal—SHG)

The LSM studies revealed the SHG signal from collagen Type I and Type II in the sample. In consistency with SEM, it was found that collagen in the GSCM was bundled into laminae with the width of about 60 μm. Laminae located at different depths have different, up to perpendicular, mutual orientation (the angle of packing is ~60–90°). Laminae consist of longitudinally positioned parallel collagen fibers (Figure 8a). At the surface of some regions, bundles of collagen in the form of cords are found (Figure 8b). Similar structures were observed by SEM, as well (Figure 7a,c).

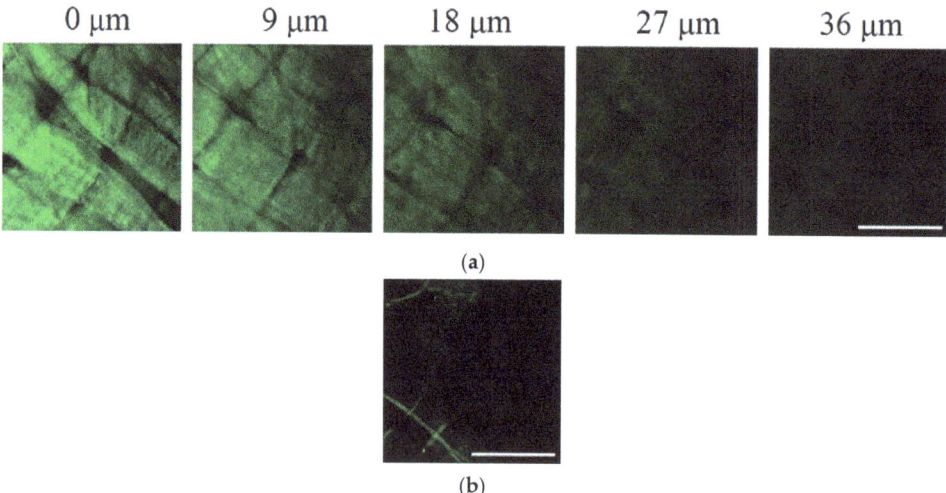

**Figure 8.** SHG images of the GSCM. (a) Collagen bundles in the form of laminae at different depths; (b) collagen in the form of cords at the sample's surface (Scale bar = 100 μm). The SHG signal from collagen is marked by green.

2.3.4. Atomic-Force Microscopy (AFM)

The microrelief of the GSCM surface was visualized using AFM. As seen from Figure 9, the GSCM surface has a fibrillar structure, with collagen fibers consisting of tightly packed longitudinally oriented fibrils.

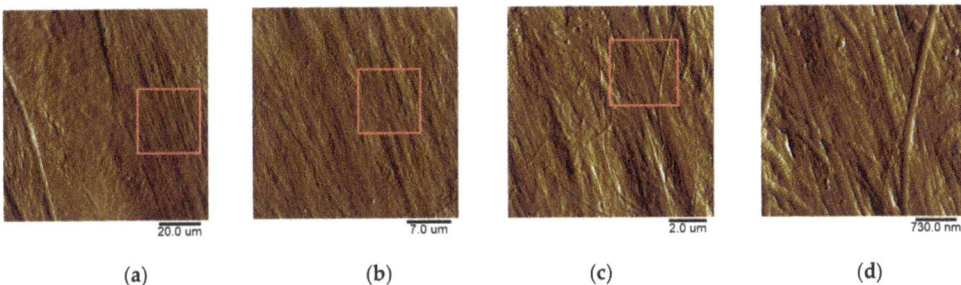

**Figure 9.** AFM topography of the GSCM with the sequential decrease of the scan size from the left to right image (increase of resolution): (**a**) 100 × 100 μm; (**b**) 30 × 30 μm; (**c**) 10 × 10 μm; (**d**) 3 × 3 μm. The samples' topography is presented using the Peak Force Error for the better detail resolution.

For comparison, we obtained the topography of the outer tunic of another squid species, *B. magister*, which has an essentially smaller size. As seen from Figure 10, the collagen structure of the outer membrane of this squid species is similar to that of the GSCM, with the corresponding scaling. The basketweave structure of both squids' reinforcing layers in the outer tunic is clearly visible in AFM images, which testifies the universal character of this structure. Since laminae comprising the reinforcing layer in the GSCM are rather wide (40–50 μm) and located at a certain angle relative to each other, AFM cannot visualize the whole laminar motif of the GSCM, even at the largest available scan size, 100 × 100 μm, so only one cell of the basketweave is seen (Figure 9a). However, for the small squid, *B. magister*, this laminar motif is clearly visible at a 50 × 50 μm scan (Figure 10a), since the *B. magister* has the proportionally smaller mantle and outer tunic thickness (Table 3).

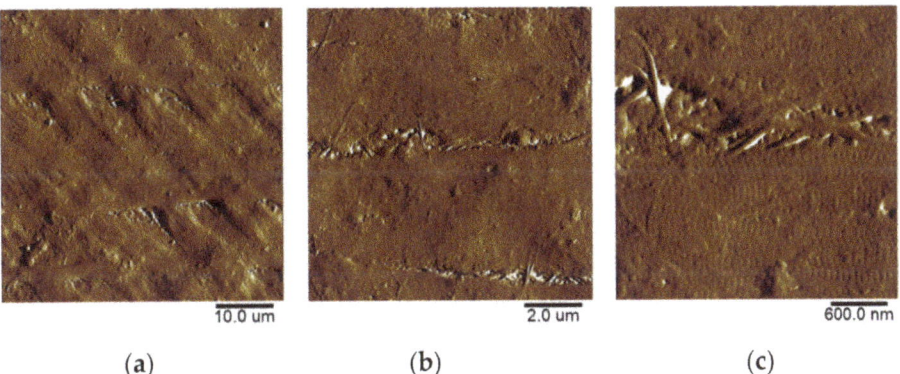

**Figure 10.** AFM topography of the collagenous membrane of a *B. magister* squid. From the left to right image (increase of resolution): (**a**) 50 × 50 μm; (**b**) 10 × 10 μm; (**c**) 3 × 3 μm. The samples' topography is presented using the Peak Force Error for the better detail resolution.

With a higher resolution (a 3 × 3 μm scan, see more on the Figure 11), one can see the characteristic striation of collagen fibrils (D-period). The D-period is equal to 67 nm, although the experimentally obtained values depend on the sample hydration [65].

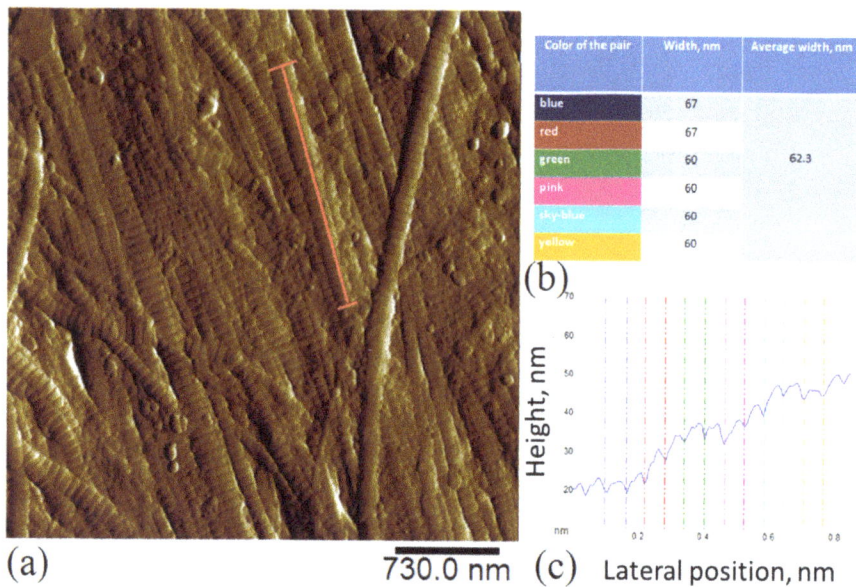

**Figure 11.** Molecular packing of collagen in the GSCM (**a**) AFM topography (Peak Force Error channel), scan size is 3 × 3 µm; (**b**,**c**) D period of an individual fibril longitudinal section (red line on the topography image). The section shows the characteristic D-period of collagen ([66,67]).

*2.4. Mechanical Properties of the GSCM*

2.4.1. Uniaxial Stretching Tests

The uniaxial stretching tests with the final sample rupture showed that the GSCM of *D. gigas* contained at least two basic directions of collagen fibers (Figure 12). The selected directions of collagen bundles may lead to the complex dependency of the GSCM mechanical properties on the deformation direction.

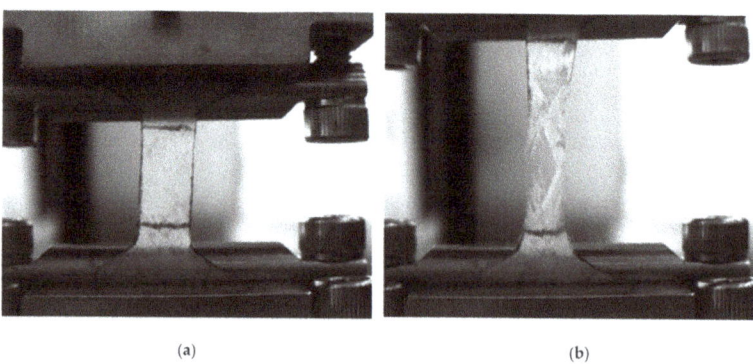

**Figure 12.** A uniaxial stretching test: (**a**)—start, (**b**)—end of test.

As seen from the results presented in Table 3, the studied samples of the GSCM of the *D. gigas* species had a rather high tensile strength for a biological material. The Young's modulus of a dry sample was $1.5 \pm 0.5$ GPa, while, after 20-min-long hydration of the material, its Young's modulus drastically dropped to $20 \pm 6$ MPa. The ultimate tensile strength of the hydrated sample also essentially decreased, however, the strain at rupture grew (to almost 50%).

For comparison, we tested the collagenous membrane of the *B. magister* squid, since it has a similar structure, as shown by AFM. The *B. magister* membrane demonstrated similar mechanical properties as well. Its Young's modulus was somewhat higher than that of the GSCM, while the ultimate tensile strength and maximum elongation at rupture were slightly lower (in the hydrated state). However, in general, the membrane from the *B. magister* squid is more deformable due to its lower thickness (20 µm).

#### 2.4.2. Micromechanical Properties Studied by AFM

As a result of the AFM-based nanoindentation studies at the micro- and nanoscale, the Young's modulus of the GSCM surface was measured as $4.1 \pm 0.5$ MPa. The corresponding value for the *B. magister* squid was slightly higher, $6.1 \pm 0.5$ MPa. The observed difference between the values at the macro- and microscale is related to the different packing and thickness of collagen structures at different levels. However, the values belong to the same order of magnitude.

**Table 3.** Mechanical properties of the GCSM and collagenous membranes from other squid species.

| Type of Squid | DML, cm | T, µm | W, µm | E(w), MPa | UTS(w), MPa | Max ε(w), % | E(d), GPa | UTS(d), MPa | Max ε(d), % | E(w), MPa |
|---|---|---|---|---|---|---|---|---|---|---|
| | | | | | Macromechanical Properties | | | | | Micromechanical Properties |
| Dosidigus gigas | 1500–2000 | 50–70 | 40–50 | $20 \pm 6$ | $20 \pm 8$ | $47 \pm 9$ | $1.5 \pm 0.5$ | $80 \pm 20$ | $20 \pm 15$ | $4.1 \pm 0.5$ |
| Loligo peale [68] | 30–50 | 20–35 | 2–7 | No data | No data | No data | No data | No data | No data | No data |
| Berryteuthis magister | 25 | 20 | 4–7 | $54 \pm 17$ | $10 \pm 3$ | $27 \pm 7$ | $0.4 \pm 0.2$ | $28 \pm 9$ | $16 \pm 5$ | $6.5 \pm 0.5$ |

DML—dorsal mantle length of squid; T—thickness of GSCM; W—width of lamina GSCM; E(w)—Young's modulus of wet GSCM; UTS(w)—ultimate tensile strength of wet GSCM; Max ε(w)—maximum elongation of wet GSCM; E(d)—Young's modulus of dry GSCM; UTS(d)—ultimate tensile strength of dry GSCM; Max ε(d)—maximum elongation of dry GSCM.

### 2.5. Cytotoxicity and Biodegradability of the GSCM

#### 2.5.1. Viability Test

To assess the potential GSCM cytotoxicity, cell viability and proliferation assays were performed. The MSC primary culture was chosen because MSCs are commonly applied in tissue engineering [69–71] and were shown to be more sensitive to toxic agents than 3T3 or L929 cell lines [72–74]. MSCs seeded at a concentration of 5000 cells per well and exposed to the GSCM extracts at any dilution showed neither reduction in the cell viability nor a decrease in the proliferation rate (Figure 13A). In contrast, both of the assays showed a significant drop (to 20% of the cell viability compared to the control cells) in the cell viability in the presence of SDS at a concentration of 0.05 mg/mL and higher (Figure 13B). Hence, the GSCM does not contain any cytotoxic compounds that could be released during cultivation. The adhesive properties of the GSCM were also shown to be appropriate—MSCs successfully adhered to GSCM films, remained viable during 3 days of cultivation, and proliferated on them. The metabolic activity of cells cultured on the surface of the GSCM was slightly higher than that of the monolayer control (Figure 13C). However, proliferation of collagen-cultivated cells was inhibited in comparison to the monolayer cell culture grown on culture plastic, probably due to the different mechanical properties of the surface. The Live/Dead assay of the GSCM revealed normal MSC spindle-shaped morphology and outnumbering living cells relative to the dead ones (Figure 13D–G). Overall, despite the decreased proliferation rates of cells, the GSCM was shown to maintain the normal cell metabolic activity, proliferation capacity, and morphology both by the extraction and contact cytotoxicity test.

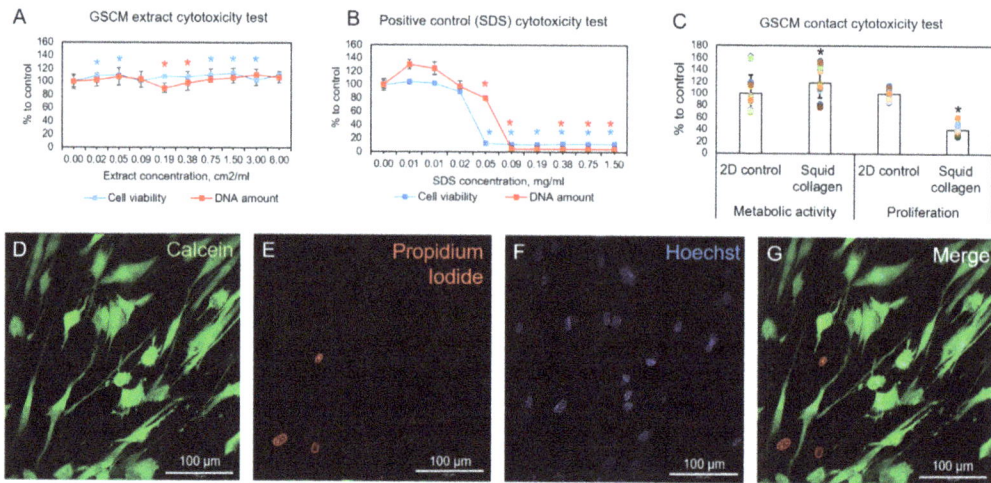

**Figure 13.** (**A**)—Elution test: AlamarBlue cytotoxicity assay and PicoGreen DNA assay of the GSCM extracts, 3 days of MSCs' cultivation, 5000 cells per well. (**B**)—AlamarBlue cytotoxicity assay and PicoGreen DNA assay of SDS (positive control), 3 days of MSCs cultivation, 5000 cells per well. (**C**)—AlamarBlue contact cytotoxicity assay and PicoGreen DNA assay of cells adhered to culture plastic (2D control) or GSCM, 3 days of cell cultivation, 20,000 cells per well. * $p < 0.05$ relative to other groups. (**D–G**)—Live/Dead cell viability assay with nuclei staining (Hoechst, blue); live cells are stained with Calcein AM (green), and dead are stained with propidium iodide (red). At 7 days of cultivation, laser scanning confocal microscopy, scale bar is 100 µm.

### 2.5.2. Resistance to Collagenase

The sensitivity to collagenase was studied in order to estimate the biodegradability of the GSCM. The collagenase cleavage study showed that in 6 h the GSCM was digested by $85 \pm 5\%$ from the initial weight.

The histological study of the GSCM samples treated with collagenase showed signs of their destruction in the form of the loss of the typical structure, as well as changes in the tinctorial and optical properties of the laminar material (see Section 2.3, Figure 4(A2,B2,C2,D2)). These signs included homogenization with lysis and appearing basophilic (Figure 4(A2)) and picrinophilic regions (Figure 4(B2)), as well as loosening and loss of orientation of collagen fibers (Figure 4(C2)) with the disappeared anisotropy (Figure 4(D2)). At the same time, in the picrosirius red-stained samples, the remaining material represented a homogenic picrinophilic mass, in which few chaotically located destroyed collagen fibers were seen.

### 2.5.3. LAL Test

To further assess the GSCM biosafety, we tested its pyrogenicity. The most common pyrogens are endotoxins derived from the cell walls of gram-negative bacteria. The LAL test is commonly applied to assess their concentration and is one of the two assays recognized by the U.S. Pharmacopeia (USP) for medical devices. For the GSCM extract, we revealed that the endotoxin level was 0.28 EU/mL, which does not exceed the concentration permitted (0.5 EU/mL) [75,76]. Therefore, the GSCM did not contain endotoxins able to induce a notable pyrogenic reaction. We also performed preliminary in vivo testing of GSCM samples implanted in rats (see Supplementary Information). It showed that the intact GSCM was still poorly compatible with the host tissues and caused notable inflammatory reaction. However, the GSCM treatment with supercritical carbon dioxide before implantation solved this problem, reducing the inflammatory reaction to only insignificant.

## 3. Discussion

The results of the biochemical and structural studies confirm that collagen is a basic component of the GSCM material. The amino acid analysis showed a high content of Hyp, which is known as a detector for the presence of collagen [77]. Its weight percentage in the samples was 10.13%, while the content of Pro and Hyp in the extracted collagen from the GSCM was 10.9% and 2.8%, respectively [43]. The presence of Cys might indicate that the GSCM possibly contains traces of elastin [78]. Gauza-Włodarczyk et al. (2017) found a similar amino acid composition for bone collagen in [79].

The comparative SDS-PAGE analysis of the GSCM with collagen Type I and Type II revealed the similarity of the GSCM collagen to collagen Type I, based on the characteristic bands. Nam et al. (2008), in the study [80], described collagen extracted from a squid's skin and compared its physicochemical properties with those of collagen prepared from bovine tendons. The similarity between the two was found, and the squid collagen was classified as Type I.

FTIR demonstrated the presence of collagen Type II, also, in the GSCM. The DSC study showed that the GSCM collagen behaved similarly to both collagen types. The characteristic shrinkage temperature also confirmed the collagenous nature of the GSCM.

The extensive morphology study, including histology, SEM, LSM, and AFM, showed the presence of ordered collagen structures at various levels of organization. From the ultrastructure of fibrils to fibers and fiber bundles, they are characterized by tight packing, orientation, and formation of a basketweave from larger collagen units, laminae. Such a sophisticated arrangement of collagen structures is apparently related to the mechanical properties of the GSCM, such as high strength and Young's modulus.

Based on the SEM study, we have deduced a possible concept of the collagen arrangement in the studied material, displayed in Figure 14. The arrows in Figure 14 indicate which SEM-revealed feature corresponds to each component of the schematic structure. The structure and packing of laminae revealed by SEM are confirmed by the other structural techniques.

We have not found any published studies on the structure of the collagenous membrane from the Giant squid of the *D. gigas* species, based either on SEM or on any other visualization technique. However, the squid mantle is known to consist of three layers: muscle fibers and two collagenous membranes surrounding them (outer and inner tunic). There is one literature source in which Otwell et al. (1980) presented a sketch of the *Loligo peale* squid mantle with the specifics of all the three layers, as well as the corresponding SEM images [68].

The structural information, especially the unique architecture of collagen fibers in the GSCM, is of special importance in regard to its mechanical properties. The SEM, AFM, and LSM data show that the collagen laminae are arranged in a basketweave manner. We also have studied the structure of the same part from another squid species, *B. magister*. This small squid is easily available as a food product. Its mantle was separated from the muscle layer and studied with AFM. The AFM studies demonstrated a similar structure of the outer tunic for both squid species, despite a significant difference in their sizes. The characteristic features of the GSCM are repeated in the outer tunic of *B. magister* at a smaller scale. It is the structure that was observed in [68] for the *Loligo peale* species. In spite of essential differences in sizes, these squid species have similar morphological and structural features, as well as comparable mechanical characteristics (Table 3).

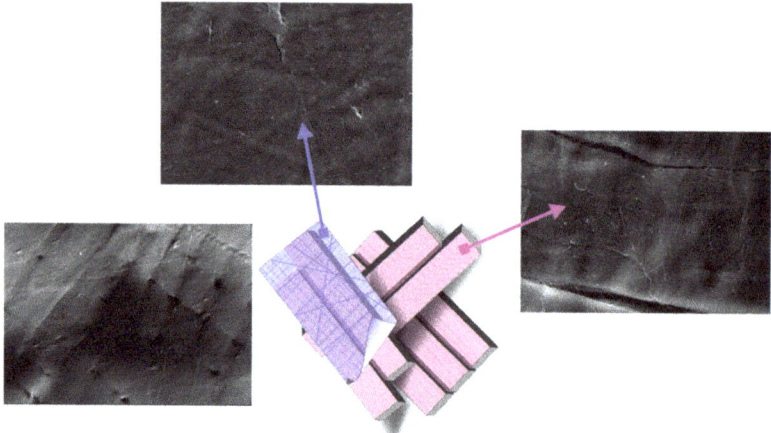

**Figure 14.** A possible concept of the arrangement of collagen fibers in the GSCM based on the SEM findings.

As the basic component of the squid mantle, collagen is related to the mechanism of the animal's locomotion. The collagenous membrane of the cephalopod has a basketweave structure that must work as a reinforcing frame in the squid's body, providing the appropriate strength and stiffness and allowing it to function at high depths.

Indeed, the data of the mechanical tests show rather high values of the tensile strength and Young's modulus for a biological collagen-based material [41,42,81]. A high value of strain at rupture is also notable. The GSCM mechanical characteristics at the microlevel measured by AFM are also high, which is associated with the tight collagen packing in the material in the form of a basketweave revealed by the microscopical visualization (SEM, LSM, ASM, histological staining). These findings are very important from the viewpoint of the potential GSCM applications in regenerative medicine.

A surgical material must have a good compatibility with the host organism tissues. Our cell experiments with gingival MSC and AlamarBlue, Live/Dead, and PicoGreen assays, as well as the LAL test and preliminary in vivo studies, have demonstrated that the GSCM does not exhibit any cytotoxic properties that testify its good biocompatibility.

The collagenase digestion experiment has additionally confirmed the collagenous nature of the material and proven that it can undergo almost complete destruction in vitro in as soon as 6 h. After the treatment, a non-collagenous amorphous component is left, which binds to picric acid and hematoxylin, but it does not bind to picrosirius red and does not show birefringence. Most likely, this component consists of glycoproteins that bind collagen fibers together, thus providing their corresponding orientation and packing in each layer-lamina and also binding together laminae themselves. However, the presence of this non-collagenous component does not prevent the enzymatic action on collagen fibers in the material that may lead to its biodegradation in vivo.

Thus, the collagen nature, basketweave layered structure, good mechanical properties, absence of cytotoxicity, and ability to biodegrade make the GSCM a prospective candidate for tissue engineering applications.

## 4. Materials and Methods
### 4.1. Material

In this study, we used a commercial material—Aksolagen membrane—provided by the Akses Swiss company (Zug, Switzerland). Aksolagen membrane is a specially treated GSCM of *Dosidicus gigas*. The squid mantle consists of several layers (Figure 15), with the central muscle layer surrounded by two collagenous membranes (outer and inner tunics); the GSCM represents the outer tunic of the mantle.

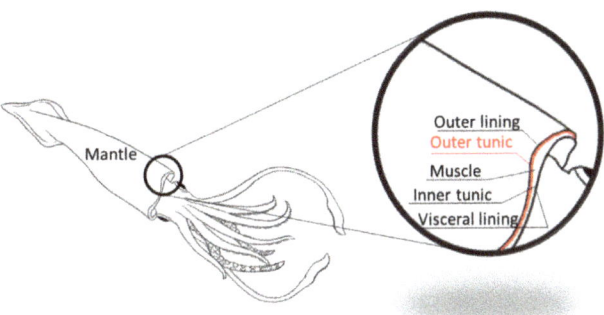

Figure 15. The *D. gigas* mantle and its inner structure.

We also studied the structure of the collagenous membrane of another squid species, a small squid *B. magister*. A frozen squid *B. magister* was purchased in a supermarket, thawed, and the collagenous membrane (outer tunic) was mechanically separated from the muscle layer of the mantle.

The thickness of the GSCM of *D. gigas* measured with a micrometer (a 5–10 N load) was $50 \pm 5$ µm, and the thickness of the *B. magister* membrane was $25 \pm 5$ µm.

### 4.2. Amino Acid Analysis

To study the GSCM composition, we conducted the amino acid analysis. The analysis was performed by ion-exchange chromatography, with the post column derivatization, using an L-8800 amino acid analyzer (Hitachi, Ltd., Tokyo, Japan) with a steel Hitachi Ion-Exchange Column 2622SC(PH) (Hitachi, Ltd., Tokyo, Japan) 4.6 × 80 mm. The column temperature was 57 °C, the flow rate was 0.4 mL/min, the charge volume was 50 µL, and the elution regime involved a stepwise gradient of eluents A (AAA PH-1 Buffer—AN0-8706 Merck Hitachi, Tokyo, Japan), B (AAA PH-2 Buffer—AN0-8707 Merck Hitachi, Tokyo, Japan), C (AAA PH-3 Buffer—AN0-8708 Merck Hitachi, Tokyo, Japan), D (AAA PH-4 Buffer—AN0-8709 Merck Hitachi, Tokyo, Japan), and E (0.2 M NaOH solution). As a calibration mixture, standard concentrated amino acid mixtures in ampoules were used (Amino Acid Standard Sigma Aldrich, St. Louis, MI, USA).

To prepare the studied solution, a dry sample was placed in a molybdenum glass ampoule, and 0.3 mL of a freshly prepared hydrolyzing mixture (concentrated hydrochloric and trifluoroacetic acids in a 2:1 ratio with the addition of 0.1% β-mercaptoethanol Sigma Aldrich, St. Louis, MI, USA) was added. The sample was frozen, and the ampoule was evacuated and sealed. The hydrolysis was conducted at 155 °C for 1 h. After the hydrolysis, the ampoule was cooled, opened, and the content was quantitatively transferred (0.1 mL of water twice) in a plastic 1.5 mL tube, then the hydrolyzing mixture was completely removed with a CentriVap vacuum concentrator (Labconco corporation, Kansas, MO, USA) at 50 °C. The residual acids were removed by repeating twice the procedure of evaporation of small water portions (0.1 mL) added to the dry residue at 50 °C. Then, 0.1 N HCl was added to the dry residue, the mixture was centrifugated, and 0.1 N HCl was added to the supernatant in a 10:1 ratio.

### 4.3. Collagen Molecular Weight Estimation (SDS-PAGE)

Following the collagen extraction, the protein concentration was evaluated by the gravimetric analysis. The sample was ≈100-fold concentrated by ultrafiltration on a Microcon Centrifugal filter unit with a 10 kDa molecular cut-off (MRCPRT010, Millipore, Burlington, MA, USA) to obtain the final collagen at 10 mg/mL. Collagen from GSCM and Type I collagen from the cattle dermis were isolated using a protocol described in [82], while Type II collagen was isolated from the tracheal cartilage by a protocol described in [83] omitting the use of pepsin. An amount of 10 µg of the proteins were diluted with an SDS-loading buffer supplemented with 100 mM DTT (20710, SERVA, Heidelberg, Germany) and heated at 95 °C for 5 min. The samples were resolved by denaturing polyacrylamide gel electrophoresis in 5% stacking and 8% separating gel using a Mini-PROTEAN Electrophoresis System (Bio-Rad, Hercules, CA, USA). The electrophoresis running conditions were as follows: at 15 mA, until samples reached the separating gel, then at 30 mA until the front reached 0.5 cm from the gel edge. The gel was stained with Coomassie Blue R-250 (35051, SERVA, Heidelberg, Germany) and scanned with a ChemiDoc Imaging System (Bio-Rad, Hercules, CA, USA). The molecular weights of the visual bands were calculated in the ImageLab software against the molecular weight standards (Spectra Multicolor High Range Protein Ladder, SM1851, Fermentas, Waltham, MA, USA).

*4.4. IR-Spectroscopy*

The FTIR analysis of the initial components was carried out using a Spectrum Two FT-IR Spectrometer (PerkinElmer, Waltham, MA, USA) in the Attenuated Total Reflectance (ATR) mode. The spectrometer features were as follows: a high-performance, room-temperature LiTaO3 MIR detector, a standard optical system with KBr windows for the data collection over a spectral range of 8300–350 $cm^{-1}$ at a resolution of 0.5 $cm^{-1}$. All the spectra were initially collected in the ATR mode and converted into the IR transmittance mode. The spectra of collagens were normalized using the intensity of the Amid I band as the internal standard.

*4.5. Differential Scanning Calorimetry (DSC)*

Differential scanning calorimetry (DSC) measurements were performed using an STA 6000 simultaneous thermal analyzer (PerkinElmer, Waltham, MA, USA). Samples for DSC experiments (about 10 mg) were encapsulated in standard PerkinElmer pans and heated in a nitrogen medium at a gas flow rate of 20 mL/min and a linear heating rate of 10 °C/min.

*4.6. Shrinkage Temperature*

A sample with the sizes of 3 × 15 mm was placed in a special calibrated glass tube and immersed in a vessel filled with distilled water. The vessel was placed in a water bath. The water bath was heated from room temperature to the moment of the sample shrinkage (~60 °C). The shrinkage temperature was determined as the temperature at which the beginning of the sample shrinkage was detected. The experiment was repeated thrice.

*4.7. Histological Study*

Intact and collagenase-treated fragments of the GSCM of *D. gigas* were fixed in a 10% solution of neutral formalin, and 4 µm-thick histological sections were prepared using a standard technique.

The prepared sections were stained with hematoxylin and eosin and picrosirius red to reveal the collagen composition. The prepared slides were studied by optical (bright-field, phase contrast and polarized light) microscopy, and the images were captured with a LEICA DM4000 B LED microscope equipped with a LEICA DFC7000 T digital camera, using the LAS V4.8 software (Leica Microsystems, Heerbrugg, Switserland).

*4.8. Scanning Electron Microscopy (SEM)*

The GSCM structure was visualized using an EVO LS10 scanning electron microscope (Carl Zeiss Microscopy GmbH Jena, Germany). Two techniques for sample preparation and visualization were used.

The first protocol allowed general images of the samples in the most native state. Naturally dried samples were attached to the microscope stage with a special carbon adhesive tape. The observations were conducted in the low vacuum regime (EP, 70 Pa) at the accelerating voltage of 20 kV and the current of 94 pA per sample. A detector for back-scattered electrons (BSE) was used. The images were obtained with the resolutions of 473.1 nm/px and 508.8 nm/px. To achieve a satisfactory resolution during back-scattered electrons observations, a working distance of 4.5 mm was used.

For detailed evaluation of the structure, samples were fixed in neutral glutaric aldehyde, dehydrated (battery of alcohols from 20% to 97% and acetone), dried bypassing the critical point of $CO_2$, and coated with an Au-Pd alloy. The so-prepared samples were attached to the microscope stage providing the charge outflow from the coated surface. The observations were conducted in the high vacuum regime at the accelerating voltage of 21 kV and the sample current of 19 pA. The microtopography images were obtained using the detector for secondary electrons (SE). The 3072 × 2304 px images were captured with the resolutions of 89.89 nm/px and 2697 nm/px.

*4.9. Laser Scanning Microscopy (Second Harmonics Generation, SHG Signal)*

The study was performed using a LSM 880 NLO laser scanning microscope (Carl Zeiss Microscopy GmbH Jena, Germany) equipped with a tunable Ti:Sa MaiTai HP laser (Spectra-Physics, Milpitas, CA, USA) with a pulse duration of less than 100 fs. The wavelength of 800 nm was used for the study, and the registration of the SHG signal was performed in the range of 370–420 nm. The power of the probing radiation was about 9 mW. The images were obtained using an oil immersion objective with the 40× magnification and numerical aperture of 1.3. The field of view was 212 × 212 µm, and the resolution of images was 1024 × 1024 pixels. A series of images (z-stack) was acquired from the sample surface into the depth with the step of 9 µm, the orientation being parallel to the surface. For the convenience of perception, the acquired images were presented in the green palette.

*4.10. Atomic Force Microscopy (AFM)*

The morphological AFM studies of the surface were performed using an atomic force microscope (BioScope Resolve, Bruker, Billerica, MA, USA) combined with an Axio Observer inverted optical microscope (Carl Zeiss Microscopy GmbH Jena, Germany). A ScanAsyst Air cantilever (Bruker, Billerica, MA, USA) was used with a nominal spring constant k = 0.4 N/m and a nominal tip radius r = 2 nm, and scanning was performed on air in the PeakForce QNM regime. The collagen structures' periodicity was estimated with the Section function of the NanoScope Analysis v1.9 software (Bruker, Billerica, MA, USA).

*4.11. Uniaxial Stretching Test*

The uniaxial stretching tests for dry and hydrated samples were conducted using a Mach-1 v500c mechanical tester (Biomomentum, Laval, QC, Canada). For the hydration, samples were immersed in distilled water for 20 min. The measurements were also performed in distilled water. Dumbbell-shaped fragments of the dry and hydrated GSCM were cut both in the tangential and radial directions in respect to the whole material area (with the circle diameter of 30 cm). The working area of the fragments had the length of 15 mm and width of 5 mm. The dry material thickness was 45 µm, while the thickness of the hydrated material was 60 µm. Before the test, the mechanical tester was calibrated using a standard sample provided by the manufacturer. Both ends of the experimental sample were tightly gripped in the clamps followed by gradual elongation at room temperature (25 °C) at a constant rate of 0.1 mm/s until rupture. The mechanical parameters were calculated from the stress-strain curves according to the manufacturer's protocol. The data were averaged over 3 or more tests.

*4.12. Micromechanics by AFM*

The mechanical properties of the samples' surface were studied in fluid (distilled water) at room temperature (25 °C), after 20 min of hydration, using an atomic force microscope (BioScope Resolve, Bruker, Billerica, MA, USA). The sample micromechanics was obtained in the regime of nanoindentation over a preset map of 50 × 50 µm with the 32 × 32 pixels resolution, as described in [84]. A ScanAsyst Fluid cantilever (Bruker, Billerica, MA, USA) with a nominal spring constant of 0.95 N/m and a nominal tip radius of 50 nm was precalibrated using a standard titanium sample. The deflection sensitivity was calibrated in the same conditions using a sapphire standard sample. The data were processed using the NanoScope Analysis v1.9 software(Bruker, Billerica, MA, USA) and averaged over 12 measurements.

### 4.13. In Vitro Cytotoxicity Assays

The biocompatibility and cytotoxicity tests were performed using the primary culture of mesenchymal stromal cells (MSCs) isolated from human gingival mucosa as described in [85]. The cells were cultivated in the medium that contained Dulbecco's Modified Eagle's Medium (DMEM)/F12 (1:1, Biolot, St. Petersburg, Russia), 10% fetal calf serum (HyClone, Logan, UT, USA), L-glutamine (5 mg/mL, Gibco, Gaithersburg, MD, USA), insulin–transferrin–sodium selenite (1:100, Biolot, St. Petersburg, Russia), bFGF (20 ng/mL, ProSpec, Rehovot, Israel), and gentamycin (50 µg/mL, Paneco, Moscow, Russia). Isolated cells were routinely checked with a SH800S microfluidic flow cytometer (Sony Biotechnology, San Jose, CA, USA) for the presence of mesenchymal surface markers (CD90, CD73, CD105) and absence of hematopoietic and endothelial markers (CD45, CD34, CD11b, CD19 and HLA-DR), according to [86]. The cells were cultivated in the standard conditions of 37 °C and 5% $CO_2$.

The cytotoxicity was analyzed via the elution and contact tests. In the first case, the extracts of the GSCM were prepared according to recommendations of ISO 10993-12. Briefly, 5000 cells per well of a 96-well plate were seeded 24 h before adding the extracts. To prepare extracts, GSCM films were incubated in the culture medium for 24 h at 37 °C. The thickness of a film was less than 0.5 mm, and, therefore, in accordance with ISO 10993-12, the required sample's area to be treated in a volume of 1 mL is 6 $cm^2$. Cells were exposed to the maximum concentration of the extract (6 $cm^2$/mL) and its serial twofold dilutions. We used serial two-fold dilutions of 1.5 mg/mL sodium dodecyl sulphate (SDS) in a standard culture medium as a positive control. Cells cultivated in the standard culture medium were applied as a negative control. After 24 h of cultivation with the extract, SDS, or culture medium, the cell viability was assessed either with the AlamarBlue cell viability reagent (Invitrogen, Waltham, MA, USA) or with the Quant-iT PicoGreen kit (Invitrogen, Waltham, MA, USA). For the AlamarBlue metabolic activity assay, the cell culture medium was replaced with a 10% reagent solution and incubated for 2 h. Then, the fluorescence of samples was measured using a Victor Nivo spectrofluorometer (PerkinElmer, Waltham, MA, USA) at a 530 nm excitation wavelength and a 590 nm emission wavelength. The DNA amount was evaluated with the PicoGreen assay after 3 freeze-thaw cycles aimed at releasing DNA, following the manufacturer's instructions. The samples' fluorescence was estimated with the spectrofluorometer at a 480-nm excitation wavelength and a 520-nm emission wavelength.

For the contact cytotoxicity, 20,000 cells were seeded on a surface of the 1 $cm^2$ GSCM films and cultivated for 3 days. Cells seeded on the culture plastic (monolayer culture) served as a control. Afterwards, the metabolic activity and DNA amount were measured as described above.

The morphology and viability of the cells seeded on the GSCM was visualized with the Live/Dead assay. Briefly, live cells were stained with calcein-AM (Sigma-Aldrich, St. Lois, MO, USA), dead cells were stained with propidium iodide (Thermofisher, Waltham, MA, USA), and nuclei were stained with Hoechst 33,258 (Thermofisher, Waltham, MA, USA). The images were obtained by laser confocal scanning microscopy using a LSM 880 instrument with Airyscan (Carl Zeiss Microscopy GmbH Jena, Germany).

All the samples were triplicated (plate wells for extract cytotoxicity and film samples for the contact cytotoxicity and Live/Dead assay).

*4.14. Resistance to Collagenase*

The susceptibility to proteolytic degradation was studied in a Collagenase A (from C histolyticum) solution. Approximately 4 mg (dry weight in triplicates) of the sample were weighed. To the weighed samples, 0.5 mL aliquots of a 2.5 mg/mL Collagenase A solution in the Tris buffer (50 mmol/L, pH 7.5) containing 10 mmol/L calcium chloride and 0.02 mg/mL sodium azide (Paneco, Moscow, Russia) were added. The samples were incubated at 37 °C for 6 h. Then, the samples were centrifuged at 605 g (3000 RPM) for 90 s (a MiniSpin microcentrifuge by Eppendorf Corporation, Hamburg, Germany). We used a low rotation speed and a short time of centrifugation in order to better preserve the structure integrity for the following histological analysis. Then, the material was washed from the residual collagenase with distilled water. The precipitate was carefully transferred using a micropipette to a coverslip for the following drying in an oven at 50 °C for 20 h. Then, the dry residue was weighed using a WXTE ultramicrobalance (Mettler Toledo GmbH Urdorf, Switzerland). Finally, the weight loss was calculated by a paired comparison before and after the treatment.

*4.15. LAL Test*

The GSCM film was cut into 5*5-mm pieces under aseptic conditions. The extracts were prepared in 1 mL of endotoxin-free water by continuous shaking for 24 h at 50 °C. The endotoxin concentrations were measured using the Chromogenic Endotoxin Quantitation Kit (Thermo Fisher Scientific, Waltham, MA, USA) in accordance with the manufacturer's instruction. Briefly, we mixed 50 µL of the extract or the endotoxin standard dilution (0.1, 0.25, 0.5, 0.1 U/mL) and 50 µL of endotoxin-specific Limulus Amebocyte Lysate (LAL) reagent in a well of a 96-well plate. The mixture was incubated for 10 min at 37 °C and then 100 µL of the chromogenic substrate was added and incubated for 6 min at 37 °C. The reaction was inhibited by adding 100 µL of 25% acetic acid. The absorbance was measured at a wavelength of 405 nm using a microplate Victor Nivo spectrofluorometer (PerkinElmer, Waltham, MA, USA). The minimal detection level of the kit used was 0.1 EU/mL (EU—unit of measurement for endotoxin activity).

## 5. Conclusions

The literature analysis shows that the GSCM material has been very poorly studied, and no application in tissue engineering has been discussed so far. The results of our studies on the GSCM composition, structure, mechanical characteristics, cytotoxicity, and biodegradability testify that the GSCM of *D. gigas* is characterized by a high tensile strength and elasticity, along with a peculiar basketweave collagen structure and biocompatibility that allows the assumption that this material may be applicable in a number of tissue engineering fields (e.g., wound care materials, scaffolds for restoration of the musculoskeletal system, repair of hernias and the prolapse of pelvic organs, dental membranes, and other applications requiring good mechanical properties and slow degradation of the implanted material).

Upon the comparison with other squid species (in particular, *B.magister*), one may conclude that the GSCM structure is represented by a typical reinforcing mesh consisting of collagen structures and providing the high strength and Young's modulus. However, since the Giant squid *D. gigas* has a large size of the mantle and, respectively, a large lateral size of the GSCM, this material is more advantageous from the processing viewpoint.

**Supplementary Materials:** The following are available online at https://www.mdpi.com/1660-3397/19/12/679/s1, Table S1: Band positions for the GSCM, collagen Type I and II; Figure S1: Morphological and optical characteristics of the implanted intact GSCM; Figure S2: Morphological and optical characteristics of the implanted GSCM after the scCO$_2$-treatment.

**Author Contributions:** Conceptualization, P.T. and S.K.; methodology, S.K., A.F. and E.I.; validation, P.T. and S.K.; formal analysis, A.M., E.G., P.B., V.E. and E.I.; investigation, A.F., N.A., I.N., A.M., E.G., Y.E., P.B., V.E. and A.K.; resources, A.F., N.A., I.N., A.M., E.G., Y.E., P.B., V.E., A.K., S.K., E.I., A.S.,

E.Z. and P.T.; data curation, A.F., S.K., E.I., A.S., E.Z. and P.T.; writing—original draft preparation, A.F., N.A., I.N., A.M., E.G., Y.E., P.B., V.E., A.K., S.K. and A.S.; writing—review and editing, A.F., A.S., S.K., E.I., E.Z. and P.T.; visualization, A.F., N.A., I.N., V.E., A.K. and A.S.; supervision, P.T.; project administration, P.T.; funding acquisition, P.T. All authors have read and agreed to the published version of the manuscript.

**Funding:** The study was financially supported by the Russian Science Foundation (18-15-00401).

**Data Availability Statement:** All the data supporting the conclusions of this article are included in this article.

**Acknowledgments:** The study was carried out using the unique scientific facility Transgenebank. The authors thank Anton Murashko (Moscow State University, Faculty of Physics) for drawing the graphical abstract. The authors are thankful to Anastasia Shpichka for her kind assistance with the cell experiments.

**Conflicts of Interest:** The authors declare no conflict of interest.

## References

1. Fayzullin, A.L.; Shekhter, A.B.; Istranov, L.P.; Istranova, E.V.; Rudenko, T.G.; Guller, A.E.; Aboyants, R.K.; Timashev, P.S.; Butnaru, D.V. Bioresorbable collagen materials in surgery: 50 years of success. *Sechenov Med. J.* **2020**, *11*, 59–70. [CrossRef]
2. Cen, L.; Liu, W.; Cui, L.; Zhang, W.; Cao, Y. Collagen tissue engineering: Development of novel biomaterials and applications. *Pediatr. Res.* **2008**, *63*, 492–496. [CrossRef] [PubMed]
3. Parenteau-Bareil, R.; Gauvin, R.; Berthod, F. Collagen-based biomaterials for tissue engineering applications. *Materials* **2010**, *3*, 1863–1887. [CrossRef]
4. Rekulapally, R.; Udayachandrika, K.; Hamlipur, S.; Sasidharan Nair, A.; Pal, B.; Singh, S. Tissue engineering of collagen scaffolds crosslinked with plant based polysaccharides. *Prog. Biomater.* **2021**, *10*, 29–41. [CrossRef]
5. Blackstone, B.N.; Gallentine, S.C.; Powell, H.M. Review collagen-based electrospun materials for tissue engineering: A systematic review. *Bioengineering* **2021**, *8*, 39. [CrossRef]
6. Huang, J.; Chen, L.; Gu, Z.; Wu, J. Red Jujube-Incorporated Gelatin Methacryloyl (GelMA) Hydrogels with Anti-Oxidation and Immunoregulation Activity for Wound Healing. *J. Biomed. Nanotechnol.* **2019**, *15*, 1357–1370. [CrossRef]
7. Nourissat, G.; Berenbaum, F.; Duprez, D. Tendon injury: From biology to tendon repair. *Nat. Rev. Rheumatol.* **2015**, *11*, 223–233. [CrossRef] [PubMed]
8. Kannus, P. Structure of the tendon connective tissue. *Scand. J. Med. Sci. Sport.* **2000**, *10*, 312–320. [CrossRef]
9. Mienaltowski, M.J.; Birk, D.E. Structure, Physiology, and Biochemistry of Collagens. In *Progress in Heritable Soft Connective Tissue Diseases*; Halper, J., Ed.; Springer: Dordrecht, The Netherlands, 2014; pp. 5–29.
10. Amiel, D.; Frank, C.; Harwood, F.; Fronek, J.; Akeson, W. Tendons and Ligaments: A Morphological and Biochemical Comparison A historical review of the evolution of the use of tendons as ligament substitutes reveals that these. *J. Orthop. Res.* **1984**, *1*, 251–265.
11. Frank, C.; Amiel, D.; Woo, S.L.Y.; Akeson, W. Normal ligament properties and ligament healing. *Clin. Orthop. Relat. Res.* **1985**, *196*, 15–25. [CrossRef]
12. Duthon, V.B.; Barea, C.; Abrassart, S.; Fasel, J.H.; Fritschy, D.; Ménétrey, J. Anatomy of the anterior cruciate ligament. *Knee Surgery, Sport. Traumatol. Arthrosc.* **2006**, *14*, 204–213. [CrossRef]
13. Franchi, M.; Fini, M.; Quaranta, M.; De Pasquale, V.; Raspanti, M.; Giavaresi, G.; Ottani, V.; Ruggeri, A. Crimp morphology in relaxed and stretched rat Achilles tendon. *J. Anat.* **2007**, *210*, 1–7. [CrossRef]
14. Bottagisio, M.; D'Arrigo, D.; Talò, G.; Bongio, M.; Ferroni, M.; Boschetti, F.; Moretti, M.; Lovati, A.B. Achilles tendon repair by decellularized and engineered xenografts in a rabbit model. *Stem Cells Int.* **2019**, *2019*. [CrossRef]
15. Song, Y.J.; Hua, Y.H. Tendon allograft for treatment of chronic Achilles tendon rupture: A systematic review. *Foot Ankle Surg.* **2019**, *25*, 252–257. [CrossRef]
16. Smith, L.T.; Holbrook, K.A.; Byers, P.H. Structure of the dermal matrix during development and in the adult. *J. Invest. Dermatol.* **1982**, *79*, 93–104. [CrossRef]
17. Armour, A.D.; Fish, J.S.; Woodhouse, K.A.; Semple, J.L. A comparison of human and porcine acellularized dermis: Interactions with human fibroblasts in vitro. *Plast. Reconstr. Surg.* **2006**, *117*, 845–856. [CrossRef] [PubMed]
18. Prasertsung, I.; Kanokpanont, S.; Bunaprasert, T.; Thanakit, V.; Damrongsakkul, S. Development of acellular dermis from porcine skin using periodic pressurized technique. *J. Biomed. Mater. Res. Part B Appl. Biomater.* **2008**, *85*, 210–219. [CrossRef]
19. Shoulders, M.D.; Raines, R.T. Collagen structure and stability. *Annu. Rev. Biochem.* **2009**, *78*, 929–958. [CrossRef]
20. Silver, F.H.; Freeman, J.W.; Devore, D. Viscoelastic properties of human skin and processed dermis. *Ski. Res. Technol.* **2001**, *7*, 18–23. [CrossRef] [PubMed]
21. Silver, F.H. *Biological Materials: Structure, Mechanical Properties, and Modeling of Soft Tissues*; NYU Press: New York, NY, USA, 1987; ISBN 9780814778609.
22. Wilkes, G.L.; Brown, I.A.; Wildnauer, R.H. The biomechanical properties of skin. *CRC Crit. Rev. Bioeng.* **1973**, *1*, 453–495. [PubMed]

23. Ní Annaidh, A.; Bruyère, K.; Destrade, M.; Gilchrist, M.D.; Otténio, M. Characterization of the anisotropic mechanical properties of excised human skin. *J. Mech. Behav. Biomed. Mater.* **2012**, *5*, 139–148. [CrossRef]
24. Ruszczak, Z. Effect of collagen matrices on dermal wound healing. *Adv. Drug Deliv. Rev.* **2003**, *55*, 1595–1611. [CrossRef] [PubMed]
25. Gullbrand, S.E.; Ashinsky, B.G.; Lai, A.; Gansau, J.; Crowley, J.; Cunha, C.; Engiles, J.B.; Fusellier, M.; Muehleman, C.; Pelletier, M.; et al. Development of a standardized histopathology scoring system for intervertebral disc degeneration and regeneration in rabbit models-An initiative of the ORSspine section. *JOR Spine* **2021**, *4*, 1–12. [CrossRef]
26. Hiroshi, Y. *Strength of Biological Materials*; Williams & Wilkins: Baltimore, MD, USA, 1970.
27. Huang, K.; Liu, G.; Gu, Z.; Wu, J. Tofu as excellent scaffolds for potential bone regeneration. *Chinese Chem. Lett.* **2020**, *31*, 3190–3194. [CrossRef]
28. Huang, K.; Hou, J.; Gu, Z.; Wu, J. Egg-White-/Eggshell-Based Biomimetic Hybrid Hydrogels for Bone Regeneration. *ACS Biomater. Sci. Eng.* **2019**, *5*, 5384–5391. [CrossRef]
29. Gallagher, A.J.; Ní Annaidh, A.; Bruyère, K.; Ottenio, M.; Xie, H.; Gilchrist, M.D. Dynamic Tensile Properties of Human Skin. In Proceedings of the 2012 IRCOBI Conference, Dublin, Ireland, 12–14 September 2012; pp. 1–6.
30. Dunn, M.; Tria, A.; Kato, P.; Bechler, J.; Ochner, R.; Zawadsky, J.; Silver, F.H. Anterior cruciate using a composite collagenous prosthesis histologic study in rabbits. *Am. J. Sports Med.* **1992**, *20*, 507–515. [CrossRef]
31. Butler, D.L.; Grood, E.S.; Noyes, F.R.; Zernicke, R.F.; Brackett, K. Effects of structure and strain measurement technique on the material properties of young human tendons and fascia. *J. Biomech.* **1984**, *17*, 579–596. [CrossRef]
32. Huang, C.Y.; Wang, V.M.; Pawluk, R.J.; Bucchieri, J.S.; Levine, W.N.; Bigliani, L.U.; Mow, V.C.; Flatow, E.L. Inhomogeneous mechanical behavior of the human supraspinatus tendon under uniaxial loading. *J. Orthop. Res.* **2005**, *23*, 924–930. [CrossRef]
33. Shen, W.; Chen, J.; Yin, Z.; Chen, X.; Liu, H.; Heng, B.C.; Chen, W.; Ouyang, H.W. Allogenous tendon stem/progenitor cells in silk scaffold for functional shoulder repair. *Cell Transplant.* **2012**, *21*, 943–958. [CrossRef] [PubMed]
34. Arya, S.; Kulig, K. Tendinopathy alters mechanical and material properties of the Achilles tendon. *J. Appl. Physiol.* **2010**, *108*, 670–675. [CrossRef]
35. Currey, J. *The Structure and Mechanical Properties of Bone*; Woodhead Publishing Limited: Sawston, UK, 2008; ISBN 9781845692049.
36. Rubod, C.; Boukerrou, M.; Brieu, M.; Jean-Charles, C.; Dubois, P.; Cosson, M. Biomechanical properties of vaginal tissue: Preliminary results. *Int. Urogynecol. J.* **2008**, *19*, 811–816. [CrossRef]
37. Zeng, Y.; Yang, J.; Huang, K.; Lee, Z.; Lee, X. A comparison of biomechanical properties between human and porcine cornea. *J. Biomech.* **2001**, *34*, 533–537. [CrossRef]
38. Grebenik, E.A.; Istranov, L.P.; Istranova, E.V.; Churbanov, S.N.; Shavkuta, B.S.; Dmitriev, R.I.; Veryasova, N.N.; Kotova, S.L.; Kurkov, A.V.; Shekhter, A.B.; et al. Chemical cross—linking of xenopericardial biomeshes: A bottom—up study of structural and functional correlations. *Xenotransplantation* **2019**, *26*, e12506. [CrossRef] [PubMed]
39. Powell, H.M.; McFarland, K.L.; Butler, D.L.; Supp, D.M.; Boyce, S.T. Uniaxial strain regulates morphogenesis, gene expression, and tissue strength in engineered skin. *Tissue Eng. Part A* **2010**, *16*, 1083–1092. [CrossRef] [PubMed]
40. Bose, S.; Li, S.; Mele, E.; Silberschmidt, V.V. Dry vs. wet: Properties and performance of collagen films. Part I. Mechanical behaviour and strain-rate effect. *J. Mech. Behav. Biomed. Mater.* **2020**, *111*, 103983. [CrossRef] [PubMed]
41. Koide, T.; Daito, M. Effects of Various Collagen Crosslinking Techniques on Mechanical Properties of Collagen Film. *Dent. Mater. J.* **1997**, *16*, 1–9. [CrossRef]
42. Habermehl, J.; Skopinska, J.; Boccafoschi, F.; Sionkowska, A.; Kaczmarek, H.; Laroche, G.; Mantovani, D. Preparation of ready-to-use, stockable and reconstituted collagen. *Macromol. Biosci.* **2005**, *5*, 821–828. [CrossRef]
43. Uriarte-Montoya, M.H.; Arias-Moscoso, J.L.; Plascencia-Jatomea, M.; Santacruz-Ortega, H.; Rouzaud-Sández, O.; Cardenas-Lopez, J.L.; Marquez-Rios, E.; Ezquerra-Brauer, J.M. Jumbo squid (*Dosidicus gigas*) mantle collagen: Extraction, characterization, and potential application in the preparation of chitosan-collagen biofilms. *Bioresour. Technol.* **2010**, *101*, 4212–4219. [CrossRef] [PubMed]
44. Wu, Y.; Liu, A.; Wang, W.; Ye, R. Improved mechanical properties and thermal-stability of collagen fiber based film by crosslinking with casein, keratin or SPI: Effect of crosslinking process and concentrations of proteins. *Int. J. Biol. Macromol.* **2017**, *109*, 1319–1328. [CrossRef]
45. Theodoridis, K.; Müller, J.; Ramm, R.; Findeisen, K.; Andrée, B.; Korossis, S.; Haverich, A.; Hilfiker, A. Effects of combined cryopreservation and decellularization on the biomechanical, structural and biochemical properties of porcine pulmonary heart valves. *Acta Biomater.* **2016**, *43*, 71–77. [CrossRef]
46. Ward, D.V.; Wainwright, S.A. Locomotory aspects of squid mantle structure. *J. Zool.* **1972**, *167*, 437–449. [CrossRef]
47. FAO. *The State of World Fisheries and Aquaculture 2018 Meeting the Sustainable Development Goals*; FAO: Rome, Italy, 2018.
48. Ibáñez, C.M.; Sepúlveda, R.D.; Ulloa, P.; Keyl, F.; Pardo-Gandarillas, M.C. The biology and ecology of the jumbo squid *Dosidicus gigas* (*Cephalopoda*) in Chilean waters: A review. *Lat. Am. J. Aquat. Res.* **2015**, *43*, 402–414. [CrossRef]
49. Nagai, T.; Izumi, M.; Ishii, M. Fish scale collagen. Preparation and partial characterization. *Int. J. Food Sci. Technol.* **2004**, *39*, 239–244. [CrossRef]
50. Torres-Arreola, W.; Pacheco-Aguilar, R.; Sotelo-Mundo, R.R.; Rouzaud-Sández, O.; Ezquerra-Brauer, J.M. Partial characterization of collagen from mantle, fin, and arms of jumbo squid (*Dosidicus gigas*). *Cienc. y Tecnol. Aliment.* **2008**, *6*, 101–108. [CrossRef]

51. Li, P.H.; Lu, W.C.; Chan, Y.J.; Ko, W.C.; Jung, C.C.; Le Huynh, D.T.; Ji, Y.X. Extraction and characterization of collagen from sea cucumber (*Holothuria cinerascens*) and its potential application in moisturizing cosmetics. *Aquaculture* **2020**, *515*, 734590. [CrossRef]
52. Adamowicz, J.; Kloskowski, T.; Stopel, M.; Gniadek, M.; Rasmus, M.; Balcerczyk, D. Materials Science & Engineering C The development of marine biomaterial derived from decellularized squid mantle for potential application as tissue engineered urinary conduit. *Mater. Sci. Eng. C* **2021**, *119*, 111579. [CrossRef]
53. De Melo Oliveira, V.; Assis, C.R.D.; Costa, B.D.A.M.; de Araujo Neri, R.C.; Monte, F.T.D.; da Costa Vasconcelos, H.M.S.; França, R.C.P.; Santos, J.F.; de Souza Bezerra, R.; Porto, A.L.F. Physical, biochemical, densitometric and spectroscopic techniques for characterization collagen from alternative sources: A review based on the sustainable valorization of aquatic by-products. *J. Mol. Struct.* **2021**, *1224*, 129023. [CrossRef]
54. Rýglová, Š.; Braun, M.; Hříbal, M.; Suchý, T.; Vörös, D. The proportion of the key components analysed in collagen-based isolates from fish and mammalian tissues processed by different protocols. *J. Food Compos. Anal.* **2021**, *103*. [CrossRef]
55. Benayahu, D.; Benayahu, Y. A Unique Marine-Derived Collagen: Its Characterization towards Biocompatibility Applications for Tissue Regeneration. *Mar. Drugs* **2021**, *19*, 419. [CrossRef] [PubMed]
56. Riaz, T.; Zeeshan, R.; Zarif, F.; Ilyas, K.; Muhammad, N.; Safi, S.Z.; Rahim, A.; Rizvi, S.A.A.; Rehman, I.U. FTIR analysis of natural and synthetic collagen. *Appl. Spectrosc. Rev.* **2018**, *53*, 703–746. [CrossRef]
57. Martínez Cortizas, A.; López-Costas, O. Linking structural and compositional changes in archaeological human bone collagen: An FTIR-ATR approach. *Sci. Rep.* **2020**, *10*, 1–14. [CrossRef]
58. Belbachir, K.; Noreen, R.; Gouspillou, G.; Petibois, C. Collagen types analysis and differentiation by FTIR spectroscopy. *Anal. Bioanal. Chem.* **2009**, *395*, 829–837. [CrossRef] [PubMed]
59. Petibois, C.; Gouspillou, G.; Wehbe, K.; Delage, J.P.; Déléris, G. Analysis of type I and IV collagens by FT-IR spectroscopy and imaging for a molecular investigation of skeletal muscle connective tissue. *Anal. Bioanal. Chem.* **2006**, *386*, 1961–1966. [CrossRef]
60. De Campos Vidal, B.; Mello, M.L.S. Collagen type I amide I band infrared spectroscopy. *Micron* **2011**, *42*, 283–289. [CrossRef] [PubMed]
61. Ghodbane, S.A.; Dunn, M.G. Physical and mechanical properties of cross-linked type I collagen scaffolds derived from bovine, porcine, and ovine tendons. *J. Biomed. Mater. Res.—Part A* **2016**, *104*, 2685–2692. [CrossRef] [PubMed]
62. Shanmugasundaram, N.; Ravikumar, T.; Babu, M. Comparative physico-chemical and in vitro properties of fibrillated collagen scaffolds from different sources. *J. Biomater. Appl.* **2004**, *18*, 247–264. [CrossRef]
63. Budrugeac, P.; Carşote, C.; Miu, L. Application of thermal analysis methods for damage assessment of leather in an old military coat belonging to the History Museum of Braşov—Romania. *J. Therm. Anal. Calorim.* **2017**, *127*, 765–772. [CrossRef]
64. Samouillan, V.; Delaunay, F.; Dandurand, J.; Merbahi, N.; Gardou, J.-P.; Yousfi, M.; Gandaglia, A.; Spina, M.; Lacabanne, C. The Use of Thermal Techniques for the Characterization and Selection of Natural Biomaterials. *J. Funct. Biomater.* **2011**, *2*, 230–248. [CrossRef]
65. Flint, M.H.; Merrilees, M.J. Relationship between the axial periodicity and staining of collagen by the Masson trichrome procedure. *Histochem. J.* **1977**, *9*, 1–13. [CrossRef]
66. Kotova, S.L.; Shekhter, A.B.; Timashev, P.S.; Guller, A.E.; Mudrov, A.A.; Timofeeva, V.A.; Panchenko, V.Y.; Bagratashvili, V.N.; Solovieva, A.B. AFM study of the extracellular connective tissue matrix in patients with pelvic organ prolapse. *J. Surf. Investig.* **2014**, *8*, 754–760. [CrossRef]
67. Baselt, D.R.; Revel, J.P.; Baldeschwieler, J.D. Subfibrillar structure of type I collagen observed by atomic force microscopy. *Biophys. J.* **1993**, *65*, 2644–2655. [CrossRef]
68. Otwell, W.; Giddings, G. Scanning electron microscopy of squid, Loligo pealei: Raw, cooked, and frozen mantle. *Mar. Fish. Rev.* **1980**, *42*, 67–72.
69. Han, Y.; Li, X.; Zhang, Y.; Han, Y.; Chang, F.; Ding, J. Mesenchymal Stem Cells for Regenerative Medicine. *Cells* **2019**, *8*, 886. [CrossRef] [PubMed]
70. Freeman, F.E.; Kelly, D.J. Tuning alginate bioink stiffness and composition for controlled growth factor delivery and to spatially direct MSC Fate within bioprinted tissues. *Sci. Rep.* **2017**, *7*, 1–12. [CrossRef]
71. Bikmulina, P.Y.; Kosheleva, N.V.; Shpichka, A.I.; Efremov, Y.M.; Yusupov, V.I.; Timashev, P.S.; Rochev, Y.A. Beyond 2D: Effects of photobiomodulation in 3D tissue-like systems. *J. Biomed. Opt.* **2020**, *25*, 1. [CrossRef] [PubMed]
72. Paterson, T.E.; Shi, R.; Tian, J.; Harrison, C.J.; De Sousa Mendes, M.; Hatton, P.V.; Li, Z.; Ortega, I. Electrospun scaffolds containing silver-doped hydroxyapatite with antimicrobial properties for applications in orthopedic and dental bone surgery. *J. Funct. Biomater.* **2020**, *11*, 58. [CrossRef] [PubMed]
73. Sindhu, K.R.; Bansode, N.; Rémy, M.; Morel, C.; Bareille, R.; Hagedorn, M.; Hinz, B.; Barthélémy, P.; Chassande, O.; Boiziau, C. New injectable self-assembled hydrogels that promote angiogenesis through a bioactive degradation product. *Acta Biomater.* **2020**, *115*, 197–209. [CrossRef]
74. Merlin Rajesh Lal, L.P.; Suraishkumar, G.K.; Nair, P.D. Chitosan-agarose scaffolds supports chondrogenesis of Human Wharton's Jelly mesenchymal stem cells. *J. Biomed. Mater. Res.—Part A* **2017**, *105*, 1845–1855. [CrossRef] [PubMed]
75. Keane, T.J.; Saldin, L.T.; Badylak, S.F. *Decellularization of Mammalian Tissues: Preparing Extracellular Matrix Bioscaffolds*; Elsevier Ltd.: Amsterdam, The Netherlands, 2016; ISBN 9781782420958.

76. Food and Drug Administration. *Guideline on Validation of the Limulus ameobocyte Lysate Test as an End-Product Endotoxin Test for Human and Animal Parenteral Drugs, Biological Products, and Medical Devices*; U.S. Department of Health & Human Services: Washington, DC, USA, 1987; pp. 1–30.
77. Stoilov, I.; Starcher, B.C.; Mecham, R.P.; Broekelmann, T.J. Measurement of elastin, collagen, and total protein levels in tissues. In *Methods in Cell Biology*; Mecham, R.P., Ed.; Elsevier Inc.: Amsterdam, The Netherlands, 2018; Volume 143, pp. 133–146. ISBN 978-0-12-812297-6.
78. Xiong, Y.L. Structure-Function Relationships of Muscle Proteins. In *Food Proteins and Their Applications*; CRC Press: Boca Raton, FL, USA, 2017; p. 52. ISBN 9780203755617.
79. Gauza-Włodarczyk, M.; Kubisz, L.; Włodarczyk, D. Amino acid composition in determination of collagen origin and assessment of physical factors effects. *Int. J. Biol. Macromol.* **2017**, *104*, 987–991. [CrossRef]
80. Nam, K.A.; You, S.G.; Kim, S.M. Molecular and physical characteristics of squid (*Todarodes pacificus*) skin collagens and biological properties of their enzymatic hydrolysates. *J. Food Sci.* **2008**, *73*, 249–255. [CrossRef]
81. Barocas, V.H.; Ph, D.; Hubel, A. Collagen Film-Based Corneal Stroma Equivalent. *Tissue Eng.* **2006**, *12*, 1565–1575.
82. Bardakova, K.N.; Grebenik, E.A.; Istranova, E.V.; Istranov, L.P.; Gerasimov, Y.V.; Grosheva, A.G.; Zharikova, T.M.; Minaev, N.V.; Shavkuta, B.S.; Dudova, D.S.; et al. Reinforced Hybrid Collagen Sponges for Tissue Engineering. *Bull. Exp. Biol. Med.* **2018**, *165*, 142–147. [CrossRef]
83. Akram, A.N.; Zhang, C. Extraction of collagen-II with pepsin and ultrasound treatment from chicken sternal cartilage; physicochemical and functional properties. *Ultrason. Sonochem.* **2020**, *64*, 105053. [CrossRef] [PubMed]
84. Efremov, Y.M.; Bakhchieva, N.A.; Shavkuta, B.S.; Frolova, A.A.; Kotova, S.L.; Novikov, I.A.; Akovantseva, A.A.; Avetisov, K.S.; Avetisov, S.E.; Timashev, P.S. Mechanical properties of anterior lens capsule assessed with AFM and nanoindenter in relation to human aging, pseudoexfoliation syndrome, and trypan blue staining. *J. Mech. Behav. Biomed. Mater.* **2020**, *112*, 104081. [CrossRef] [PubMed]
85. Zorin, V.L.; Pulin, A.A.; Eremin, I.I.; Korsakov, I.N.; Zorina, A.I.; Khromova, N.V.; Sokova, O.I.; Kotenko, K.V.; Kopnin, P.B. Myogenic potential of human alveolar mucosa derived cells Vadim. *Cell Cycle* **2017**, *16*, 545–555. [CrossRef] [PubMed]
86. Dominici, M.; Le Blanc, K.; Mueller, I.; Slaper-Cortenbach, I.; Marini, F.C.; Krause, D.S.; Deans, R.J.; Keating, A.; Prockop, D.J.; Horwitz, E.M. Minimal criteria for defining multipotent mesenchymal stromal cells. The International Society for Cellular Therapy position statement. *Cytotherapy* **2006**, *8*, 315–317. [CrossRef] [PubMed]

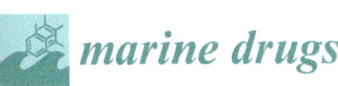

Article

# A 3D-Printed Polycaprolactone/Marine Collagen Scaffold Reinforced with Carbonated Hydroxyapatite from Fish Bones for Bone Regeneration

Se-Chang Kim [1,2], Seong-Yeong Heo [3], Gun-Woo Oh [4], Myunggi Yi [1,5] and Won-Kyo Jung [1,2,5,*]

1. Major of Biomedical Engineering, Division of Smart Healthcare, College of Information Technology and Convergence and New-Senior Healthcare Innovation Center (BK21 Plus), Pukyong National University, Busan 48531, Korea; tpckd181q@pukyong.ac.kr (S.-C.K.); myunggi@pknu.ac.kr (M.Y.)
2. Marine Integrated Biomedical Technology Center, The National Key Research Institutes in Universities, Pukyong National University, Busan 48513, Korea
3. Jeju Marine Research Center, Korea Institute of Ocean Science & Technology (KIOST), Jeju 63349, Korea; syheo@kiost.ac.kr
4. National Marine Biodiversity Institute of Korea (MABIK), Seochun, Chungcheongnam 33662, Korea; ogwchobo@mabik.re.kr
5. Research Center for Marine Integrated Bionics Technology, Pukyong National University, Busan 48513, Korea
* Correspondence: wkjung@pknu.ac.kr; Tel.: +82-51-629-5775

**Abstract:** In bone tissue regeneration, extracellular matrix (ECM) and bioceramics are important factors, because of their osteogenic potential and cell–matrix interactions. Surface modifications with hydrophilic material including proteins show significant potential in tissue engineering applications, because scaffolds are generally fabricated using synthetic polymers and bioceramics. In the present study, carbonated hydroxyapatite (CHA) and marine atelocollagen (MC) were extracted from the bones and skins, respectively, of *Paralichthys olivaceus*. The extracted CHA was characterized using Fourier transform infrared (FTIR) spectroscopy and X-ray diffraction (XRD) analysis, while MC was characterized using FTIR spectroscopy and sodium dodecyl sulfate-polyacrylamide gel electrophoresis (SDS-PAGE). The scaffolds consisting of polycaprolactone (PCL), and different compositions of CHA (2.5%, 5%, and 10%) were fabricated using a three-axis plotting system and coated with 2% MC. Then, the MC3T3-E1 cells were seeded on the scaffolds to evaluate the osteogenic differentiation in vitro, and in vivo calvarial implantation of the scaffolds was performed to study bone tissue regeneration. The results of mineralization confirmed that the MC/PCL, 2.5% CHA/MC/PCL, 5% CHA/MC/PCL, and 10% CHA/MC/PCL scaffolds increased osteogenic differentiation by 302%, 858%, 970%, and 1044%, respectively, compared with pure PCL scaffolds. Consequently, these results suggest that CHA and MC obtained from byproducts of *P. olivaceus* are superior alternatives for land animal-derived substances.

**Keywords:** marine collagen; carbonated hydroxyapatite; fishery by-product; 3D scaffold; bone regeneration

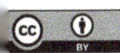

## 1. Introduction

Bone is a dense, complex, hierarchically structured connective tissue composed of calcified matrix, which includes 65% inorganic materials, 25% organic materials, and 10% water, cells (osteoblasts, osteoclasts, and osteocytes), and various proteins, such as osteocalcin, osteopontin, and osteoprotegerin [1,2]. Bone is one of the most important tissues in the human body and provides mechanical strength, protects vital body organs, and stores and releases minerals; also, bone is continuously subjected to various defects, injuries, and diseases [3]. Some bone-related issues cannot be self-repaired and require special treatments, such as bone grafts including autografts, allografts, and tissue-engineered bone substitutes that promote bone tissue regeneration [4]. Bioceramics including bioactive glass, hydroxyapatite (HA), and calcium phosphate are promising bioactive materials that were successfully used for bone tissue regeneration applications [5].

HA ($Ca_{10}(PO_4)_6(OH)_2$) is the main component of bone and accounts for approximately 60–70% of total bone mass [6,7]. Hence, HA was reported to be a potential therapeutic material and was applied in spinal fusion surgery, bone defect treatment, bone-related surgery, and bone mass augmentation [8,9]. Although HA is a bioactive material that induces bone regeneration, this material has a lack of mechanical stability, high brittleness, and low interaction with cells. Thus, many studies are currently being conducted to composite HA with various synthetic and natural materials to improve its mechanical properties and cellular functions such as cell adhesion, migration, and differentiation [10,11].

Collagen is the main protein in the extracellular matrix (ECM), accounting for approximately one-quarter of total body protein [12,13]. Collagen is a structural protein with a triple-helical structure that is composed of repeated G-X-Y peptide units. There are 29 types of collagen, and the majority are type I, II, and III. Collagen is a particularly promising biomaterial that promotes cell adhesion, proliferation, and differentiation by providing an ECM-mimicking environment [14,15]. However, collagen isolated from land animals, such as pigs and cows, has various barriers to application in medical products, due to religious reasons and zooanthroponoses. Marine-derived collagen is a highly potent alternative to land animal-derived collagen, since there are no religious barriers or reported zooanthroponoses [16–18]. In addition, marine-derived collagen has shown a lower immune response, higher water solubility, and lower production costs than land animal-derived collagen [19,20]. Among marine organisms, *Paralichthys olivaceus* may be a good substitute for land animal-derived collagen, because of its good accessibility and availability as a byproduct in the seafood industry in the Republic of Korea [21]. However, investigations of bone regenerative scaffolds fabricated with *P. olivaceus*-derived biomaterials were rarely reported. In addition, unlike jellyfish containing a large amount of collagen type 2 and a marine sponge containing a large amount of collagen type 4, fish skins contain a large amount of collagen type 1, so it can be used as a raw material for biomaterials for tissue regeneration [22].

Polycaprolactone (PCL) is a biocompatible, biodegradable synthetic polymer that was approved by the United States Food and Drug Administration (FDA) and is widely used in the fabrication of tissue-engineered substitutes for bone regeneration applications [23,24]. Moreover, PCL has good mechanical properties such as high stiffness and strength, and slow biodegradation time (2–4 years); these properties play key roles in maintaining the appropriate mechanical strength in tissue-engineered bone substitutes fabricated with natural polymers and bioceramics [25–27].

A three-axis plotted scaffold provides a three-dimensional (3D) structural environment to facilitate osteocyte adhesion, migration, and differentiation; these scaffolds are subjects of bone regeneration research [28,29]. In particular, 3D printing is an immerging technology that can be applied to fabricate complex and personalized structures; this technique is highly reproducible, compared with other techniques such as gas foaming, hydrogel usage, and electrospinning [30]. Moreover, organic substances, such as alginate, chitosan, gelatin, and collagen, and inorganic substances, such as HA, tricalcium phosphate, and whitlockite are widely used to fabricate bone regenerative scaffolds using 3D printing technology [5,31,32]. Therefore, 3D-printed scaffolds offer benefits for patient treatment through personalization.

In this study, we fabricated a composite 3D-printed scaffold using PCL and carbonated HA (CHA), and enhanced the biological properties using a coating of marine atelocollagen (MC). MC and CHA were extracted from the skin and bones, respectively, which are byproducts of *P. olivaceus*. Sodium dodecyl sulfate-polyacrylamide gel electrophoresis (SDS-PAGE), Fourier transform infrared (FTIR) spectroscopy, and amino acid composition analyses were used to evaluate the characteristics of MC, and FTIR spectroscopy, X-ray diffraction (XRD) analysis, and energy dispersive spectroscopy (EDS) were performed to evaluate the characteristics of CHA. The fabricated CHA/MC/PCL scaffolds were then analyzed to determine their potential for facilitating osteogenic differentiation and bone tissue regeneration through in vitro and in vivo investigations.

## 2. Results

### 2.1. Extraction and Characterization of MC

One simple method to identify collagen is to scan collagen samples on a UV spectrum (200–400 nm), because the triple helical structure of collagen has absorption at 230 nm. As shown in Figure 1A, commercial atelocollagen and MC have a maximum absorption peak at 230 nm, which is associated with $COO^-$, $CONH_2$, and C=O groups in the polypeptides of collagen. Collagen has a few tryptophan, histidine, tyrosine, and phenylalanine components that absorb UV at 250 nm and 280 nm.

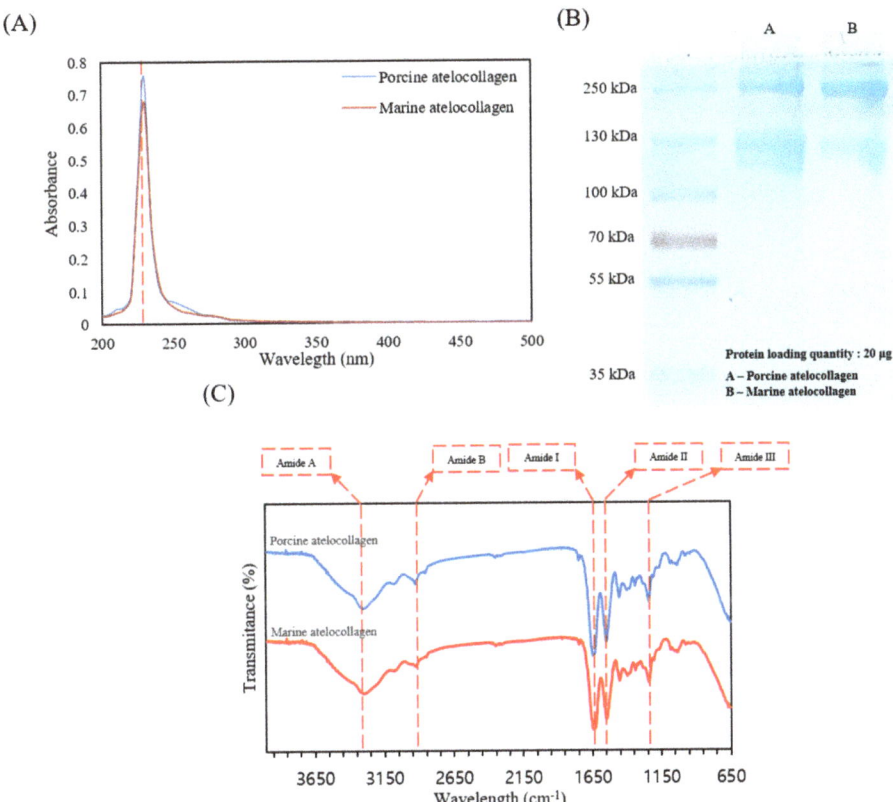

**Figure 1.** Characterization of collagen extracted from skins of *P. olivaceus* and of porcine commercial atelocollagen. (**A**) UV-Vis spectra of the two types of collagen; (**B**) Sodium dodecyl sulfate-polyacrylamide electrophoresis evidences the molecular structure and organization of two collagen; (**C**) Fourier transform infrared spectra of collagens exhibits the main vibrations of collagen molecular organization.

Figure 1B represents the SDS-PAGE components of commercial atelocollagen and MC. Commercial atelocollagen and MC both consist of $\alpha_1$ and $\alpha_2$ chains and high molecular weight β and γ components. Thus, the extracted commercial atelocollagen and MC correspond to type I collagen.

The FTIR spectra of commercial atelocollagen and MC from the skins of *P. olivaceus*, which can be used to identify information on the secondary structure of collagen, are shown in Figure 1C. The changes in the spectral peaks were shown to include changes in the amide A and B bands as well as the amide I–III regions. The amide A band at 3300 cm$^{-1}$ and the amide B band peaks at 2972 cm$^{-1}$ are associated with N–H stretching vibrations and the asymmetrical stretching of $CH_2$. In addition, the amide I peak at 1635 cm$^{-1}$ is mainly associated with the stretching vibrations of C=O, along with the polypeptide backbone or COO$^-$. The amide II region of collagen type I appears at approximately 1549 cm$^{-1}$ from N–H bending vibration coupled with C=N stretching vibrations. The amide III region at 1239 cm$^{-1}$ represents the peaks between C=N stretching vibrations and N–H deformation from amide linkages of $CH_2$ groups of the glycine backbone and proline side-chain. As shown in Figure 1C, the intensity and positions of the amide A, B, and I–III bands are similar for the commercial atelocollagen and MC, as well as type I collagen.

## 2.2. Amino Acid Components

Table 1 shows the amino acid components of commercial atelocollagen and MC from *P. olivaceus*. Commercial atelocollagen and MC were found to have glycine (238.3 and 247.3 per 1000, respectively) and to be low in tyrosine, histidine, methionine, and cysteine. The imino acid content of the extracted collagen was 264.3 and 208.6 per 1000 for porcine atelocollagen and marine atelocollagen, respectively. Based on these differences, the mechanical properties of MC are weaker than commercial collagen. Collagen with a greater imino acid content is more stable in the helix structure, due to the contents of proline and hydroxyproline.

**Table 1.** Amino acid composition of atelocollagen obtained from the skins of *P. olivaceus* and of porcine commercial atelocollagen (per 1000 residues).

| Amino Acid | Porcine Atelocollagen | Marine Atelocollagen |
|---|---|---|
| Asp | 53.6 | 56.2 |
| Thr | 17.9 | 27.4 |
| Ser | 33.1 | 44.8 |
| Glu | 96.0 | 95.6 |
| Gly | 238.3 | 247.3 |
| Ala | 91.0 | 108.2 |
| Cys | 1.6 | 2.0 |
| Val | 18.3 | 16.6 |
| Met | 5.7 | 11.0 |
| Iie | 9.4 | 6.9 |
| Leu | 28.8 | 23.7 |
| Tyr | 1.2 | 2.1 |
| Phe | 18.4 | 20.5 |
| Lys | 35.9 | 36.9 |
| His | 6.4 | 7.3 |
| Arg | 80.0 | 84.8 |
| Hypro | 126.0 | 96.9 |
| Pro | 138.3 | 111.7 |
| Total | 1000.0 | 1000.0 |

## 2.3. Extraction and Characterization of CHA

The FTIR spectra of raw fishbones and HA and CHA from the bones of *P. olivaceus* are shown in Figure 2A. The FTIR bands of raw fishbones were observed at 1047 cm$^{-1}$, 1644–1740 cm$^{-1}$, 2911 cm$^{-1}$, and 2977 cm$^{-1}$; these bands are both minerals and organic compound of fishbones. HA has bands at 878 cm$^{-1}$, 1000–1100 cm$^{-1}$, 1400–1500 cm$^{-1}$, 3447 cm$^{-1}$, and 3571 cm$^{-1}$. The strongest band from 1000–1100 cm$^{-1}$ is the stretching of $PO_4^{3-}$ vibrations. The band at approximately 1400–1500 cm$^{-1}$ corresponds to the carbonate group of HA and CHA. The band of OH stretching of HA appears from 1000–1100 cm$^{-1}$. CHA also shows all of the bands of $PO_4^{3-}$, $CO_3^{2-}$, and OH, and because CHA was extracted by alkaline lysis, the band of $CO_3^{2-}$ for CHA is more prominent than that for HA (Figure 2A).

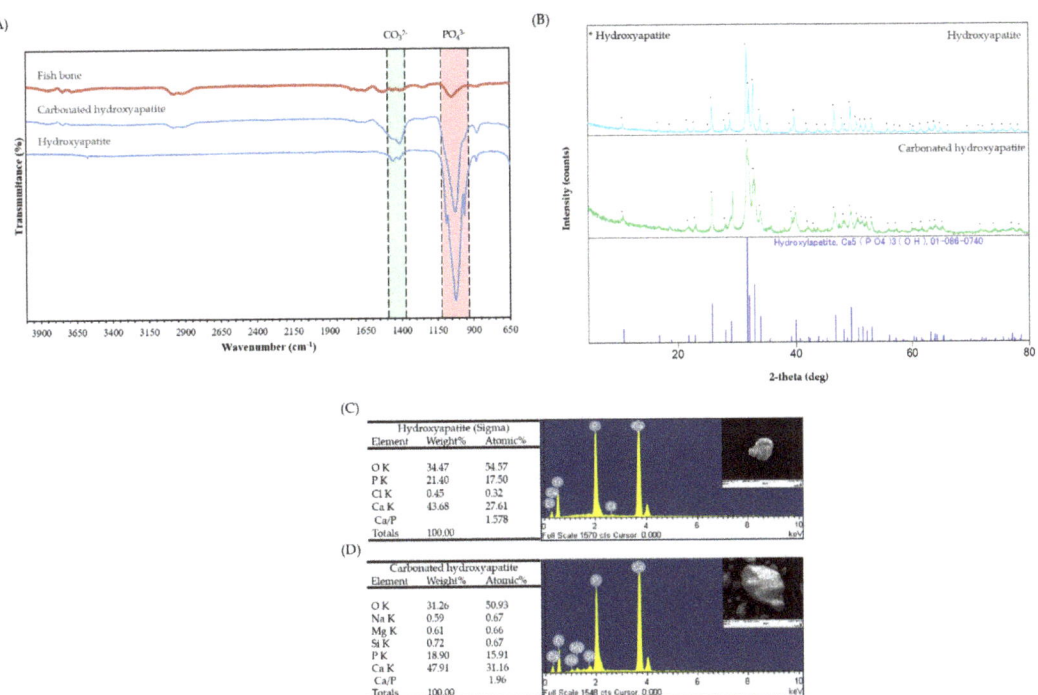

**Figure 2.** Characterization of hydroxyapatite isolated from frame of *Paralichthys olivaceus* and sigma. (**A**) Fourier transform infrared spectra of HA and CHA; (**B**) X-ray diffraction spectra of HA and CHA. The energy dispersive spectrometer of (**C**) HA and (**D**) CHA.

XRD analysis is a reliable method for investigating the phase purity and crystallinity of a compound and determining the quantitative and qualitative aspects of a solid compound. Results of XRD are mainly evaluated through comparison with the International Center for Diffraction Data (ICDD) standards. The crystallinity and purity of HA and CHA were defined by XRD analysis. The XRD peaks of the standard and the HA and CHA from the bones of *P. olivaceus* are shown in Figure 2B. The obtained peaks of HA and CHA at 2-theta were identical to 01-086-0740 from the ICDD. The peaks of HA and CHA matched with those of the standard ICDD 01-086-0740 (Hydroxyapatite; $Ca_5(PO_4)_3OH$) (Figure 2B).

### 2.4. Energy Dispersive Spectrometer (EDS)

Figure 2C,D displays the EDS data that confirm the content of C, O, Na, Mg, Cl, P, and Ca in the powder. The ratio of Ca/P for the HA powder was 1.578, and that for the CHA powder was 1.96. These results show that CHA has carbonate groups, because it was extracted by alkaline hydrolysis.

### 2.5. Characterization of the CHA-Reinforced Scaffolds

The mean strut diameter of the CHA-reinforced scaffolds was controlled by adjusting the extruding temperature, nozzle diameter, and speed of the extruder. Based on SEM observations, the strut diameters of PCL, 2.5% CHA/PCL, 5% CHA/PCL, 10% CHA/PCL, 10% HA/PCL, MC/PCL, 2.5% CHA/MC/PCL, 5% CHA/MC/PCL, 10% CHA/MC/PCL, and 10% HA/MC/PCL scaffolds were 518.54 ± 5.72 µm, 607.27 ± 3.34 µm, 571.37 ± 16.43 µm,

561.03 ± 16.5 µm, 484.57 ± 19.68 µm, 508.17 ± 11.62 µm, 599.42 ± 2.94 µm, 526.28 ± 15.34 µm, 539.12 ± 15.34 µm, and 466.67 ± 16.04 µm, respectively. For these results, the strut diameter and pore size of the CHA-reinforced scaffolds were fabricated under the same conditions, but slight differences were observed between the scaffolds (Figure 3A, Table 2).

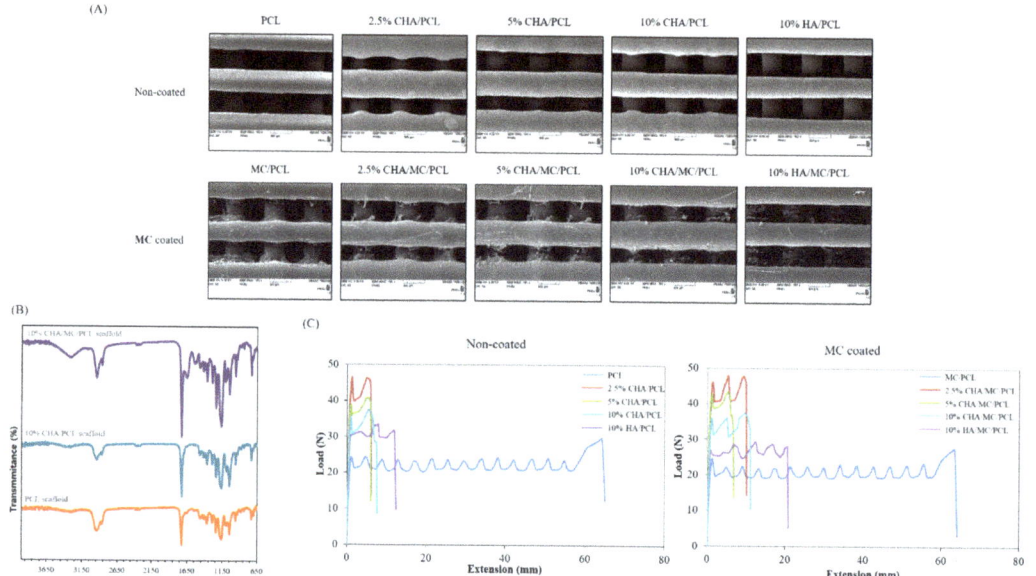

**Figure 3.** Morphology and characterization of the CHA-reinforced scaffolds. (**A**) SEM image of non-coated group and MC coated group; (**B**) FTIR analysis of non-coated group and MC coated group; (**C**) load-extension curve of non-coated group and MC coated group.

**Table 2.** Strut diameter and elastic modulus of CHA-reinforced scaffolds.

| Scaffolds | Strut Diameter (µm) | Elastic Modulus (MPa) |
|---|---|---|
| PCL | 518.54 ± 5.72 | 6.29 ± 0.28 |
| 2.5% CHA/PCL | 607.27 ± 3.34 | 10.19 ± 0.01 |
| 5% CHA/PCL | 571.37 ± 16.43 | 9.26 ± 0.33 |
| 10% CHA/PCL | 561.03 ± 16.5 | 6.85 ± 0.55 |
| 10% HA/PCL | 484.57 ± 19.68 | 7.76 ± 0.37 |
| MC/PCL | 508.17 ± 11.62 | 6.37 ± 0.16 |
| 2.5% CHA/MC/PCL | 599.42 ± 2.94 | 9.38 ± 0.45 |
| 5% CHA/MC/PCL | 526.28 ± 15.34 | 9.1 ± 0.12 |
| 10% CHA/MC/PCL | 539.12 ± 15.34 | 7.08 ± 0.52 |
| 10% HA/MC/PCL | 466.67 ± 16.04 | 7.77 ± 0.42 |

The FTIR spectra of the CHA-reinforced scaffolds were in the spectral range of 4000–650 cm$^{-1}$. The FTIR spectrum of the PCL scaffold was observed at 2860 cm$^{-1}$ (C-H) and 1720 cm$^{-1}$ (C=O) stretching peaks, and the FTIR spectrum of the 10% CHA/PCL scaffold was observed at the same peaks. For the 10% CHA/MC/PCL scaffold, in addition to the peaks of the PCL scaffold, the amide peaks (amide A, B, I–III) of MC were also identified (Figure 3B).

The mechanical properties of the CHA-reinforced scaffolds were evaluated using tensile mechanical testing in a universal testing machine. As shown in Figure 3C, the elastic modulus values of PCL, 2.5% CHA/PCL, 5% CHA/PCL, 10% CHA/PCL, 10% HA/PCL, MC/PCL, 2.5% CHA/MC/PCL, 5% CHA/MC/PCL, 10% CHA/MC/PCL, and

10% HA/MC/PCL scaffolds were 6.29 ± 0.28 MPa, 10.19 ± 0.01 MPa, 9.26 ± 0.33 MPa, 6.85 ± 0.55 MPa, 7.76 ± 0.37 MPa, 6.37 ± 0.16 MPa, 9.38 ± 0.45 MPa, 9.1 ± 0.12 MPa, 7.08 ± 0.52 MPa, and 7.77 ± 0.42 MPa, respectively. The elastic modulus value tended to increase in the scaffolds containing CHA and HA, compared with that of PCL; furthermore, the elastic modulus value decreased as the content of CHA and HA increased. These results may be due to the diameter of the strut and the size of CHA and HA (Figure 3C, Table 2).

### 2.6. Cell Viability on the CHA-Reinforced Scaffolds

Cytotoxicity to the CHA-reinforced scaffolds was evaluated using a cell live/dead assay 7 days after cell seeding on the scaffolds. At 7 days after cell seeding, the contents of the CHA and HA did not affect cytotoxicity and cell distribution. In addition, on the 7th day, the presence of an MC coating on the CHA-reinforced scaffold did not affect the cell distribution. However, the detection amount of PI in the MC-coated scaffolds was lower than that of the MC-uncoated scaffolds (Figure 4A). As a result of the cell viability for 3, 5, and 7 days, it was possible to confirm a larger number of living cells in the MC-coated scaffold group.

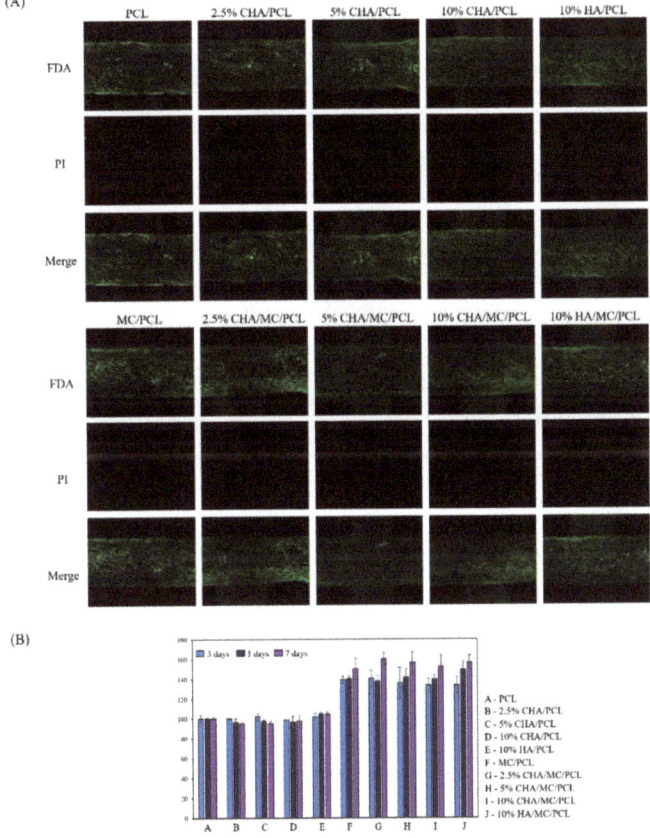

**Figure 4.** Cell viability of non-coated and MC-coated scaffolds on MC3T3-E1. (**A**) cell fluorescence image stained FDA/PI; and (**B**) cell viability for 3, 5, and 7 days.

### 2.7. Alkaline Phosphatase Activity of the CHA-Reinforced Scaffolds

The ALP activities of PCL, 2.5% CHA/PCL, 5% CHA/PCL, 10% CHA/PCL, 10% HA/PCL, MC/PCL, 2.5% CHA/MC/PCL, 5% CHA/MC/PCL, 10% CHA/MC/PCL, and

10% HA/MC/PCL scaffolds were 100 ± 5.08, 104.63 ± 4.91, 110.78 ± 3.28, 100.59 ± 1.27, 111.31 ± 1.81, 152.20 ± 5.09, 154.74 ± 2.59, 153.75 ± 3.26, 152.50 ± 2.62, and 153.05 ± 2.38, respectively. These results confirm that the ALP activity was increased in the MC-coated group on the scaffold (Figure 5A).

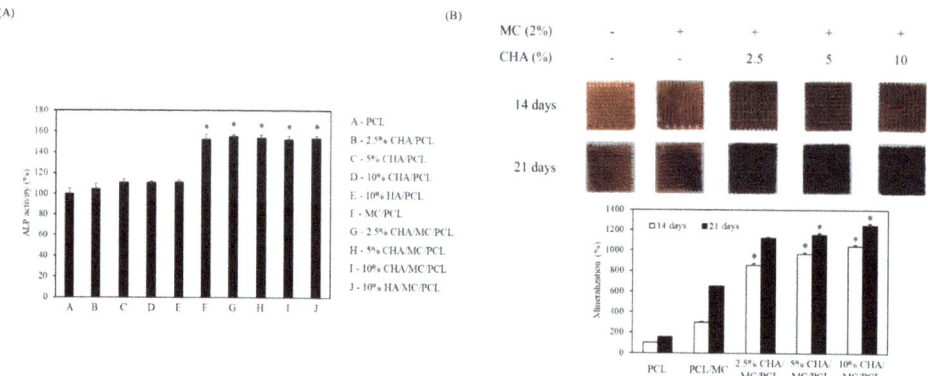

Figure 5. In vitro effect of scaffolds on (A) ALP activity and (B) mineralization activity during osteogenic differentiation of MC3T3-E1 cells. * $p < 0.05$ was considered to indicate a statistically significant difference compared with non-coated scaffolds.

### 2.8. Mineralization of the CHA-Reinforced Scaffolds

The PCL, MC/PCL, 2.5% CHA/MC/PCL, 5% CHA/MC/PCL, and 10% CHA/MC/PCL scaffolds were stained with Alizarin Red S stain, and calcium deposition on the scaffolds was observed. Along with the increasing concentration of CHA, the scaffolds created calcium in a dose-dependent manner. At 21 days, the 10% CHA/MC/PCL scaffold showed eight times more mineralization than the PCL scaffold (Figure 5B).

### 2.9. In Vivo Experiments

To confirm the bone regeneration ability of the scaffolds, the PCL, 10% CHA/MC/PCL, and 10% HA/MC/PCL scaffolds were implanted into a defect in the mouse calvarial defect model.

In the defect site, a difference in bone regeneration was confirmed by micro-CT between the non-treatment, PCL, CHA, and HA reinforced scaffolds. Twenty weeks after surgery, the area of the bone defect was determined by micro-CT. The 10% CHA/MC/PCL and 10% HA/MC/PCL scaffolds showed better regeneration, due to the synergistic effects of their 3D structure with CHA and MC for promoting bone regeneration, than the non-treatment group. Further investigation of the 3D reconstruction was conducted by analyzing the bone defect areas. This analysis showed that the bone volume of the 10% CHA/MC/PCL and 10% HA/MC/PCL scaffold groups have a greater quantity of bone volume regenerated than those of the non-treatment group (Figure 6A).

Histological analysis was performed with hematoxylin and eosin (HE), picrosirius red, and Masson's trichrome (MT) staining of the bone defect area. At low magnification, the new bone and host bone were separated to define a 3-mm bone defect. Although the bone defect did not completely regenerate, the CHA- and HA-reinforced scaffold groups showed better regeneration than the non-treatment and PCL scaffold groups. As shown in the HE and MT staining images (Figure 6B), both CHA- and HA-reinforced scaffold groups formed regenerative tissue around the scaffolds. In addition, picrosirius red staining confirmed that the collagen formation around the scaffold was improved.

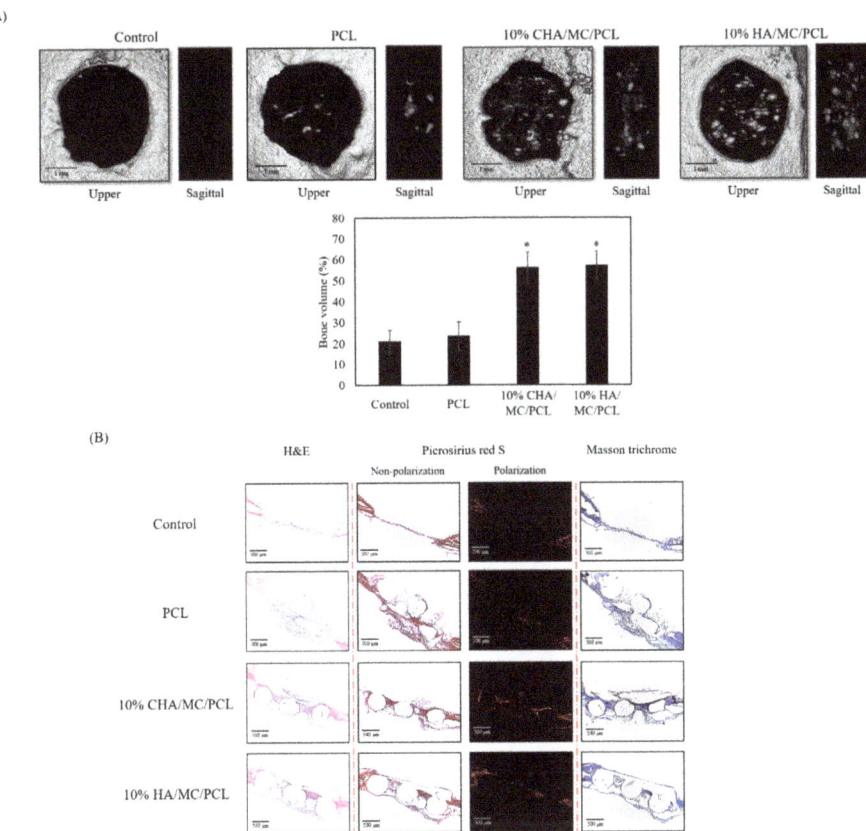

**Figure 6.** In vivo performance evaluation. (**A**) 3D reconstruction images of bone defect areas and (**B**) histological analysis of the effect of scaffolds on bone regeneration in vivo. Note: "S" represents scaffold; "black arrow" indicates new bone; "white arrow" indicates new type I collage. * $p < 0.05$ was considered to indicate a statistically significant difference compared with PCL group.

## 3. Discussion

The increasing global demand for fish has caused an increase in fish byproducts, such as fish scales, bones, and skins. Studying these byproducts as biomaterials can reduce the number of fish byproducts and increase their value [33]. Although not conducted in this study, it is necessary to study the selection of materials suitable for tissue engineering by comparing the characteristics of the collagen derived from terrestrial organisms and the collagen derived from marine organisms. In the present study, we isolated and characterized MC and CHA from *P. olivaceus* using pepsin hydrolysis and alkaline hydrolysis, respectively [34]. Numerous studies have reported about HA and collagen extracted and isolated from different fish species, such as *Oncorhynchus keta*, *Thunnus obesus*, and *Oreochromis* [35–37]. Unlike thermally extracted HA, HA extracted through alkaline hydrolysis retains its carbonate groups, because carbonate cannot be separated without heat treatment [36]. Furthermore, CHA was reported to have a similar chemical composition to that of HA present in natural bone tissue [38]. According to previous studies, the HA derived from fish bones shows improved biocompatibility and osteogenic differentiation activity, and enhanced potential for bone formation on scaffolds fabricated with HA. Thus, CHA is a potential biomaterial that can be employed with various synthetic or natural polymers to fabricate tissue-engineered bone substitutes for bone tissue regeneration applications [39].

XRD, FTIR spectroscopy, and EDS analyses of isolated CHA and commercially available HA were performed to compare and determine the crystallinity, chemical composition, and atomic percentage, respectively. The XRD analysis of CHA showed the same peak international standard as HA (ICDD 01-086-0740) at 002, 211, 112, 202, 310, 222, 213, 321, and 004 of Bragg's reflection in the standard [35]. In addition, the results of both FTIR spectroscopy and EDS clearly indicated that the isolated CHA has a carbonate group attached to the HA unit, as shown in Figures 2A and 3. In Figure 2A, a larger band value of CHA was confirmed at 1400–1500 cm$^{-1}$, which appears to be because the carbonate group increased [40]. The relatively large value of these two bands (1400–1500 cm$^{-1}$) is because CHA has a relatively higher carbonate group than HA. EDS analysis was performed to evaluate the presence of trace elements, such as Ca and P, belonging to the isolated CHA and commercial HA, and the results showed a Ca/P weight ratio of 1.96 and 1.578 for CHA and HA, respectively (Figure 3), indicating that the extraction process (alkaline hydrolysis) of CHA has affected the Ca/P ratio. However, according to previous studies, the Ca/P ratios of both CHA and HA are not significantly different, and they were within the accepted range for hydroxyapatite [39].

Collagen was extensively used to fabricate various tissue regenerative substitutes, because it is one of the main components of the ECM and is an excellent biomaterial that provides exceptional biological and functional properties, without an associated inflammatory response or cytotoxicity [21]. In particular, MC is an alternative and attractive type of collagen over land animal-derived collagen for tissue engineering applications, since it does not have religious restrictions and is not associated with a risk of disease transmission to humans. Hence, we extracted MC from *P. olivaceus* and characterized it using UV/Vis spectra, SDS-PAGE, FTIR spectroscopy, and amino acid composition analysis. The UV/Vis spectra recorded a relatively low absorption value at approximately 280 nm compared with general proteins, because collagen contains a relatively lesser amount of tyrosine and phenylalanine than general proteins (Figure 1A). Moreover, the SDS-PAGE results showed two distinguishable bands at approximately 130 kDa, corresponding to the α1 and α2 chains, and two bands at 250 kDa and 310 kDa, corresponding to the larger β and γ chains, respectively, suggesting that extracted *P. olivaceus* skin collagen is type I collagen, which is in agreement with the findings of previous studies [21]. The FTIR spectra of the extracted MC showed five characteristic peaks at 3300 cm$^{-1}$, 2972 cm$^{-1}$, 1635 cm$^{-1}$, 1549 cm$^{-1}$, and 1239 cm$^{-1}$, which correspond to amide A, amide B, amide I, amide II, and amide III, respectively, similar to that of commercial collagen and the findings of previous publications [41]. Type I collagen forms a triple-helix structure with 20 different amino acids and is stabilized by its high content of glycine repeated every three residues, proline, and hydroxyproline. Moreover, proline and hydroxyproline showed lower values in MC, which is in agreement with the findings of previous reports [42]. Overall, the results suggested that MC and CHA were successfully extracted and characterized from *P. olivaceus*.

According to previous reports, various synthetic and natural biocompatible materials were employed to fabricate 3D-printed scaffolds and demonstrated good bone tissue regeneration effects. Among them, many researchers have focused on improving biological activities including cell adhesion, proliferation, migration, and differentiation through surface modifications including surface coating with natural or chemically modified biocompatible materials [43]. In the present study, we fabricated a 3D-printed porous PCL scaffold reinforced with CHA and surface-coated with MC to enhance osteogenic differentiation. To evaluate the osteogenic activity of the fabricated scaffolds, MC3T3-E1 cell-seeded scaffolds were analyzed, using ALP assay and Alizarin Red S staining. According to the results, the CHA/MC/PCL scaffolds significantly enhanced the mineral deposition through differentiation of MC3T3-E1 pre-osteoblasts to osteoblasts compared with the pure PCL scaffold, indicating that MC and CHA have excellent osteogenic activities and excellent synergetic effects on bone tissue regeneration. Moreover, the bone tissue regeneration effects of the fabricated scaffolds were evaluated using an in vivo calvarial defect mouse model. Micro-CT and histological analysis indicated that the 10% CHA/MC/PCL- and 10%

HA/MC/PCL-treated groups had prominent bone tissue reconstruction effects, compared with the non-treatment and PCL-treated groups (Figure 6). Overall, these results suggest that materials obtained from marine byproducts have considerable potential for bone tissue regeneration and are attractive alternatives for terrestrial or synthetic materials. Based on this study, the possibility was evaluated of MC- and CHA-derived byproducts from *P. olivaceus* used as a substitute material for bone tissue. Furthermore, we will proceed with research on bone mimic scaffold containing MC and CHA. 4.

## 4. Materials and Methods

### 4.1. Materials

The by-product from *P. olivaceus* was provided by EUNHA Marine Co., Ltd. (Busan, Korea). The α-minimum Eagle's medium (α-MEM), fetal bovine serum (FBS), trypsin (250 U/mg), penicillin/streptomycin, and other materials used in cell culture experiments were purchased from GIBCO™ (Gaithersburg, MD, USA). Polycaprolactone (PCL), 1-Step p-nitrophenyl phosphate (pNPP), and Alizarin Red S were purchased from Sigma-Aldrich (St. Louis, MO, USA). The other chemical reagents and materials that were used were commercially available and analytical grade.

### 4.2. Extraction and Characterization of Pepsin Soluble MC

#### 4.2.1. Extraction of Pepsin Soluble MC

*P. olivaceus* skin was descaled and desalted by washing with cold water at 4 °C for one day and cut into small pieces. Pepsin-soluble MC was extracted from the prepared skin, following the method described by [44] with slight modifications. All steps of the procedure were carried out at 4 °C with gentle stirring. Non-collagenous proteins were removed with 0.1 M NaOH at small pieces to a solution ratio of 1:10 (w/v) for 2 days. The skins were then washed with ultrapure water until they became a neutral pH. The skins were defatted with acetone with a pieces to solution ratio of 1:10 (w/v) for 2 days with a changing to new acetone solution every 12 h, and then thoroughly washed with ultrapure water. Then the skins were suspended in 0.5 M acetic acid with a pieces to solution ratio of 1:20 (w/v) for 1 day. After pretreatment, the fish skin was hydrolyzed by pepsin to extract collagen. The skin was dissolved in 0.5 M acetic acid with pepsin (pepsin 1:3000, Sigma, St. Louis, MO, USA) for 24 h at 4 °C, then centrifuged at 15,000 rpm for 30 min. The supernatant was salted out by adding NaCl until a final concentration of 0.9 M. The resultant precipitate was collected by centrifugation at 15,000 rpm for 1 h and then dissolved in 0.5 M acetic acid. The solution was then dialyzed against 0.1 M acetic acid for 1 day and ultrapure water for 3 days. The resultant dialysate was lyophilized and was referred to as MC (Figure 7).

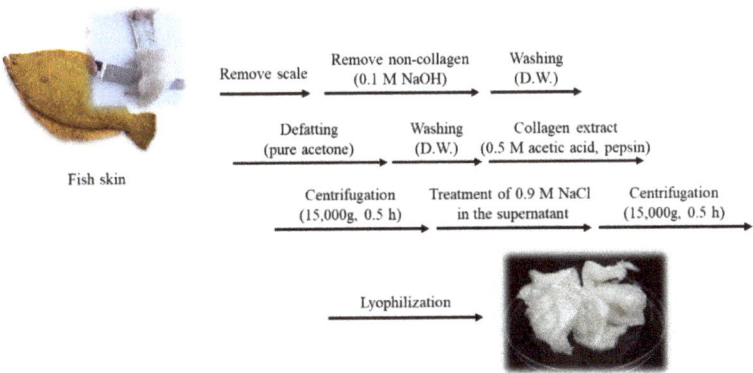

**Figure 7.** MC extraction methods from *P. olivaceus* (pepsin hydrolysis).

### 4.2.2. Sodium Dodecyl Sulfate Polyacrylamide-Gel Electrophoresis (SDS-PAGE)

SDS-PAGE was performed, following the method of [45] with slight modifications, using 7.5% separating and 5% stacking gel. The collagen samples were dissolved in the sample buffer and the obtained mixture (1 mg/mL) was heated at 100 °C for 5 min. The mixture was centrifuged at 4000 rpm for 5 min using a microcentrifuge at room temperature to remove debris. A total of 20 µg of the sample was loaded onto a polyacrylamide gel and subjected to electrophoresis at a constant voltage (100 V) for 1 h using MiniProtein II unit (Bio-Rad Laboratories, Inc. Richmond, CA, USA). The resultant gel was stained with 0.1% (w/v) Coomassie blue R-250 in 50% (v/v) methanol and 10% (v/v) acetic acid for 2 h and destained with 40% (v/v) methanol and 10% (v/v) acetic acid. High molecular weight markers were loaded alongside the collagen to estimate the molecular weight of MC, and commercial atelocollagen (Atelocollagen, Dalim Tissen, Korea) was loaded next to the protein marker as standard collagen.

### 4.2.3. UV Absorbance Analysis

The UV absorption spectra of MC from the skin of *P. olivaceus* were studied, following the method reported elsewhere with slight modifications [46]. The MC and commercial atelocollagen samples (1 mg) were dissolved in 1 mL of 0.5 M acetic acid and the collagen solutions were centrifuged at 15,000 rpm for 10 min at 4 °C. The collagen solution was placed in a quartz cell with a path length of 1 mm. The collagen solutions were subjected to absorbance at wavelengths between 200 and 500 nm at a scan speed of 2 nm per second with an interval of 1 nm. All spectra were obtained using a UV–visible spectrometer (Epoch 2 Microplate reader, Biotek, Winooski, VT, USA).

### 4.2.4. Amino Acid Contents

Amino acid compositions were analyzed using an automatic analyzer (Hitachi Model 835-50, Tokyo, Japan) with a C18 column (5 µm, 4.6 × 250 nm, Watchers, MA, USA). The reaction was carried out at 38 °C, with the detection wavelength at 254 nm and flow rate of 1.0 mL/min. All chemical analyses (from each tank) were carried out in triplicate.

### *4.3. Isolation and Characterization of Carbonated Hydroxyapatite*

#### 4.3.1. Isolation of Carbonated Hydroxyapatite from *P. Olivaceus*

*P. olivaceus* bones were cut into small pieces using a bladed cutter. The bone pieces were boiled in 100 °C purified water for 1 h to remove unnecessary parts. Then, the bone pieces were boiled in 10 mL of acetone and 2% NaOH for 1 h, and the water was completely removed at 100 °C. The dried bone pieces were crushed using a homogenizer. CHA was extracted by boiling the crushed bone pieces for 1 h in 200 °C 2 M NaOH to completely remove the organic materials. Collected CHA was washed with purified water to adjust the pH to neutrality and to remove all of the moisture from the dry oven (Figure 8).

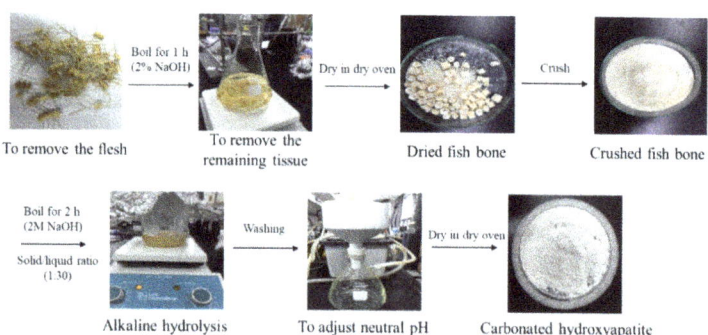

**Figure 8.** CHA extraction methods from *P. olivaceus* (Alkaline hydrolysis).

### 4.3.2. Fourier Transform Infrared (FTIR) Spectroscopy

FTIR spectroscopy (Perkin Elmer, Waltham, MA, USA) data were collected from raw fishbones, CHA, HA, MC, and commercial atelocollagen to determine the functional groups of hydroxyapatite and collagen. The IR spectra represent the average of 30 scans between 500 cm$^{-1}$ and 4000 cm$^{-1}$, at a resolution of 4 cm$^{-1}$.

### 4.3.3. X-ray Diffraction (XRD) Analysis

XRD analysis was conducted on the fishbones, HA and CHA using an Ultima IV system (Rigaku Co., Tokyo, Japan) with Cu-K$\alpha$ radiation. The X-ray diffraction intensities were recorded within the range of 5 to 80°, at a scanning rate of 2° min$^{-1}$.

## 4.4. Fabrication and Characterization of 3D Scaffolds

In this study, we used a computer-controlled three-axis robot system (EZ-ROBO-5GX ST2520, Iwashita Engineering Inc., Fukuoka, Japan), supplemented with a dispenser to fabricate the PCL, HA/PCL, and CHA/PCL structure. The PCL struts were melted at 100 °C in a heating barrel and were extruded through a heated 21G nozzle at a constant pressure (500 ± 25 kPa). Following this condition, the PCL struts were built in a layer-by-layer manner to make a 3D structure with uniform height and porosity. After fabricating the multilayered structure, the fabricated scaffold was sterilized in 70% EtOH. After fabricating the PCL, the HA/PCL and CHA/PCL scaffolds were coated with MC on the surface through 1-ethyl-(3-3-dimethylaminopropyl) carbodiimide hydrochloride (EDC) coupling reaction (Figure 9).

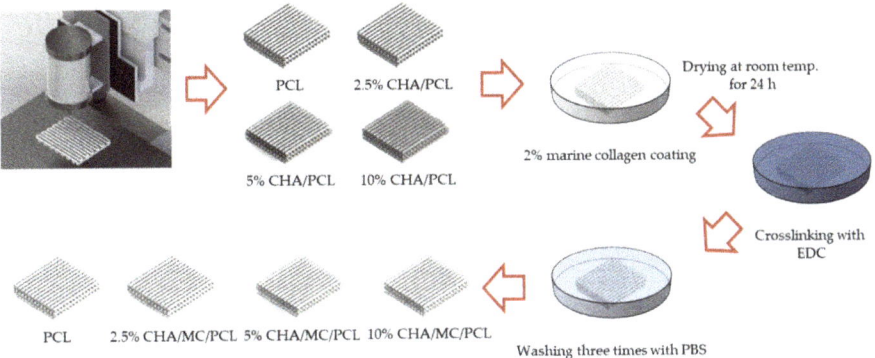

**Figure 9.** Schematic diagram of CHA-reinforced PCL scaffold and coated collagen.

### 4.4.1. Scanning Electron Microscope (SEM) Analysis

The structural morphologies of PCL, 2.5% CHA/PCL, 5% CHA/PCL, 10% CHA/PCL, 10% HA/PCL, MC/PCL, 2.5% CHA/MC/PCL, 5% CHA/MC/PCL, 10% CHA/MC/PCL, and 10% HA/MC/PCL scaffolds were examined using a field emission scanning electron microscope (SEM, Tescan, Czech, VEGA II LSU) at 15 kV. The diameter of the 3D scaffolds was measured from the SEM image using image analysis software (Image J, National Institutes of Health, Bethesda, MD, USA).

### 4.4.2. Tensile Properties

The tensile properties of PCL, 2.5% CHA/PCL, 5% CHA/PCL, 10% CHA/PCL, 10% HA/PCL, MC/PCL, 2.5% CHA/MC/PCL, 5% CHA/MC/PCL, 10% CHA/MC/PCL, and 10% HA/MC/PCL scaffold (2.5 × 2.5 mm$^2$) were measured using a universal tensile machine (Top-tech 2000, Chemilab, Kimpo, Korea). The PCL scaffolds were mounted and subjected to a crosshead speed of 0.2 mm/s at room temperature until failure. The elastic modulus was investigated by the average of three runs for each scaffold.

## 4.5. In Vitro Study on Fabricated Scaffolds

### 4.5.1. Cell Culture and Cell Viability

The MC3T3-E1 subclone 4 cells were purchased from the American Type of Culture Collection (Rockville, MD, USA). The MC3T3-E1 cells were cultured in α-MEM without ascorbic acid, supplemented with 10% fetal bovine serum (FBS), 100 μg/mL streptomycin, and 100 U/mL penicillin. The MC3T3-E1 cells were incubated in 5% $CO_2$ humidified atmosphere and at 37 °C and sub-cultured every 2–3 days.

The MC3T3-E1 cells were seeded onto the scaffolds by dropping them onto scaffolds at a density of $1 \times 10^5$ per scaffold. Before the cells were seeded, the scaffolds were sterilized with 70% ethyl alcohol (EtOH) and UV light.

The cell viability and distribution of the MC3T3-E1 pre-osteoblasts cultured on the CHA-reinforced scaffolds were determined by Cell Counting Kit-8 (CCK-8) assay (Dojindo, Kumamoto, Japan) and live/dead fluorescence staining. Cell viability at 3, 5, and 7 days via CCK-8 assay was evaluated, according to the manufacturer's protocol. A total of 10 μL of CCK-8 solution along with 100 μL of α-MEM were added to each well; the mixture was incubated at 37 °C. for 2 h. The cell viability was evaluated at 450 nm by using a microplate reader (Biotek, Winooski, VT, USA). The cell viability was evaluated using a fluorescence microscope through the Live/Dead assay. After 7 days, the MC3T3-E1 seeded on the CHA-reinforced scaffolds were stained with fluorescein diacetate (8 μg/mL) and propidium iodide (20 μg/mL) for 15 min at room temperature after washing three times with PBS. The stained MC3T3-E1 on the scaffolds were qualitatively examined under a fluorescence microscope (Axio Observer A1, Zeiss, Jena, Germany).

### 4.5.2. ALP Activity and Mineralization Analysis on 3D Scaffolds

MC3T3-E1 cells were cultured in α-MEM containing 50 μg/mL ascorbic acid and 10 mM β-glycerophosphate for the osteogenic differentiation. For the incubation, the osteogenic differentiation media was changed every 2 days.

After 7 days, the 1-StepTM PNPP reagent (100 μL) was added to wells and incubated for 30 min. The 2N NaOH solution was added to stop reactions. The absorbance was measured at 405 nm with a microplate reader. Mineralization in the scaffolds was calculated by subtracting the Alizarin Red values, which were stained by the HA and CHA contained in the cell-free scaffolds.

After 14 and 21 days, the MC3T3-E1 cells were fixed with 10% formalin and stained with Alizarin Red S (40 mM). After staining with Alizarin Red S, the Alizarin Red S was removed and washed three times with D.W. The staining was dissolved through cetylpyridinium chloride and the absorbance of the dissolved stain was measured at 550 nm using a microplate reader.

## 4.6. In Vivo Study in Mouse Calvarial Defect Model

The experimental protocol was approved by the Animal Care and Experiment Committee of Pukyong National University and performed following relevant guidelines and regulations for the care and use of laboratory animals. To determine the bone regeneration ability of the containing MHA and MC, Male CrljOri:CD1 (ICR) mice (approximate weight of 35 g) were used as an in vivo bone defect model. The experiment was conducted according to the protocols approved by the Institutional Animal Care and Use Committee. The ICR mice were maintained on a 12 h light/dark cycle in a controlled environment (relative humidity: 40–70%; temperature: 20–24 °C).

### 4.6.1. Mouse Calvarial Defect Model and Implantation of 3D Scaffolds

Anesthesia of ICR mice was performed by intraperitoneal injection of Zoletil 50. After brightening and disinfecting the upper part of the head, the surgical site was vertically incised and the soft tissue was removed to expose the calvarium. Two 3 mm diameter defects created on both side in the exposed calvarium and PCL, 10% HA/MC/PCL, and

10% CHA/MC/PCL scaffolds were implanted into the bone defect site. The non-treated group was used as a control group.

#### 4.6.2. Micro-Computed Tomography Analysis

After the calvarial defect was created, it was implanted with PCL, 10% HA/MC/PCL, and 10% CHA/MC/PCL scaffolds. After 20 weeks of operation, ICR mice were euthanatized and the calvarial specimens were harvested and fixed in 10% formalin for further characterization and analysis. Micro-CT (NFR Polaris-G90, NanoFocusRay Co., Ltd., Korea) was firstly used to detect the defect area with the settings (80 kV, 0.06 mA). The 3D structures of calvarium were reconstructed through Mimic software (Radiant, Poznan, Poland).

#### 4.6.3. Histological Analysis

Calvarial specimens were fixed in 10% formalin for 5 days at room temperature and decalcified in 8% formic acid and 8% hydrochloric acid, frozen in mounting media. The frozen blocks were cut into 5 μm-thick sections across the center of the defect area and stained with HE, picrosirius red, and MT staining to evaluate the bone regeneration.

### 4.7. Statistical Analysis

All quantitative data are presented as means ± standard deviation (SD) with at least three individual experiments that were conducted using fresh reagents. Significant differences among the groups were determined using the unpaired Student's $t$-test. The differences were considered statistically significant at $p < 0.05$.

## 5. Conclusions

In this study, MC and CHA were extracted from *P. olivaceus* byproducts (skin and bone), and a 3D scaffold reinforced with CHA and coated with MC was fabricated to evaluate bone regeneration. First, CHA and MC extracted from the *P. olivaceus* byproducts were analyzed to determine that they had the characteristics of HA and collagen. By fabricating a 3D scaffold, osteogenic differentiation was confirmed using MC3T3-E1 cells, and bone regeneration was confirmed in a mouse calvarial defect model. Micro-CT and histological analysis revealed that the tissue regeneration of the defect site in the 10% HA/MC/PCL and 10% CHA/MC/PCL groups was superior to that in the non-treatment and PCL scaffold groups. These results suggest that marine byproduct-derived materials can be valuable alternatives for land animal-derived materials. Based on the results, further study is needed to develop bone mimic scaffold with blood vessels, in order to understand bone regenerative mechanism.

**Author Contributions:** Conceptualization and methodology, S.-C.K. and S.-Y.H.; Technical execution, S.-C.K., S.-Y.H. and G.-W.O.; Discussion of results, S.-C.K., M.Y. and W.-K.J.; Writing—Original Draft Preparation, S.-C.K. and S.-Y.H.; Writing—Review and Editing, S.-C.K., M.Y. and W.-K.J.; Funding Acquisition, W.-K.J. All authors have read and agreed to the published version of the manuscript.

**Funding:** This research was supported by the Basic Science Research Program through the National Research Foundation of Korea (NRF) funded by the Ministry of Education (2021R1A6A1A03039211) and NRF grant funded by the Ministry of Science and ICT (2019R1A2C1007218). This research was also supported by Development of technology for biomaterialization of marine fisheries by-products of Korea institute of Marine Scinece & Technology Promotion (KIMST) funded by the Ministry of Oceans and Fisheries (KIMST-20220128).

**Institutional Review Board Statement:** All experimental procedures were approved by the institutional animal care and utilization committee of Pukyong National University (Number PKNUIACUC-2018-07).

**Data Availability Statement:** Not applicable.

**Conflicts of Interest:** The authors declare no conflict of interest.

## References

1. Zhu, L.; Luo, D.; Liu, Y. Effect of the nano/microscale structure of biomaterial scaffolds on bone regeneration. *Int. J. Oral Sci.* **2020**, *12*, 6. [CrossRef] [PubMed]
2. Raghavendra, S.S.; Jadhav, G.R.; Gathani, K.M.; Kotadia, P. Bioceramics in endodontics—A review. *J. Istanb. Univ. Fac. Dent.* **2017**, *51*, S128. [CrossRef]
3. Xu, S.; Wang, Y.; Lu, J.; Xu, J. Osteoprotegerin and RANKL in the pathogenesis of rheumatoid arthritis-induced osteoporosis. *Rheumatol. Int.* **2012**, *32*, 3397–3403. [CrossRef] [PubMed]
4. Berner, A.; Reichert, J.C.; Müller, M.B.; Zellner, J.; Pfeifer, C.; Dienstknecht, T.; Nerlich, M.; Sommerville, S.; Dickinson, I.C.; Schütz, M.A. Treatment of long bone defects and non-unions: From research to clinical practice. *Cell Tissue Res.* **2012**, *347*, 501–519. [CrossRef] [PubMed]
5. Tang, D.; Tare, R.S.; Yang, L.-Y.; Williams, D.F.; Ou, K.-L.; Oreffo, R.O. Biofabrication of bone tissue: Approaches, challenges and translation for bone regeneration. *Biomaterials* **2016**, *83*, 363–382. [CrossRef]
6. Islam, M.T.; Felfel, R.M.; Abou Neel, E.A.; Grant, D.M.; Ahmed, I.; Hossain, K.M.Z. Bioactive calcium phosphate–based glasses and ceramics and their biomedical applications: A review. *J. Tissue Eng.* **2017**, *8*, 2041731417719170. [CrossRef]
7. Hu, Y.-Y.; Rawal, A.; Schmidt-Rohr, K. Strongly bound citrate stabilizes the apatite nanocrystals in bone. *Proc. Natl. Acad. Sci. USA* **2010**, *107*, 22425–22429. [CrossRef]
8. Gomes, D.; Santos, A.; Neves, G.; Menezes, R. A brief review on hydroxyapatite production and use in biomedicine. *Cerâmica* **2019**, *65*, 282–302. [CrossRef]
9. Venkatesan, J.; Qian, Z.J.; Ryu, B.; Thomas, N.V.; Kim, S.K. A comparative study of thermal calcination and an alkaline hydrolysis method in the isolation of hydroxyapatite from Thunnus obesus bone. *Biomed. Mater.* **2011**, *6*, 035003. [CrossRef]
10. Palmer, L.C.; Newcomb, C.J.; Kaltz, S.R.; Spoerke, E.D.; Stupp, S.I. Biomimetic systems for hydroxyapatite mineralization inspired by bone and enamel. *Chem. Rev.* **2008**, *108*, 4754–4783. [CrossRef]
11. Wang, T.; Yang, X.; Qi, X.; Jiang, C. Osteoinduction and proliferation of bone-marrow stromal cells in three-dimensional poly (ε-caprolactone)/hydroxyapatite/collagen scaffolds. *J. Transl. Med.* **2015**, *13*, 152. [CrossRef]
12. Qi, X.; Huang, Y.; Han, D.; Zhang, J.; Cao, J.; Jin, X.; Huang, J.; Li, X.; Wang, T. Three-dimensional poly (ε-caprolactone)/hydroxyapatite scaffolds incorporating bone marrow mesenchymal stem cells for the repair of bone defects. *Biomed. Mater.* **2016**, *11*, 025005. [CrossRef] [PubMed]
13. Shoulders, M.D.; Raines, R.T. Collagen structure and stability. *Annu. Rev. Biochem.* **2009**, *78*, 929–958. [CrossRef] [PubMed]
14. Brinckmann, J. Collagens at a glance. In *Collagen*; Springer: Berlin/Heidelberg, Germany, 2005; pp. 1–6.
15. Boudko, S.P.; Bächinger, H.P. Structural insight for chain selection and stagger control in collagen. *Sci. Rep.* **2016**, *6*, 37831. [CrossRef] [PubMed]
16. Coppola, D.; Oliviero, M.; Vitale, G.A.; Lauritano, C.; D'Ambra, I.; Iannace, S.; de Pascale, D. Marine collagen from alternative and sustainable sources: Extraction, processing and applications. *Mar. Drugs* **2020**, *18*, 214. [CrossRef] [PubMed]
17. Müller, W.E. The origin of metazoan complexity: Porifera as integrated animals. *Integr. Comp. Biol.* **2003**, *43*, 3–10. [CrossRef] [PubMed]
18. Lim, Y.-S.; Ok, Y.-J.; Hwang, S.-Y.; Kwak, J.-Y.; Yoon, S. Marine collagen as a promising biomaterial for biomedical applications. *Mar. Drugs* **2019**, *17*, 467. [CrossRef]
19. Giraud-Guille, M.-M.; Besseau, L.; Chopin, C.; Durand, P.; Herbage, D. Structural aspects of fish skin collagen which forms ordered arrays via liquid crystalline states. *Biomaterials* **2000**, *21*, 899–906. [CrossRef]
20. Nagai, T.; Yamashita, E.; Taniguchi, K.; Kanamori, N.; Suzuki, N. Isolation and characterisation of collagen from the outer skin waste material of cuttlefish (*Sepia lycidas*). *Food Chem.* **2001**, *72*, 425–429. [CrossRef]
21. Chandika, P.; Ko, S.-C.; Oh, G.-W.; Heo, S.-Y.; Nguyen, V.-T.; Jeon, Y.-J.; Lee, B.; Jang, C.H.; Kim, G.; Park, W.S. Fish collagen/alginate/chitooligosaccharides integrated scaffold for skin tissue regeneration application. *Int. J. Biol. Macromol.* **2015**, *81*, 504–513. [CrossRef]
22. Felician, F.F.; Xia, C.; Qi, W.; Xu, H. Collagen from marine biological sources and medical applications. *Chem. Biodivers.* **2018**, *15*, e1700557. [CrossRef] [PubMed]
23. Dwivedi, R.; Kumar, S.; Pandey, R.; Mahajan, A.; Nandana, D.; Katti, D.S.; Mehrotra, D. Polycaprolactone as biomaterial for bone scaffolds: Review of literature. *J. Oral Biol. Craniofacial Res.* **2020**, *10*, 381–388. [CrossRef] [PubMed]
24. Poh, P.S.P.; Hutmacher, D.W.; Holzapfel, B.M.; Solanki, A.K.; Stevens, M.M.; Woodruff, M.A. In vitro and in vivo bone formation potential of surface calcium phosphate-coated polycaprolactone and polycaprolactone/bioactive glass composite scaffolds. *Acta Biomater.* **2016**, *30*, 319–333. [CrossRef]
25. Woodruff, M.A.; Hutmacher, D.W. The return of a forgotten polymer—Polycaprolactone in the 21st century. *Prog. Polym. Sci.* **2010**, *35*, 1217–1256. [CrossRef]
26. Manoukian, O.S.; Sardashti, N.; Stedman, T.; Gailiunas, K.; Ojha, A.; Penalosa, A.; Mancuso, C.; Hobert, M.; Kumbar, S.G. Biomaterials for Tissue Engineering and Regenerative Medicine. In *Encyclopedia of Biomedical Engineering*; Narayan, R., Ed.; Elsevier: Oxford, UK, 2019; pp. 462–482.
27. Cooper, A.; Bhattarai, N.; Zhang, M. Fabrication and cellular compatibility of aligned chitosan–PCL fibers for nerve tissue regeneration. *Carbohydr. Polym.* **2011**, *85*, 149–156. [CrossRef]

28. Schmid, J.; Wallkamm, B.; Hämmerle, C.H.; Gogolewski, S.; Lang, N.P. The significance of angiogenesis in guided bone regeneration. A case report of a rabbit experiment. *Clin. Oral Implant. Res.* **1997**, *8*, 244–248. [CrossRef] [PubMed]
29. Leach, J.K.; Kaigler, D.; Wang, Z.; Krebsbach, P.H.; Mooney, D.J. Coating of VEGF-releasing scaffolds with bioactive glass for angiogenesis and bone regeneration. *Biomaterials* **2006**, *27*, 3249–3255. [PubMed]
30. Heo, S.Y.; Ko, S.C.; Oh, G.W.; Kim, N.; Choi, I.W.; Park, W.S.; Jung, W.K. Fabrication and characterization of the 3D-printed polycaprolactone/fish bone extract scaffolds for bone tissue regeneration. *J. Biomed. Mater. Res. Part B Appl. Biomater.* **2019**, *107*, 1937–1944. [CrossRef]
31. Yan, Y.; Chen, H.; Zhang, H.; Guo, C.; Yang, K.; Chen, K.; Cheng, R.; Qian, N.; Sandler, N.; Zhang, Y.S. Vascularized 3D printed scaffolds for promoting bone regeneration. *Biomaterials* **2019**, *190*, 97–110. [CrossRef]
32. Inzana, J.A.; Olvera, D.; Fuller, S.M.; Kelly, J.P.; Graeve, O.A.; Schwarz, E.M.; Kates, S.L.; Awad, H.A. 3D printing of composite calcium phosphate and collagen scaffolds for bone regeneration. *Biomaterials* **2014**, *35*, 4026–4034. [CrossRef]
33. Coppola, D.; Lauritano, C.; Palma Esposito, F.; Riccio, G.; Rizzo, C.; de Pascale, D. Fish waste: From problem to valuable resource. *Mar. Drugs* **2021**, *19*, 116. [CrossRef] [PubMed]
34. Caruso, G.; Floris, R.; Serangeli, C.; Di Paola, L. Fishery wastes as a yet undiscovered treasure from the sea: Biomolecules sources, extraction methods and valorization. *Mar. Drugs* **2020**, *18*, 622. [CrossRef] [PubMed]
35. Venkatesan, J.; Kim, S.K. Effect of temperature on isolation and characterization of hydroxyapatite from tuna (*Thunnus obesus*) bone. *Materials* **2010**, *3*, 4761–4772. [CrossRef] [PubMed]
36. Venkatesan, J.; Lowe, B.; Manivasagan, P.; Kang, K.-H.; Chalisserry, E.P.; Anil, S.; Kim, D.G.; Kim, S.-K. Isolation and characterization of nano-hydroxyapatite from salmon fish bone. *Materials* **2015**, *8*, 5426–5439. [CrossRef] [PubMed]
37. Zainol, I.; Adenan, N.; Rahim, N.; Jaafar, C.A. Extraction of natural hydroxyapatite from tilapia fish scales using alkaline treatment. *Mater. Today Proc.* **2019**, *16*, 1942–1948. [CrossRef]
38. Landi, E.; Celotti, G.; Logroscino, G.; Tampieri, A. Carbonated hydroxyapatite as bone substitute. *J. Eur. Ceram. Soc.* **2003**, *23*, 2931–2937. [CrossRef]
39. Latif, A.F.A.; Mohd Pu'ad, N.A.S.; Ramli, N.A.A.; Muhamad, M.S.; Abdullah, H.Z.; Idris, M.I.; Lee, T.C. Extraction of Biological Hydroxyapatite from Tuna Fish Bone for Biomedical Applications. In *Materials Science Forum*; Trans Tech Publications Ltd.: Bäch, Switzerland, 2020; pp. 584–589.
40. Ravarian, R.; Moztarzadeh, F.; Hashjin, M.S.; Rabiee, S.; Khoshakhlagh, P.; Tahriri, M. Synthesis, characterization and bioactivity investigation of bioglass/hydroxyapatite composite. *Ceram. Int.* **2010**, *36*, 291–297. [CrossRef]
41. Kozlowska, J.; Sionkowska, A.; Skopinska-Wisniewska, J.; Piechowicz, K. Northern pike (*Esox lucius*) collagen: Extraction, characterization and potential application. *Int. J. Biol. Macromol.* **2015**, *81*, 220–227. [CrossRef]
42. Carvalho, A.M.; Marques, A.P.; Silva, T.H.; Reis, R.L. Evaluation of the potential of collagen from codfish skin as a biomaterial for biomedical applications. *Mar. Drugs* **2018**, *16*, 495. [CrossRef]
43. Martin, V.; Ribeiro, I.A.; Alves, M.M.; Gonçalves, L.; Claudio, R.A.; Grenho, L.; Fernandes, M.H.; Gomes, P.; Santos, C.F.; Bettencourt, A.F. Engineering a multifunctional 3D-printed PLA-collagen-minocycline-nanoHydroxyapatite scaffold with combined antimicrobial and osteogenic effects for bone regeneration. *Mater. Sci. Eng. C* **2019**, *101*, 15–26. [CrossRef]
44. Singh, P.; Benjakul, S.; Maqsood, S.; Kishimura, H. Isolation and characterisation of collagen extracted from the skin of striped catfish (*Pangasianodon hypophthalmus*). *Food Chem.* **2011**, *124*, 97–105. [CrossRef]
45. Laemmli, U.K. Cleavage of structural proteins during the assembly of the head of bacteriophage T4. *Nature* **1970**, *227*, 680–685. [CrossRef] [PubMed]
46. Zhang, F.; Wang, A.; Li, Z.; He, S.; Shao, L. Preparation and characterisation of collagen from freshwater fish scales. *Food Nutr. Sci.* **2011**, *2011*, 818–823. [CrossRef]

# Potential Biomedical Applications of Collagen Filaments derived from the Marine Demosponges *Ircinia oros* (Schmidt, 1864) and *Sarcotragus foetidus* (Schmidt, 1862)

Marina Pozzolini [1,*], Eleonora Tassara [1], Andrea Dodero [2], Maila Castellano [2], Silvia Vicini [2], Sara Ferrando [1], Stefano Aicardi [1], Dario Cavallo [2], Marco Bertolino [1], Iaroslav Petrenko [3], Hermann Ehrlich [3,4] and Marco Giovine [1]

1. Department of Earth, Environment and Life Sciences (DISTAV), University of Genova, Via Pastore 3, 16132 Genova, Italy; eleonora.tassara@edu.unige.it (E.T.); sara.ferrando@unige.it (S.F.); stefano.aicardi94@libero.it (S.A.); marco.bertolino@edu.unige.it (M.B.); mgiovine@unige.it (M.G.)
2. Department of Chemistry and Industrial Chemistry (DCCI), University of Genova, Via Dodecaneso 31, 16146 Genova, Italy; andrea.dodero@edu.unige.it (A.D.); maila@chimica.unige.it (M.C.); silvia.vicini@unige.it (S.V.); Dario.Cavallo@unige.it (D.C.)
3. Institute of Electronic and Sensor Materials, TU Bergakademie Freiberg, 09599 Freiberg, Germany; iaroslavpetrenko@gmail.com (I.P.); Hermann.Ehrlich@esm.tu-freiberg.de (H.E.)
4. Center for Advanced Technology, Adam Mickiewicz University, 61614 Poznan, Poland
* Correspondence: marina.pozzolini@unige.it

**Abstract:** Collagen filaments derived from the two marine demosponges *Ircinia oros* and *Sarcotragus foetidus* were for the first time isolated, biochemically characterised and tested for their potential use in regenerative medicine. SDS-PAGE of isolated filaments revealed a main collagen subunit band of 130 kDa in both of the samples under study. DSC analysis on 2D membranes produced with collagenous sponge filaments showed higher thermal stability than commercial mammalian-derived collagen membranes. Dynamic mechanical and thermal analysis attested that the membranes obtained from filaments of *S. foetidus* were more resistant and stable at the rising temperature, compared to the ones derived from filaments of *I. oros*. Moreover, the former has higher stability in saline and in collagenase solutions and evident antioxidant activity. Conversely, their water binding capacity results were lower than that of membranes obtained from *I. oros*. Adhesion and proliferation tests using L929 fibroblasts and HaCaT keratinocytes resulted in a remarkable biocompatibility of both developed membrane models, and gene expression analysis showed an evident up-regulation of ECM-related genes. Finally, membranes from *I. oros* significantly increased type I collagen gene expression and its release in the culture medium. The findings here reported strongly suggest the biotechnological potential of these collagenous structures of poriferan origin as scaffolds for wound healing.

**Keywords:** porifera; demosponges; biomaterial; collagen; spongin; wound healing

## 1. Introduction

Regenerative medicine currently needs innovative biomaterials characterised by low immunogenicity and toxicity and by good mechanical properties. Many biopolymers are available for their production, among them collagen—alone or combined with other ECM components, such as GAGs or elastin—is one of the most used and effective for these purposes [1]. Although skin and bones from bovine or porcine waste remain the primary source of this protein for regenerative medicine, the scientific community has recently shown a strong interest in marine collagen [2], consequently fish and various marine invertebrate collagens have been isolated and tested for tissue engineering applications [3–5]. Marine sponges in particular are one of the most promising sources among marine invertebrates for the production of collagen-derived biomaterials [6]. Marine sponge-derived collagen was tested for in vitro and in vivo studies, mainly for bone graft applications [7–11], and intact decellularized sponge 3D structures were used as bioinspired scaffolds for bone regeneration experiments [12]. Despite these several examples of the potential use of sponge collagen in regenerative medicine, there is only partial information on molecular characterisations of sponge-derived collagens [13,14], as well as on the molecular mechanisms involved in its biosynthesis [15,16].

Porifera is an extremely rich and biodiverse phylum, with more than 6,500 different species described to date [17]. These simple sessile animals are characterised by various shapes and textures supported by different structural solutions. Many species are characterised by a mineral skeleton made of silica or calcium carbonate, while others, commonly designated as keratose or horny sponges, have bodies formed exclusively by a flexible fibrous proteinaceous material commonly referred to as spongin [18,19]. The chemical-physical analyses of the abovementioned "spongin" lead back to a collagenic nature [18,20], but the co-presence of intercellular collagen fibres of smaller diameter in the same animals requires a better definition and characterisation of the various structures of collagen origin present in these sponges. Conventionally, the insoluble fibrous material isolated from the horny sponges after cell elimination by enzymatic treatment and centrifugation at low speed is designated as spongin B, while the collagenous suspension that can only be recovered through long and high-speed centrifugations is considered spongin A, or more generally, the sponges' intercellular collagen fibres [18]. A third sponge collagenic material was furthermore found only in members of the *Irciniidae* family: peculiar collagen filaments intimately connected to the fibrous spongin matrix, forming a single extremely robust and flexible support unit, specifically described in the two genera, *Ircinia* and *Sarcotragus* [21,22]. Their function remains controversial. Previously, some studies have also advanced the hypothesis of structures acquired by parasites [23]. However, their detailed morphological and chemical-physical characterisation confirmed the collagenic nature of these structures [21], attesting to their function as a skeleton specialisation typical of these genera. Depending on the species, the size of these filaments varies from a few millimetres in length to a few microns, and, in most cases, they end with an ovoid knob. Their ultrastructural analyses show that they are composed of tightly connected sets of collagen fibrils, often containing iron hydroxide granules of Lepidocrocite ($\gamma$-FeO(OH)) [24], whose function remains unknown. Unlike spongin, these filaments are surrounded by a thin amorphous cuticle whose positivity to Alcian blue strongly suggest the presence of carbohydrate components. This overall organisation shapes the tight packaging of the collagen fibrils composing the filaments, and it confers them as a relevant resistance to enzymatic digestion [21]. Ultimately, these peculiar structural features of horny sponge filaments represent something unique of their kind, and in our opinion they could have in principle relevant characteristics as a raw material for the production of 3D composites [25], as well as new devices for regenerative medicine.

The aim of this work is to develop a preliminary study to verify this hypothesis. For this purpose, two typologies of sponge-derived filaments are used: the large size ones from *Ircinia oros* (Schmidt 1864) and the small size ones from *Sarcotragus foetidus* (Schmidt 1862). 2D membranes were obtained by combining purified collagen filaments and intercellular collagen fibres from both sponge materials. Their ultrastructural, thermal and mechanical properties were analysed. Finally, their biocompatibility and ability to induce collagen and fibronectin production in fibroblast cell lines were tested to evaluate their potential as new biomaterials for skin regeneration in wound-dressing applications.

## 2. Results and Discussion

*2.1. Sponge Collagen Filaments (SCFs) Characterisation*

2.1.1. SCFs Microscopy Analysis

Microscopy analysis of fresh slices of *I. oros* and *S. foetidus* tissues showed their organic skeleton anatomy, articulated in a combination of main branched brown structures, commonly known as spongin, on which thin and clear filaments are tightly enveloped.

With slight pressure on a free edge of the tissue, these filaments can be observed to emerge from the spongin's main branch (Figure 1A,Aa,B,Ba).

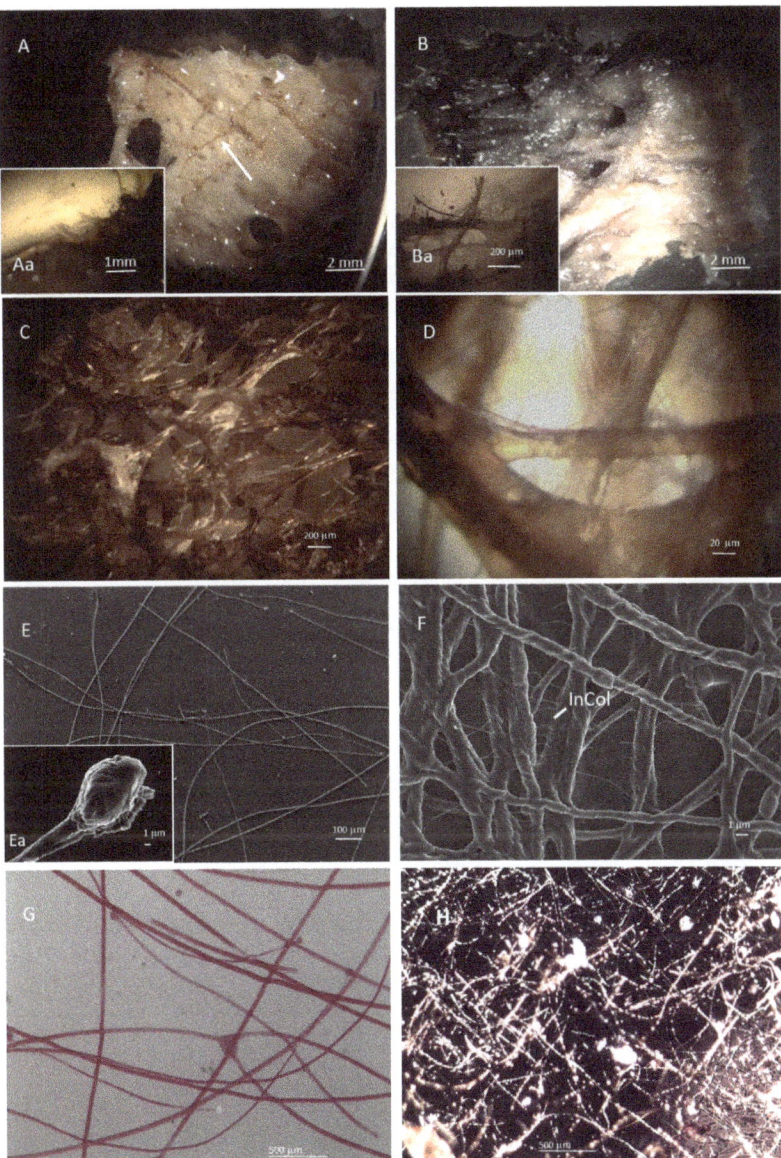

**Figure 1.** Morphology of collagen filaments derived from *I. oros* and *S. foetidus*. (**A,Aa,C,E,Ea,G**) Micrographs of collagen filaments isolated from *I. oros* tissues. (**B,Ba,D,F,H**) Collagen filaments isolated from *S. foetidus* tissues. (**A,Aa,B,Ba**) Stereo-microscopy analysis of fresh tissue. (**C,D**) Residual collagen filaments associated with spongin matrix at the end of the purification process. (**E,Ea,F**) Scanning electron microscopy analysis of isolated collagen filaments. (**G,H**) Micrograph of picro-sirius red staining of collagen filaments.

Using a tissue dissociation enzymatic procedure combined with repeated extraction cycles in distilled water starting from 20 g (wet weight) of *I. oros* tissue, up to 400 mL of an aqueous suspension of collagen filaments isolated from the brown spongin matrix at a final concentration of 2 mg/mL could be obtained. The filaments extracted during the first two extraction rounds contained sediment residues and various sponge tissue debris and were thus discarded, while those obtained in subsequent cycles were progressively cleaner. After several extraction cycles, almost all the filaments have been removed from the brown matrix and collected in water suspension, and only a residual quantity still remained tightly knotted to the spongin structure (Figure 1C). Electron microscopy analysis of isolated filaments from *I. oros* confirmed the expected forms and dimensions, according to the descriptions previously published [21,26]. They showed a diameter of 13 μm, a length of several millimetres (up to 8 mm) and they ended with an oval knob (15–22 μm). The *I. oros* filaments were also strongly positive for picro-sirius red stain (Figure 1G), confirming their collagenous origin (Figure 1G).

A similar approach was followed to extract filaments from *S. foetidus*, with some specific adaptations. The filament dimensions, lower than the *I. oros* ones, and the high presence of inorganic sediments intimately distributed in the whole inner body of *S. foetidus* were the main cause of a greater difficulty in the isolation and cleaning procedure. Differently from the *I. oros* case, the reduced dimensions of *S. foetidus* filaments prevented the exploitation of a different speed of sedimentation to remove sediment residues and cell debris. Although the animal's tissues are very rich in collagenic filaments, numerous repetitions of extraction cycles were necessary to obtain enough purified material; therefore, the first four cycles of extraction were discarded and only after the fifth cycle it was possible to obtain a filament suspension that is clean and pure enough. On the other hand, in these animals, the brown spongin structure intimately associated with filaments seemed to flake off more easily than in the previous case of *I. oros* (Figure 1D). Definitively, in *S. foetidus*, starting from 20 g of fresh tissue in our experimental conditions, it was possible to recover 200 mL of purified filament suspension with a final concentration of 2 mg/mL. Ultrastructural analyses showed filament diameters of 1–3 μm without any knobs at their ends. At a higher magnification, intercellular collagen fibres are clearly visible between the filaments, which are co-extracted during the purification steps (Figure 1F). Furthermore, *S. foetidus* filaments appeared intriguingly coated with an irregular sheath of inorganic material, formed by iron-containing compounds as shown by EDS analyses (Figure S1). This suggests that *S. foetidus* collagen filaments could contain iron-based mineral phases, as previously described in filaments of other sponges of the *Ircinia* genera [21]. The irregular distribution of these mineral sleeves found in our samples is partly a consequence of the extraction procedure, based on repeated cycles, as the ultrastructural analysis conducted on intact *S. foetidus* tissues shows that this coverage is considerably more homogeneous in origin (Figure S2). The remarkable discontinuous biomineral coatings prevent the homogeneous staining of this sample with picro-sirius red dye conversely to that obtained in *I. oros* filaments (Figure 1H). Notably, the presence of biogenic iron hydroxide intimately associated with collagenic material makes the biomaterials derived from this sponge species extremely interesting regarding biotechnological application, given the innumerable uses of composite collagen matrices with iron-based minerals [27–29].

2.1.2. SCFs Biochemical Analysis

Amino Acid Composition

Table 1 shows the amino acid composition of hydrolysed SCFs derived from *I. oros* and *S. foetidus*, expressed as residues ‰. The amino acid profile of the collagen filaments of both sponges is similar. Therefore, this suggests that despite very different sizes, these filaments are formed by similar collagen molecules. Like rat and codfish collagen, sponge collagenous filaments have glycine as their major amino acid, as shown in 359/1000 and 385.46/1000 residues, in *I. oros* and *S. foetidus* filaments, respectively. Proline contents in collagen filaments from *I. oros* and *S. foetidus* resulted in 57.06 and 67.29 residues ‰, respectively.

Together with glycine and proline, hydroxyproline and hydroxylisine are amino acid characterising collagens. In particular, the total amount of hydroxyproline residues in collagen can affect the thermal stability of collagen [30]; furthermore, its content is higher in rat collagen than sponge collagenous filaments, as it suits the higher mammalian body temperatures. Conversely, its content level is lower in codfish than in sponge collagenous filaments, due to the lower temperature in which this animal lives, compared to *I. oros* and *S. foetidus*, which typically grow in low depths of the Mediterranean Sea. As observed for proline residues, the lysine content in the collagenous filaments of sponges is also lower than in vertebrate collagens; however, its percentage of hydroxylation is higher. Highly hydroxylated collagen has been reported previously within skeletal structures of glass sponges [31]. Here, the total hydroxylysine content is remarkably higher in the sponges' filaments than in vertebrate collagen, resulting in almost double compared to codfish collagen. Hydroxylysine residues are known to be involved in crosslink reactions during fibre assembling [32], and their peculiar abundance could explain the strong insolubility of filaments themselves. Another very interesting fact that emerged in this study is the high level of aspartic acid content in sponge filaments compared to vertebrate collagen. This last feature, already described in several other poriferan collagens [21,33–35], is again something peculiar in the context of sponge collagens, and it could explain their difficulty in being solubilised in acidic conditions, contrary to the collagens of higher organisms.

**Table 1.** Amino acid composition of *I. oros* and *S. foetidus* collagen filaments compared with collagen from skin of codfish and commercial rat collagen (per 1000 residues).

| Amino Acid | I.oros | S. foetidus | Rat * | Codfish * |
|---|---|---|---|---|
| Ala+Arg | 152 | 157 | 153.4 | 121.93 |
| Aspartic acid | 100.03 | 78.83 | 45.32 | 38.82 |
| Glutamic acid | 111.90 | 114.27 | 73.33 | 56.08 |
| Glycine | 359.00 | 385.46 | 333.18 | 266.12 |
| Histidine | 0.96 | 1.34 | 3.61 | 5.01 |
| Hydroxylysine | 13.91 | 14.26 | 9.33 | 6.65 |
| Hydroxyproline | 69.29 | 61.53 | 96.09 | 39.6 |
| Isoleucine | 8.57 | 5.62 | 7.48 | 5.61 |
| Leucine | 23.19 | 18.96 | 23.29 | 6.51 |
| Lysine | 13.80 | 12.00 | 27.07 | 19.62 |
| Methionine | 1.64 | 1.80 | 8.03 | 15.04 |
| Phenylalanine | 13.31 | 10.42 | 14.62 | 12.7 |
| Proline | 57.06 | 43.56 | 109.21 | 62.69 |
| Serine | 41.65 | 61.28 | 42.74 | 53.87 |
| Threonine | 18.53 | 18.66 | 18.79 | 16.89 |
| Tyrosine | 4.99 | 5.17 | 3.76 | 2.25 |
| Valine | 10.59 | 10.18 | 17.08 | 12.02 |

* Value obtained from [36].

Amino Acids, Glycosaminoglycans (GAGs) and Iron Content

The results obtained by the quantitative analysis of total amino acids (GAGs) and iron is showed in Table 2. These data indicated that the proteinaceous component in *I. oros* filaments are double compared to *S. foetidus* filaments. Conversely, the GAGs amount obtained by Alcian blue quantitative assay were higher in *S. foetidus* filaments compared to *I. oros* counterpart, resulting in 28.49 ± 8.3 µg/mg and 12.28 ± 5.4 µg/mg, respectively.

**Table 2.** Comparison between *I.oros* collagen filaments and *S.foetidus* collagen filaments in amino acids, GAGs and iron content (µg/mg dry collagen filaments).

| | Amino Acids (µg/mg) | GAGs (µg/mg) | Iron (µg/mg) |
|---|---|---|---|
| *I. oros* | 490.3 ± 3.4 | 12.28 ± 5.4 | 2.7 ± 0.32 |
| *S. foetidus* | 250.9 ± 2.9 | 28.49 ± 8.3 | 45.32 ± 2.8 |

Finally, the quantitative evaluation of the iron component in SCFs obtained by inductively coupled plasma atomic emission (ICP–AES) confirmed the previously obtained data in *I. oros* samples [22], and provides us with a quantitative indication on the biomineral component identified in *S.foetidus* collagen filaments through EDS (Figure S1) in ultrastructural analyses.

Sodium Dodecyl Sulfate Poly Acrylamide Gel Electrophoresis (SDS-PAGE)

The electrophoretic profile of purified SCFs from *I. oros* and *S. foetidus* could be obtained only after their destruction by glass beads in 1× denaturing gel loading buffer (Figure 2). No differences in electrophoretic patterns between the sponge species were observed. In both samples, a weak band corresponding to 120 kDa, consistent with the typical size of the fibrillar collagens α-chains of higher animals [36] and other marine sponge species, was detected. In particular, a similar molecular size was observed in the SDS-PAGE analysis of fibrillar collagen extract purified from the marine sponge *Chondrosia reniformis* [37]. The presence of a single band suggests that the fibrillar collagens of these sponge filaments should be homotrimers forming homotypic fibres.

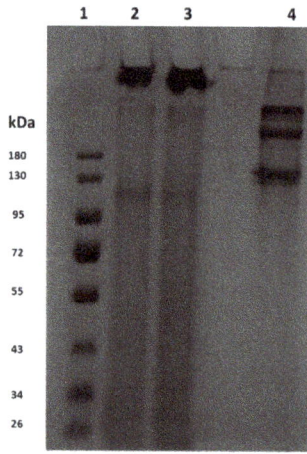

**Figure 2.** SDS-PAGE analysis of purified SCFs. A total of 40 µL of 2 mg/mL sponge filament suspensions crushed in acid-washed glass beads in 1× gel loading buffer and heated at 90 °C for 5 min were loaded in a 7% polyacrylamide gel. After electrophoresis, gel was stained with colloidal Coomassie blue staining as described in Section 4.3. Lane 1: standard molecular weight markers (kDa); Lane 2: *I. oros* collagen filaments; Lane 3: *S. foetidus* collagen filaments; Lane 4: rat tail type I collagen.

*2.2. Sponge Collagen Filament Membranes (SCFMs) Characterisation*

2.2.1. SCFM Surface Morphologies

When SCFs derived from *I. oros* and *S. foetidus* were cast and dried in silicon mods, it was possible to recover thin, light membranes that were extremely smooth to the touch (Figures 3A and 4A). The texture of *I. oros*-derived membranes was clearly visible under an optical microscope at low magnification, thanks to the larger size of its filaments (Figure 3B–D). The membrane structure appeared to be a disorganised web of filaments bound by a bright, transparent matrix. The pores delimited by the mesh of the membrane texture spanned an average value of 624.09 ± 291.49 µm². Ultrastructural analysis showed that the *I. oros* collagenic filaments in the membranes were intimately associated with intercellular collagen fibres that were co-extracted with the filaments and that, once dried, formed a whole with the filaments themselves (Figure 3E,F). At light microscopy, the network of the membranes obtained from the collagen filaments of *S. foetidus* was more compact than that derived from *I. oros* filaments (Figure 4A), and their mesh was only visible in the edge through high magnification (Figure 4B). In electronic microscopy with high magnification, these membranes were formed by a dense weave of filaments bound by intercellular collagen fibres with a smaller diameter (Figure 4C–F). Here, the pores delimited by the mesh of the membrane texture spanned an average value of $8.90 \pm 5.61$ $\mu m^2$. The remarkable differences in the filament networking and the pore texture can be justified by the different diameters of the filaments (13 µm for *I. oros* and 1–3 µm for *S. foetidus*), and by their distinct surface characteristics. *S foetidus* filaments, in particular, have a very peculiar coating of iron oxide, and this feature could play a role in the intercellular matrix protein-filament interactions in the membrane structure.

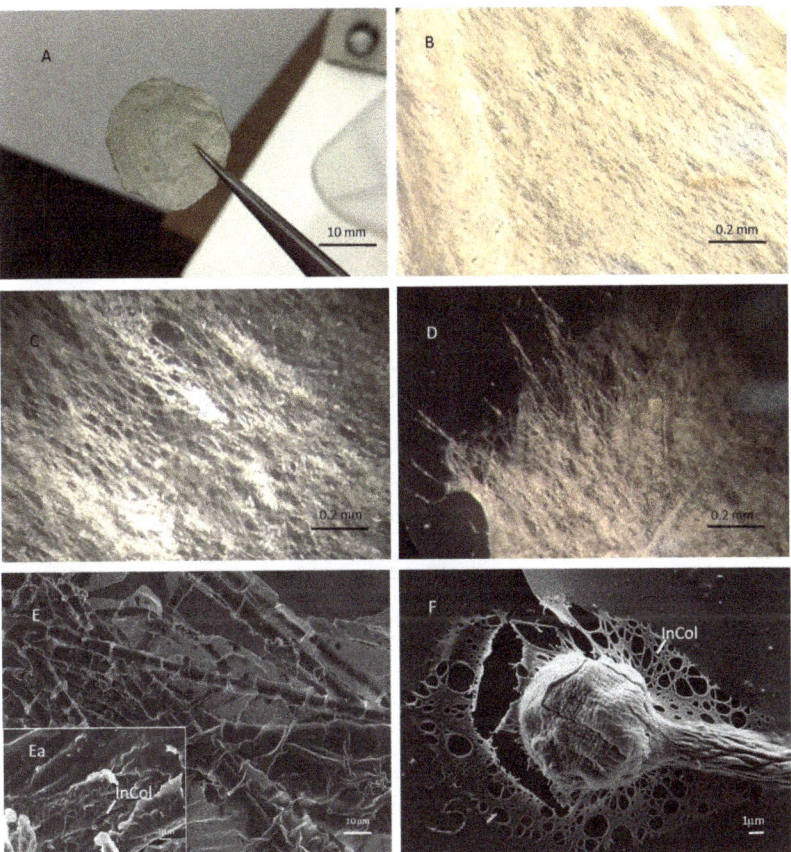

**Figure 3.** *I. oros*-derived membranes morphology. (**A**) Photograph of whole *I. oros*-derived membrane. (**B,C**) Micrographs showing the texture *I. oros*-derived membranes. (**D**) Micrograph showing the jagged edge of the *I. oros*-derived membrane. (**E,Ea**) Scanning electron microscopy analysis showing the texture of the *I. oros*-derived membrane. (**F**) Scanning electron microscopy analysis showing the filament knob embedded in intercellular collagen fibre matrix. **InCol**: intercellular collagen fibres.

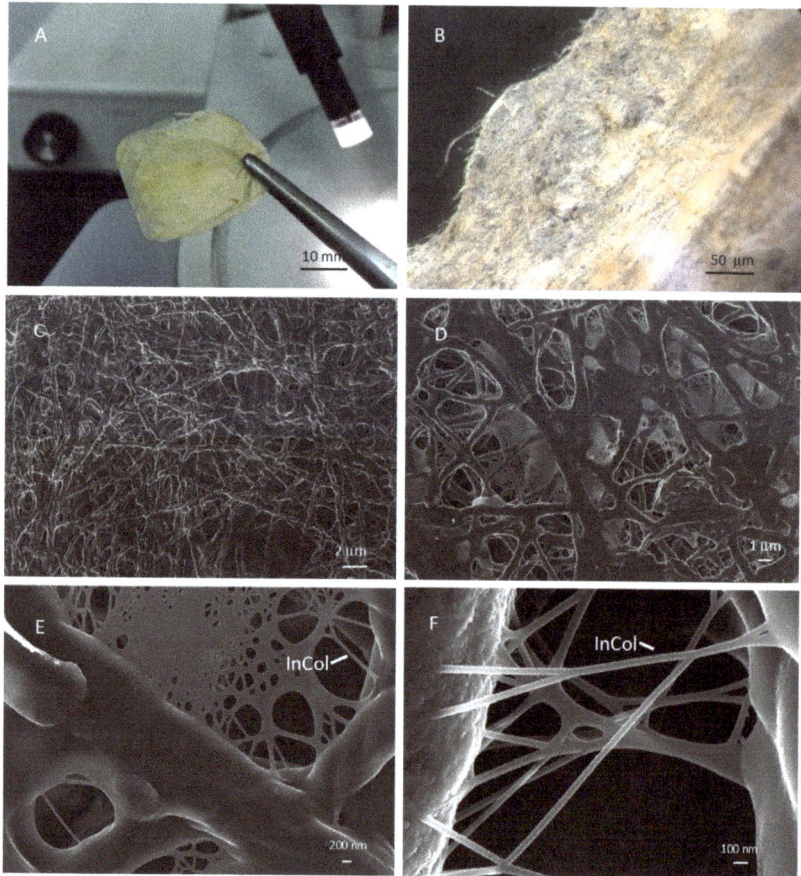

**Figure 4.** *S. foetidus*-derived membranes morphology. (**A**) Photograph of whole *S. foetidus*-derived membrane. (**B**) Micrographs showing the jagged edge of the *S. foetidus*-derived membrane. (**C–F**) Scanning electron microscopy analysis showing the texture of the *S. foetidus*-derived membranes. InCol: intercellular collagen fibres.

2.2.2. Thermal Properties

Differential scanning calorimetry (DSC) thermograms of dried SCFMs and of one commercial collagen membrane (BioGide®, chosen as comparison biomaterial) are shown in Figure 5. An endothermic peak, with a maximum temperature point (Tmax) of 71.19 and 55.79 °C, was observed for *I. oros*-derived and *S. foetidus*-derived membranes, respectively, while BioGide® commercial collagen membranes showed a Tmax at 54.17 °C. Therefore, compared to BioGide®, both SCFMs showed higher thermal stability. However, while *S. foetidus*-derived membranes differed by a few degrees, those derived from *I. oros* filaments showed a higher difference compared to commercial collagen membranes. A high thermal stability of solubilised collagen molecules is related to the high level of proline/hydroxyproline [30]. However, a small difference in the amount of these amino acids was observed in the collagen filaments isolated from both species (Table 1). Furthermore, their content is considerably lower than in mammalian collagen, where commercial membranes are formed. It is therefore evident that other chemical characteristics must come into play to ensure the high thermal stability found in the *I. oros*-derived membranes. Typically, commercial collagen membranes were obtained from controlled in vitro fibrillogenesis of solubilised tropo-collagen. Conversely, SCFMs are obtained by casting and drying the collagen filaments formed by tightly assembled intact collagen fibres that, for *I. oros* filaments, are further enveloped in Alcian blue positive sugar sheath [21]. The thermal stability of a collagen-derived biomaterial is increased by its crosslink level [38]; hence, the high thermal stability observed in *I. oros*-derived membranes could be related to the interchain cross-links involved in the association of collagen fibres. *S. foetidus* filaments are partially covered by iron biomineral; however, the presence of mineral nanoparticles does not seem to affect the thermal stability of collagen-derived scaffolds [38,39]. This could explain the low Tmax difference between commercial collagen and *S. foetidus*-derived membranes.

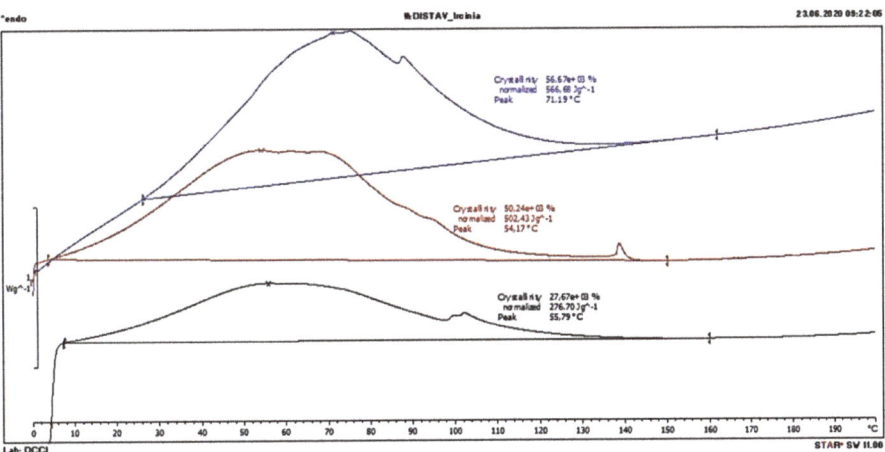

**Figure 5.** DSC analysis of SCFMs. Thermograms of 3 mg of dry *I. oros*-derived membrane (blue line), *S. foetidus*-derived membrane (black line) and commercial porcine collagen membrane Bio-Gide®(red line).

2.2.3. Mechanical Properties

DMA and DMTA were carried out on the prepared SCFMs in order to compare their overall mechanical performances. As summarised in Table 3, *S. foetidus*-derived membranes present much higher elastic (E') and loss modulus (E"), with respect to those derived from *I. oros* in the same experimental conditions. This greater mechanical stiffness may be ascribed to different reasons. First, the smaller size of the filaments' diameter from which *S. foetidus*-derived membranes are formed generates a more compact texture with smaller diameter pores, which can in turn enhance the sample rigidity [40]. Second, despite that in both types of membranes the filaments are bound by intercellular collagen fibres co-extracted with the filaments, the smaller size of the *S. foetidus* filaments could allow these filaments to interact better with the intercellular collagen fibres to form a continuous structure, while this is harder in the *I. oros*-derived membranes due to the larger size difference between the filament diameter and dispersed intercellular collagen fibres. Finally, the iron biomineral coating present in *S. foetidus* filaments is likewise responsible for a further enhancement of the sample mechanical performances with respect to the *I. oros*-derived membranes [41]. Additionally, as shown in Figure 6, it is noteworthy that both the prepared SCFMs are characterised by a high thermal stability within the investigated temperature range. However, *S. foetidus*-derived membranes appear to once again perform better compared to the *I. oros*-derived ones, presenting a lower decrease in the elastic modulus as the temperature is increased.

**Table 3.** Mechanical test of SCFMs. DMA.

| Sample | E′ @ 1 Hz, 25 °C (MPa) | St. Dev | E″ @ 1 Hz, 25 °C (MPa) | St. Dev |
|---|---|---|---|---|
| I. oros | 447.15 | 9.49 | 18.52 | 0.86 |
| S. foetidus | 819.27 | 37.88 | 44.25 | 4.50 |

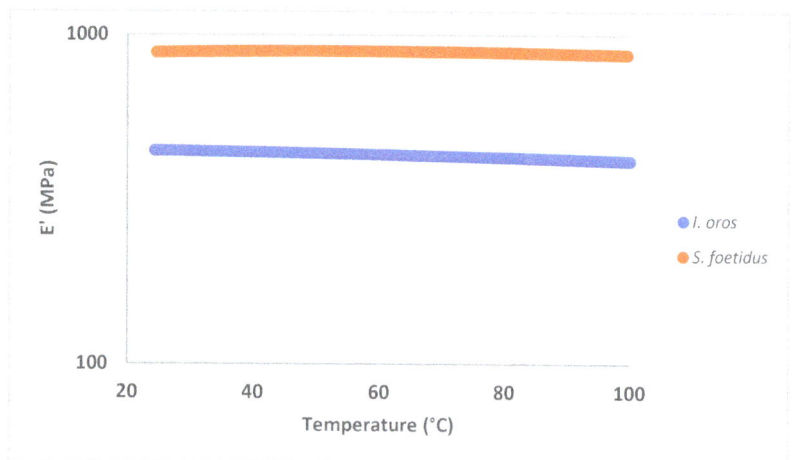

**Figure 6.** Mechanical test of SCFMs. DMTA spectra of *I. oros*-derived (blue curve) and *S. foetidus*-derived (orange curve) membranes measured in extensional configuration with a frequency of 1 Hz and an extensional stress of 0.1 MPa.

Generally speaking, both SCFMs are characterised by suitable mechanical properties for a broad range of biomedical applications, ranging from scaffolds for tissue regeneration to wound-healing patches.

2.2.4. In Vitro Degradation Evaluation

The degradation rate of SCFMs in PBS or collagenase solution was first investigated by evaluating the percentage of weight loss as a function of the degradation time. The percentage weight loss of SCFMs within 21 days in PBS (pH 7.4) is shown in Figure 7A. For each membrane type, the main weight loss was detected within seven days, while insignificant weight loss was observed after 14 and 21 days. After seven days, *I. oros*-derived membranes exhibited a weight loss rate of 36.27 ± 8.54%, while in *S. foetidus* types, the weight loss was 13.9 ± 3.25%, which was more stable than *I. oros*-derived membranes.

The weight loss of the SCFMs due to the collagenase enzymatic activity within 21 days is shown in Figure 7B. In both membrane types, the weight loss after seven days was not significantly different from the corresponding samples in PBS, resulting in 26.29 ± 5.25% and 18.03 ± 6.0%, respectively, while after 14 days in the enzyme treated cases the weight loss almost doubled. Specifically, in *I. oros*-derived membranes, a 58.93 ± 23.34% weight loss was detected, while in *S. foetidus*-derived membranes, it was 28.98 ± 0.06%. No further increase in weight loss was observed after 21 days in both samples.

The evaluation of the organic compound release in saline or in collagenase solution from SCFMs during the in vitro degradation evaluation, obtained by the 280 nm absorbance in the membrane incubation media, has shown a similar trend in SCFM degradation rate (Figure 7C,D). Compared to the previous methods, here in the presence of collagenase, significant differences with respect to the PBS were detected already after 7 days.

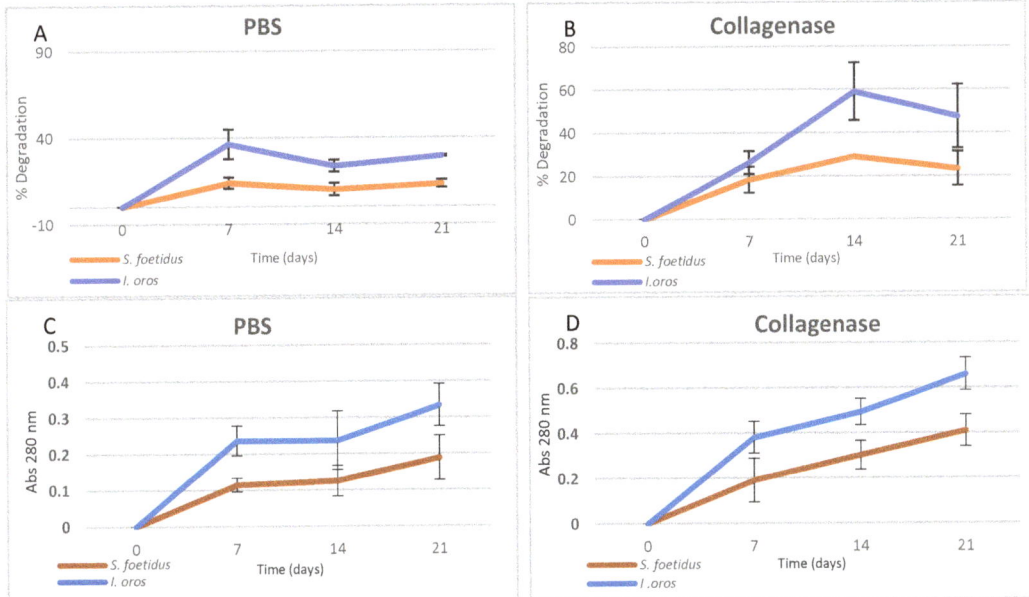

**Figure 7.** In vitro degradation test. Percentage degradation in PBS (**A**) and in 0.1 mg/mL collagenase solution (**B**) obtained as dry wight difference. Organic compound release from SCFMs in PBS (**C**) and in 0.1 mg/mL collagenase solution (**D**) obtained by 280 nm absorbance measurement of the incubation media. ($n$ = 3, mean ± standard deviation).

To evaluate the percentage of collagen released or hydrolysed from the SCFMs within 21 days in PBS or in collagenase solution, the incubation media of the in vitro degradation test was hydrolysed and the hydroxyproline content was measured. When the membranes were incubated in PBS, no detectable hydroxyproline (<0.6 mg/mL) was found in each type of membrane. In the presence of collagenase in *I. oros*-derived membranes, the level of hydroxyproline recorded in the incubation media appeared to increase over time, resulting in 6.03 ± 0.89 µg/mL after 21 days, while in *S. foetidus*-derived membranes, the level of hydroxyproline was appreciable only after 21 days, resulting in 2.30 ± 0.37 µg/mL. (Table 4). These data indicate that the membrane weight loss observed in PBS incubation was not due to collagen release, but to different organic compounds, while when the membranes were incubated in collagenase solution, considering a presence of hydroxyproline on average of 6.5% (Table 1) in the collagen, only a 26.2% and a 18.5% of the weight loss was collagen in *I. oros*-derived membranes and *S. foetidus*-derived membranes, respectively.

**Table 4.** Hydroxyproline content the incubation media of the in the vitro degradation test.

| Time (days) | *I. oros* | *S. foetidus* |
|---|---|---|
| | µg/mL | µg/mL |
| 7 | 3.64 ± 0.56 | <0.6 |
| 14 | 5.78 ± 0.28 | <0.6 |
| 21 | 6.03 ± 0.89 | 2.30 ± 0.37 |

The greater stability of the *S. foetidus*-derived membranes compared to those derived from *I. oros*, evaluated in PBS and collagenase, obtained through the dry weight difference and through the analysis of the absorption at 280 nm of the incubation media could be due to the different textures of these membranes. These results are congruent with what was previously highlighted in relation to mechanical properties. The larger pore sizes in *I. oros*-derived membranes and the discontinuity of the intercellular collagen matrix that binds the filaments make this structure more susceptible to the dispersion of some of its components in water, and more accessible to collagenase digestion. Although it has previously been shown that sponge collagen is extremely resistant to collagenase treatment [33], the membranes in this study were subjected to greater weight loss after 14 days and a higher organic compound release after 7 days, compared to the saline solution, attesting a possible enzymatic activity. However, the analysis of the hydroxyproline level in the hydrolised membrane incubation media revealed that only a low percentage of weight loss was collagen material, suggesting an intimate association between collagen fibres and other organic materials that are solubilised together to the hydrolysed collagen. Moreover, the increased resistance to collagenase digestion exhibited by *S. foetidus*-derived membranes compared to *I. oros*-derived membranes could be probably linked to the partial coating of the filaments with the biomineral material, which could limit access to the enzymes.

### 2.2.5. Swelling Test and Antioxidant Activity

The degree of swelling of SCFMs after immersion in water over a 24 h period is shown in Table 5. *I. oros*-derived membranes showed a percentage of swelling that was about double as compared to *S. foetidus* membranes (1511.44 ± 149.23% and 827.94 ± 64.40%, respectively). An extended immersion time of the membranes by an additional 24 h did not increase their weight (data not shown), showing that they had already reached their maximum swelling level after 24 h. The great difference in hydrophilicity between the two membrane types could be related to the abundant presence of iron biominerals in the surface of *S. foetidus* filaments. The addition of iron nanoparticles to collagen-derived biomaterial can in fact reduce its water affinity [42]. This inorganic component almost certainly increases the stability of the membranes in aqueous solutions, but at the same time, it reduces the surface interaction between water and the collagen fibres, and this definitively could decrease the membrane's ability to bind water. The swelling behaviour of a material is driven not only by its chemical nature but also by its structure. Compared to membranes with the same surface area obtained by collagen fibres isolated from the marine sponge *C. reniformis* [11], the membranes described in this study showed higher hydration levels. Here, the greater dimensions of the collagen's diameters increase the membrane thickness, thus improving the surface contact with water.

**Table 5.** Swelling index and antioxidant activity evaluation of SCFMs derived from *I. oros* and *S. foetidus*. (n = 3, mean ± standard deviation).

| Sample | Swelling Index (%) | Antioxidant Activity (%) |
| --- | --- | --- |
| *I. oros* | 1511.44 ± 149.23 | 4.64 ± 1.78 |
| *S. foetidus* | 827.94 ± 64.40 | 57.24 ± 8.58 |

The above described membrane features strongly suggest some uses in regenerative medicine, in particular in tissue repair approaches. In the animal kingdom, including in mammalians and human beings, wound-healing processes are mostly accompanied by a local inflammatory response, generating reactive oxygen species and cell oxidative stress [43]. Thus, biomaterials designed for these applications are often conjugated with antioxidant compounds [44]. Marine sponges are known to be rich in secondary metabolites [45]; many of which have antioxidant properties [46]; furthermore, sponge collagenic peptides seem to have, in certain instances, antioxidant properties [37]. Here, we have evaluated the radical scavenging activity of SCFMs using the DPPH assay. The results reported in Table 5 indicate that no significant antioxidant activity was detected in *I. oros*-derived membranes, while each 25 × 28 mm *S. foetidus*-derived membrane exhibited 57.24 ± 8.58% of antioxidant activity. Since both membranes are composed of collagen, in this specific case we cannot attribute a direct role of sponge collagen, but we suggest that the remarkable difference in antioxidant properties can be due to the presence of iron-based biominerals.

This assumption can also be supported by the literature evidence, where the antioxidant properties of iron oxide nanoparticles of biogenic origin are extensively documented with proposed uses in biomedicine and bioremediation [47].

### 2.3. SCFM Biocompatibility Evaluation

#### 2.3.1. Cell Adhesion and Cell Proliferation

To evaluate the biocompatibility of SCFMs, L929 fibroblasts and HaCaT keratinocytes were grown on SCF-coated plates. Subsequently, a cell adhesion rate of 16 h after plating, and cell viability at three and six days were tested using MTT assay. Rat tail collagen was used as a comparison. No significant differences in cell adhesion were observed for both cell lines used on plates coated with *I. oros* collagenous filaments, compared to the uncoated plate controls after 16 h (Figure 8). Some reduced attachment of L929 fibroblast was observed on plates coated with *S. foetidus* collagen filaments, (77.14 ± 6.94%, see Figure 8), while no significant differences compared to the control were detected for HaCaT keratinocytes. An analogous slight reduction in L929 adhesion can be observed in the case of rat tail collagen coating used as a comparison (83.28 ± 8.57% of L929 fibroblasts were attached to the plates), while no significant differences compared to the control, were detected for HaCaT keratinocytes. Overall, these data showed that except for L929 fibroblasts plated on *S. foetidus* collagen filaments, no significant differences in cell adhesion rate were observed after 16 h in the other cases.

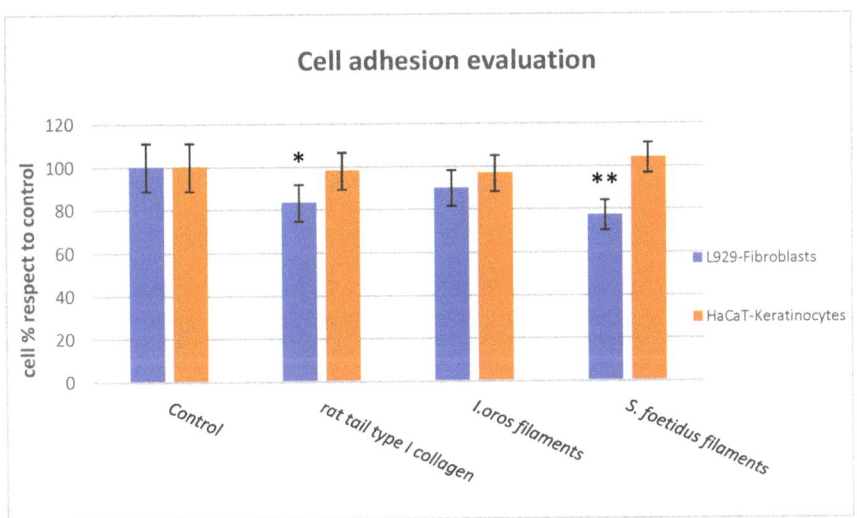

**Figure 8.** Cell adhesion evaluation. Cell adhesion quantitative evaluation, by MTT test, of L929 fibroblasts (blue bars) and HaCaT keratinocytes (orange bars) on the rat tail type I collagen, *I. oros* collagen filaments and *S. foetidus* collagen filaments pre-coated plates after 16 h of incubation. Results are expressed as cell percentages with respect to controls that were seeded on uncoated wells and are the mean ± S.D. of three experiments that were performed using eight well for each experimental condition. Statistical analysis results: one-way ANOVA, (blue bars) $p < 0.05$; (orange bars) $p < 0.05$. Asterisks indicate a significant difference versus the respective control (paired Tukey test, * $p < 0.05$, ** $p < 0.001$).

Along with adhesion, in our experimental model, cell viability results are also reported here. The L929 fibroblast viability assay of SCFMs and rat tail collagen coating three and six days after plating is shown in Figure 9 (Panel I). Compared to the control, no significant differences were observed on plates coated with *I. oros* filaments after three days, while after six days, L929 fibroblasts growth resulted in 132.48 ± 6.83% compared to the control, attesting an improved proliferation rate. Similar results were observed in fibroblasts growing on plates coated with *S. foetidus* filaments. No difference in cell viability was observed with this biomaterial after three days, in comparison with the uncoated control sample, while after six days, the L929 fibroblast viability on this biomaterial was 134.19 ± 12.82% compared to the control. Conversely, on rat tail collagen coating, the cell viability after three days was 89.74 ± 9.40% compared to the control and no significant differences were registered after six days. Therefore, in our experimental conditions, in regards to the cell growth induction, SCF coating was more effective for fibroblast cell lines than mammalian collagen coating. Micrographs of the phalloidin-stained L929 fibroblasts growing on *I. oros* and *S. foetidus* collagen filaments, respectively, are shown in Figure 9A,B. After 24 h, their shape and their interaction with the biomaterials were very similar to the cell morphology observed in the controls and cells plated on rat tail collagen (Figure 9A,B, respectively). Figure 9 also shows the HaCaT keratinocytes proliferation assay (Panel L). Here, no significant differences in viability were detected on *I. oros* collagen filament coatings three days after plating, while after six days a significative increase in viability was observed (137.18 ± 8.97%), compared to the control. On *S. foetidus* collagen filament coatings, cell growth of 141.25 ± 24.61% and 133.33 ± 5.10% was registered after three and six days, respectively, compared to their controls. Similarly, in the rat tail collagen coating, a cell viability of 129.23 ± 13.85% and 146.15 ± 10.26% was measured after three and six days, respectively. Therefore, despite different temporal kinetics, SCF coatings are also able to promote in vitro cell proliferation of keratinocytes similar to that observed in mammalian collagen coatings. The phalloidin-stained HaCaT keratinocyte cells growing on *I. oros* and *S. foetidus* collagen filaments are shown in Figure 9G,H, respectively. As previously shown for fibroblasts, no significant morphology variations were observed compared to the control and rat tail coating samples (Figure 9E,F, respectively). Similar to what has been previously reported for spongin structures [48], the *I. oros* filaments emitted weak green autofluorescence, and this peculiar histological property, combined with their large size, allows a detailed observation of how both the fibroblasts and keratinocytes are intimately associated with the biomaterial and their prolongations (Figure 9C,G). In Figure 10, the way that the cell extensions faithfully follow the filaments' shape can be observed in detail at a higher magnification (Figure 10A,C). Different to *I. oros*, *S. foetidus* filaments do not emit autofluorescence, but by superimposing the images obtained with fluorescence and light microscopy, it is still possible to observe that even with this biomaterial, both the fibroblasts and the keratinocytes are closely associated with the filaments, and their cell body often follows the filaments' direction (Figure 10B,D). Together these data show us that regardless of their size or the presence of iron biomineral coverage, both sponge-derived collagen filaments exhibited good biocompatibility, and can improve fibroblast and keratinocytes proliferation. Furthermore, the direct cell surface interactions with these marine biomaterials and their ability to drive the cell growth direction along their structure are extremely suitable to guided tissue regeneration (GTR) applications [49].

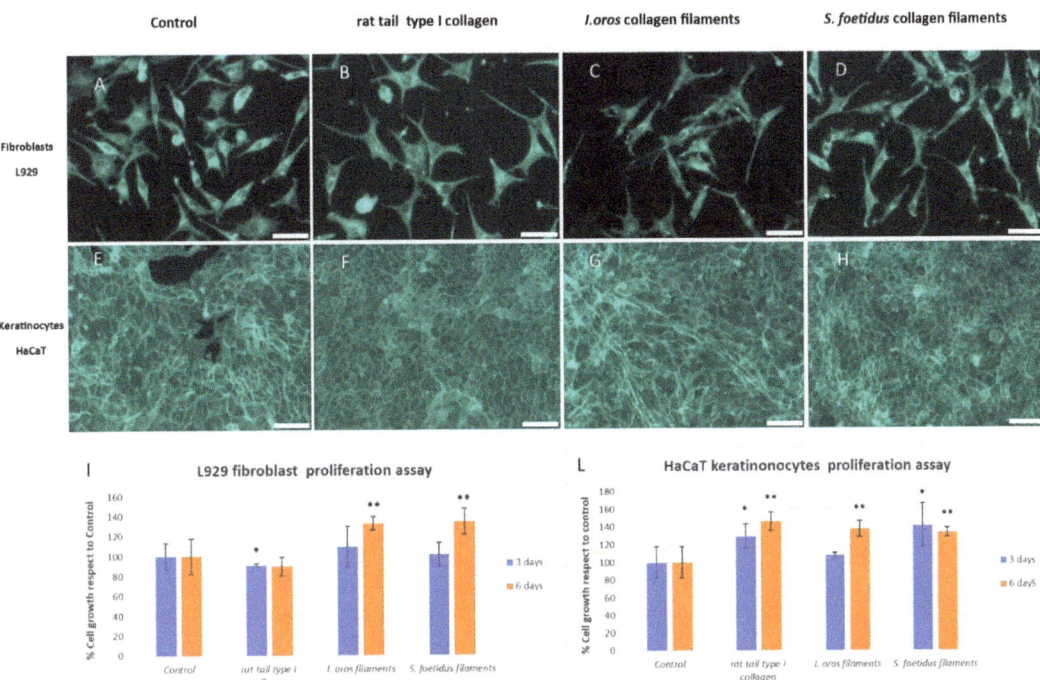

**Figure 9.** Cell proliferation evaluation. (**A–D**) Alexa Fluor 488-conjugated phalloindin stained L929 fibroblasts, epifluorescence microscope. (**A**) In control cells, the fluorescent actin cytoskeleton allows the observation of the typical aspect of fibroblast in culture, with fusiform, elongate shape, some focal adhesion (bright dots) and no preferential direction of cell and processes elongation. (**B**) Cells with rat tail type I collagen show no shape alteration. (**C**) *I. oros* collagen filaments are visible as weakly fluorescent stripes in the background. The fibroblasts clearly interact with the collagen and maintain their overall shape. (**D**) The thin collagen filaments of *S. foetidus* are not easily visible through the fluorescent filters; fibroblast have a morphology similar to the control. (**E, F**) Alexa Fluor 488-conjugated phalloindin stained HaCAT keratinocytes, epifluorescence microscope. (**E**) In control cells, the fluorescent actin cytoskeleton allows the observation of the organisation of keratinocytes that tend to interact, forming sheets. (**F–H**) The presence of collagen from rat tail, *I. oros* and *S. foetidus* does not induce detectable alterations in the morphology of cultured keratinocytes. Although covered by cells, the presence of collagen filaments of *I. oros* is detectable as two stripes from top left to the bottom right corner of the G photograph. Scale bars 50 μm. (**I–L**) Cell viability quantitative evaluation, by MTT test, of L929 fibroblasts (panel **I**) and HaCaT keratinocytes (panel **L**) on the rat tail type I collagen, *I. oros* collagen filament and *S. foetidus* collagen filament pre-coated plates after 3 days (blue bars) and 6 days (orange bars) of incubation. Results are expressed as cell percentages compared to controls that were seeded on uncoated wells, and are the mean ± S.D. of three experiments that were performed using eight well for each experimental condition. Statistical analysis results: one-way ANOVA, (I, blue bars) $p < 0.0001$, (I, orange bars) $p < 0.0001$; (L, blue bars) $p < 0.0001$, (L, orange bars) $p < 0.005$. Asterisks indicate a significant difference versus the respective control (paired Tukey test, * $p < 0.05$, ** $p < 0.001$).

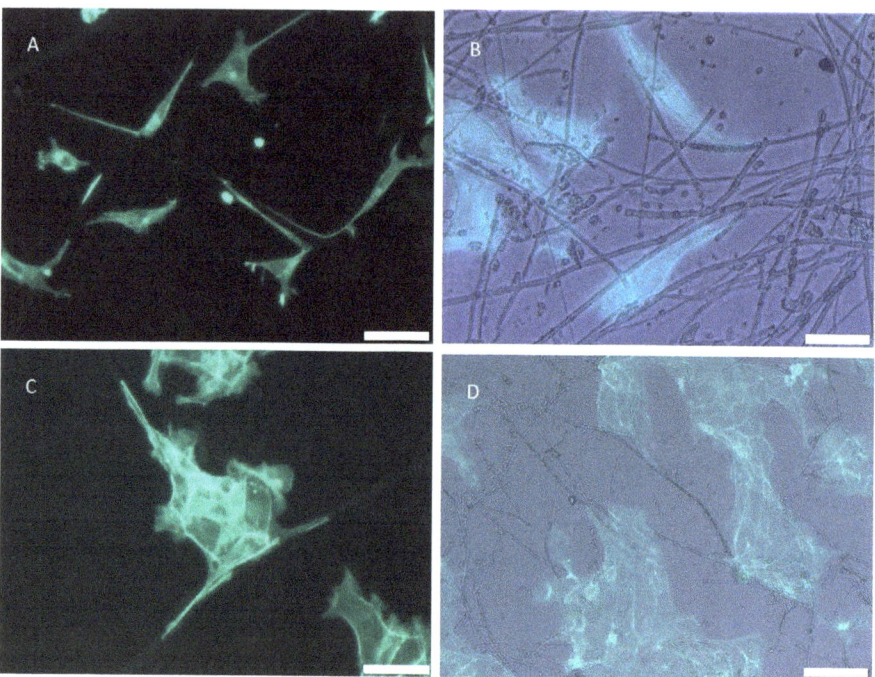

**Figure 10.** Alexa Fluor 488-conjugated phalloindin stained cell, epifluorescence microscope. (**A**) L929 fibroblasts and *I. oros* collagen filaments. Both the short and the long cell processes interact with the large collagen fibres that are visible because of a weak autofluorescence. The cell processes appear bended to adhere to the filaments. Scale bar 50 µm. (**B**) L929 fibroblasts and *S. foetidus* collagen filaments. As the thin filaments are not visible in the fluorescence photographs, the transmitted light image is overlapped to the fluorescence. Fibroblasts interact with collagen filaments. Scale bar 20 µm. (**C**) HaCAT keratinocytes and *I. oros* collagen filaments. The cells tend to form the usual sheets while interacting with the collagen filaments that are visible because of a weak autofluorescence. Scale bar 50 µm. (**D**) HaCAT keratinocytes and *S. foetidus* collagen filaments. As the thin filaments are not visible in the fluorescence photographs, the transmitted light image is overlapped to the fluorescence. The sheets of cells are in contact with the collagen filaments. Scale bar 100 µm.

2.3.2. Fibroblast Gene Expression Analysis and Collagen Expression Level

In the early phases after injury, various extracellular matrix proteins have been released during dermal reconstitution in the wound-healing process [50,51]. To assess whether SCFMs can induce ECM production-related gene up-regulation, α1 chain of collagen type I (COL1A1) and the fibronectin gene expression profile were evaluated by qPCR in L929 fibroblasts growing on plates coated with *I. oros* and *S. foetidus* collagen filaments. Rat tail collagen coating was used as a comparison. As shown in Figure 11 (Panel A), a COL1A1 and fibronectin gene expression increase of $1.91 \pm 0.23$ and $1.87 \pm 0.45$ folds, respectively, was observed in cells plated on *I. oros* filaments after 24 h compared with the control. In cells plated on *S. foetidus* filaments, no significant COL1A1 mRNA level fold increase was detected compared to the control, while a fibronectin mRNA fold increase of $1.7 \pm 1.25$ was registered, as has been observed when fibroblasts were grown on rat tail collagen coating, where no significant COL1A1 gene up-regulation was detected, while fibronectin mRNA was $2.2 \pm 0.6$ fold higher than the control sample. The positive effect on collagen production generated by the interaction of L929 fibroblasts with *I. oros* collagen filaments was further confirmed by the biochemical evaluation of the tropo-collagen expression level in the culture medium within 48 h after plating. In our experimental conditions, collagen production was significantly increased by 40% in fibroblasts growing on this biomaterial compared to the control sample, as shown in Figure 11 (Panel B). This increment of collagen secretion appears not significantly different from what was observed in fibroblasts growth on rat tail collagen coating. However, in the L929 plated on *I. oros* filaments, the increase in collagen production is clearly dependent on an up-regulation of COL1A1 gene expression level, while a different mechanism seems to be activated in the case of L929 plated on rat tail collagen, among which a possible contribution from the degradation action of the coating on which the fibroblasts are plated cannot be excluded, where no significant COL1A1 mRNA increase was observed. (Figure 11, panel A, blue bar). To date, the induction of collagen biosynthesis by sponge-derived collagen has only been reported when it is enzymatically hydrolysed into short bioactive peptides [37]. This study for the first time demonstrates a direct effect of intact collagen filaments used as growth scaffolds on the collagen expression level in in vitro fibroblasts. Microscopic analysis did not reveal evident differences with respect to controls, suggesting a possible differentiation to myofibroblasts of L929 cells plated on SCFMs, however further molecular studies may better elucidate the pathway involved in the up-regulation of collagen and fibronectin. However, it is known that fibroblasts can respond to mechanical forces by altering their expression of a specific gene or proteins involved in differentiation and growth [52]. The different response to the collagen gene expression of L929 cell line in the two types of SCFMs could be related to the different porosity of these biomaterials, inducing differences to mechanical loading.

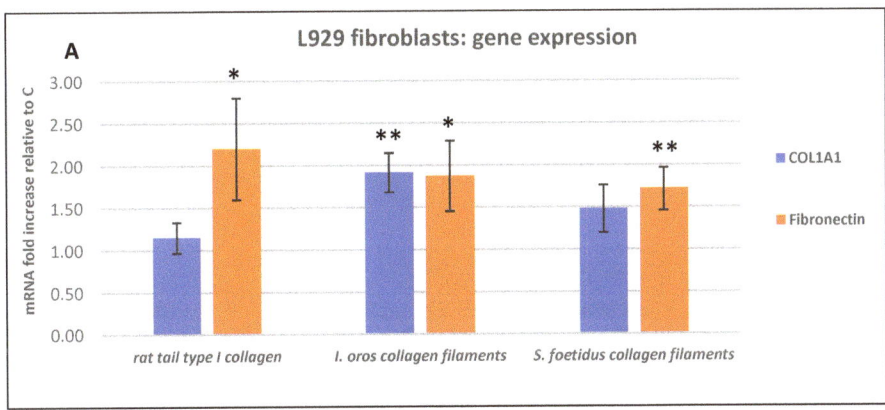

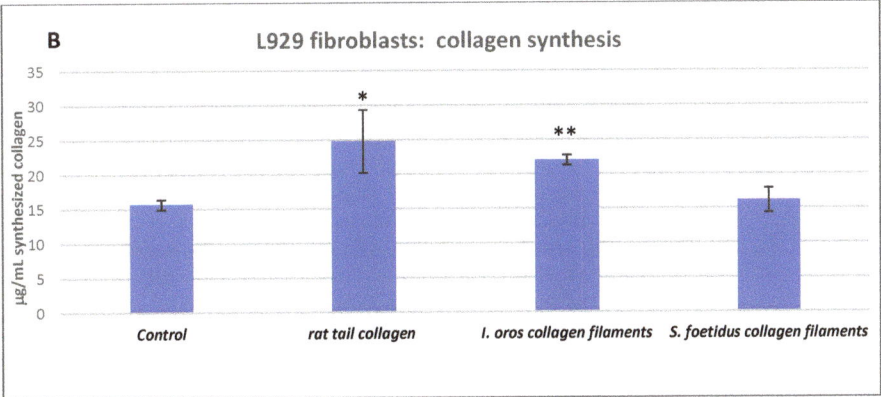

**Figure 11.** Gene expression profile of ECM production-related genes and fibrillar collagen expression level analysis in L929 fibroblast growing on SCMs. (**A**) qPCR evaluation of type I collagen (COL1A1) and fibronectin gene expression (blue and

orange bars, respectively) in L929 mouse fibroblasts growing 24 h on wells precoated with rat tail type I collagen, *I. oros* collagen filaments and *S. foetidus* collagen filaments. Data are expressed as fold increase relative to the control (uncoated wells) and normalised to GAPDH gene. Each bar represents the mean ± S.D. of two independent experiments performed in triplicate. (**B**) Fibrillar collagen synthesis quantification measured using the Sircol colorimetric method as described in Section 4.8.4 of L929 fibroblast growing 48 h on uncoated wells (control) or precoated with rat tail type I collagen, *I. oros* collagen filaments and *S. foetidus* collagen filaments. Statistical analysis results: one-way ANOVA, (**A**) $p < 0.005$; (**B**) $p < 0.001$. Asterisks indicate a significant difference versus the respective control (paired Tukey test, * $p < 0.05$, ** $p < 0.001$).

## 3. Conclusions

In this study, the biomedicine applicative potential of unique collagen structures extracted from keratose sponges belonging to the genera *Ircinia* and *Sarcotragus* has been evaluated for the first time. Their peculiarity derives from an interesting organisation of sponge collagen characterised by high species specificity, where shape and size of the filaments strongly vary in the animal species. Here, we have verified the potential use of two very different types of filaments, derived from *I. oros* and *S. foetidus*, to produce 2D membranes for cell and tissue culture. The data obtained showed that these marine biomaterials, once purified, could be particularly suitable to produce 2D films for wound-dressing applications, as they combine mechanical strength, stability in saline solutions, antioxidant properties and biocompatibility. Particularly, *I. oros*-derived membranes, compared with those derived from *S. foetidus*, showed higher thermal stability and swelling properties. Conversely, *S. foetidus*-derived membranes exhibited higher mechanical resistance, good stability in saline and collagenase solutions and antioxidant properties. Both membrane types can promote cell growth and fibronectin gene up-regulation in fibroblast cells line. *I. oros*-derived membranes could also stimulate a strong collagen production. The peculiarities of these two different marine biomaterials highlighted in this study further confirm the extraordinary applicative potential of these marine sponges in the innovative biomaterials field. The development and optimisation of effective marine aquaculture systems combined with that of the filament extraction processes would allow the large-scale creation of new materials, inspired by nature, for extremely high-performing biomedical use.

## 4. Materials and Methods

### 4.1. Chemicals

All reagents were acquired from SIGMA-ALDRICH (Milan, Italy), unless otherwise stated.

### 4.2. Sponge Sampling

Specimens of *Ircinia oros* (Schmidt, 1864) and *Sarcotragus foetidus* (Schmidt, 1862) were harvested from scuba diving in the area of the Portofino Promontory (Liguria, Italy) at depths of 10–20 m, and were transferred to a laboratory in a thermic bag maintained at 14–15 °C. The sponge specimens were frozen at −20 °C until further processing.

### 4.3. Sponge Collagenous Filaments and Intercellular Collagen Isolation

Frozen sponges were extensively washed in running tap water to remove sand residues, and finally washed with distilled water. The sponge tissues were minced in small pieces with scissors and enzymatically digested, as previously described [18]. The flowsheet of the extraction procedure is shown in Scheme 1. A total of 20 g of cut sponge tissues were treated with 0.1% trypsin in 100 mL of ammonium bicarbonate, pH 8.5, overnight at 37 °C on a horizontal shaker. Subsequently, the dark fluid was removed by filtration with a metallic strainer, and the solid material was suspended in three volumes of cool deionised water and incubated at 5 °C for three days in a rotary disc shaker aliquoted in 50 mL tubes.

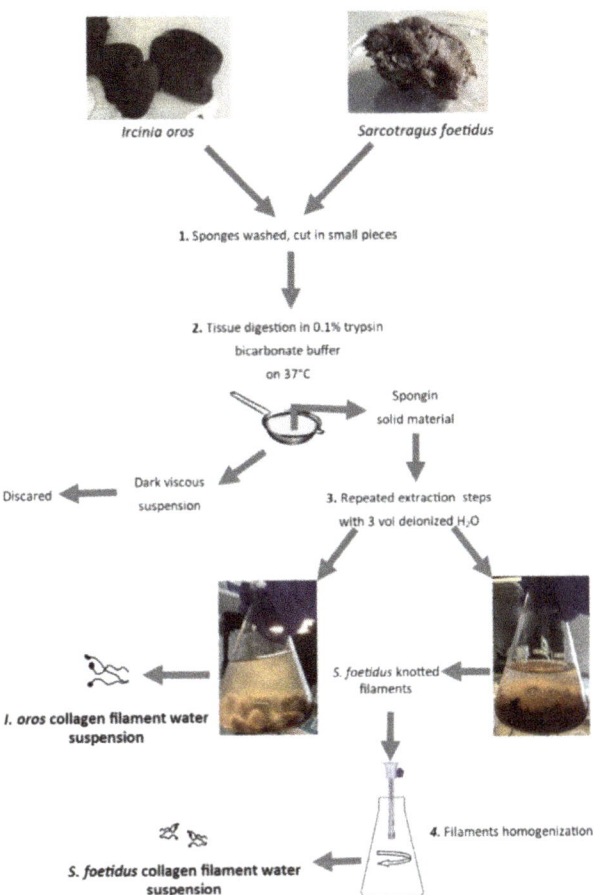

**Scheme 1.** Schematic representation of the extraction procedure used to isolate the collagen filaments from *I. oros* and *S. foetidus* tissue.

This treatment efficiently disperses the intercellular collagen fibrils in water, leaving only the brown spongin scaffold combined with the collagenous filaments in the final residue. These last structures, combined with residual intercellular collagen, were finally separated from the fibrous spongin matrix through different rounds of sedimentation steps under gravity, by mild stirring in large volumes of distilled water and repeated decantations. To obtain a homogenous suspension for *S. foetidus* collagenous filaments, the sample was subjected to a short round of homogenisation steps in ice for 15 s at the end of the extraction using Ultra Turrax T25 basic (IKA-WERKE, Staufen im Breisgau, Germany). During all the extraction phases, the filaments' suspension was never subjected to centrifugation steps to avoid knotting the filaments. The filaments were extensively washed with distilled water to allow them to settle by gravity. The extracted sponge collagenous filament suspensions were conserved at 4 °C. To establish the concentration of the sponge collagen filaments, 1 mL of each suspension was lyophilised, and the dry material was weighed.

### 4.4. Light Microscopy and Environmental Scanning Electron Microscope (ESEM) Observation

*I. oros* and *S. foetidus* tissue fragments, isolated sponge collagenous filaments and sponge collagenous filament membranes (SCFMs) were observed in light microscopy through a stereomicroscope (Nikon SMZ1000, Nikon, Tokyo, Japan) equipped with a digital camera (digital Sight DS-SM, Nikon). Isolated sponge collagenous filaments were coloured with picro-sirius red, as described in [53], in order to prove their collagen composition. For ESEM observation, isolated sponge collagenous filaments and SCFMs were firstly completely dehydrated by soaking them in a series of alcoholic solutions with an increasing concentration of ethanol up to 100%, then graphite was covered and examined. Images of the samples were observed and acquired with an ESEM Vega3–Tescan, type LMU (Tescan Brno s.r.o., Brno, Czech Republic) provided with a microanalyser system EDS-Apollo_x and EDS texture and elemental analytical microscopy software (TEAM™ Analysis System, version 1.0, Coherent Scientific, Thebarton SA). Observation and acquisition of the four SCFMs images were performed with a FESEM Zeiss SUPRA 40 VP (Carl Zeiss AG, Oberkochen, Germany) and its associated software. The fibrillar diameter and the pore areas observed in the collagen membranes were analysed by performing physical measurements on the images of the various membranes acquired with the FESEM, using the ImageJ free software (version 1.53 Rasband, W.S., ImageJ, U.S. National Institutes of Health, Bethesda, MD, USA, https://imagej.nih.gov/ij/, 1997–2016). Means ± S.D. were calculated on at least 40 random measurements of fibril diameter or pore areas performed on each membrane.

### 4.5. SCFs Biochemical Characterisation

#### 4.5.1. Amino Acid Composition

Amino acid analysis was performed using a Jasco X- LC system equipped with an autosampler, Xtreme high pressure pumps, degasser, column oven compartment, fluorescence detector connected to a HP ProDesk processor, as described in [54]. In total, 0.5 mL of each sponge collagenous filament suspensions at 2 mg/mL were hydrolysed in NaOH 2 N for 20 min a 121 °C at 1 Atm and neutralised with equal volume of HCl 2N.

Hydrolysed amino acids were then derivatised by ortho-phthalaldehyde (OPA) and fluorenylmethylchloroformate (FMOC), leading to the formation of derivatives from primary amino acids and secondary amino acids, respectively. Derivatisation was performed accordingly wiyh Jasco autosampler program. The derivatives were detected with a fluorometric detector (emission $\lambda$ = 446 nm – excitation $\lambda$ = 340 nm for OPA derivatives and emission $\lambda$ = 268 nm – excitation $\lambda$ = 308 nm for FMOC derivatives). Amino acid identification was performed via elution times of the obtained derivatives and compared to a mixture of standard amino acids submitted to derivation in identical test conditions. Data processing software (ChromNav, version 2.0, JASCO, Inc., Easton, MD, USA) allowed integration of peak areas for the assessment of the amount of amino acids occurring in the sample.

#### 4.5.2. Glycosaminoglycans (GAGs) Quantification

The quantitative evaluation of the GAGs content in sponge collagen filaments was obtained using the Alcian blue assay as described in [11] and expressed as µg of dry weight of collagen filaments.

#### 4.5.3. Quantitative Analysis of Iron Content

The µg of iron present in sponge collagen filaments was obtained by inductively coupled plasma atomic emission (ICP–AES), as described in [55].

#### 4.5.4. Sodium Dodecyl Sulfate Poly Acrylamide Gel Electrophoresis (SDS-PAGE)

Protein patterns of sponge collagenous filament samples were analysed by SDS–PAGE using Mini-Protean 3 (Bio-Rad Laboratories, Hercules, CA, USA), according to the method previously described [56]. A total of 0.5 mL of each sponge collagen filament suspension normalised at 4 mg/mL were added to an equal to volume of acid-washed glass beads (0.5 mm diameter) and vortexed 3 times for 30 s. Samples were mixed at 1:1 (*v/v*) ratio with 2× gel loading buffer (1 M Tris–HCl buffer (pH 6.8), 10% 2-mercaptoethanol, 40% glycerol, 0.2% bromophenol blue and 20% Sodium Dodecyl Sulfate solution) and was heated at 90 °C for 5 min, and 40 µL were loaded in a 7% of polyacrylamide gel and run at 60 mA with constant amperage. After electrophoresis, the gel was fixed for 1 h a room temperature in a solution containing 10% (*v/v*) acetic acid and 40% (*v/v*) ethanol), washed twice for 10 min at room temperature with distilled water and stained over night at room temperature with a staining solution obtained combing 80 mL of colloidal Coomassie solution (0.1% (*w/v*) Coomassie Brilant blue G250, 2% (*w/v*) ortho-phosphoric acid, 10 (*w/v*) ammonium sulphate) with 20 mL of methanol. Finally, the gel was destained with 5% acetic acid solution and acquired with ChemiDoc Imaging System (Bio-Rad, Milan, Italy). Rat tail type I collagen (0.5 mg/mL) was run alongside as control.

### 4.6. SCFMs Production

SCFMs were obtained by casting 2 mg/mL of sponge collagenous filament suspension in silicone moulds as rectangular (25 × 28 mm) sheets that were filled with 3.3 mL of 2 mg/mL of each suspension, and as rectangular (10 × 45 mm) sheets for mechanical tests, filled with 2.25 mL of 2 mg/mL of each SCF suspension and let completely dry at 37 °C overnight. For DSC analysis, 3 mg of sponge collagenous filaments were left to dry directly on metallic melting pot. For biocompatibility tests, 2 mg/mL of sponge collagenous filament suspension derived from each sponge species and a standard rat tail collagen were used to directly coat 24-well and 96-well plates. In total, 300 µL (for 24-well plates) or 50 µL (for 96-well plates) were placed on the plates and were left to dry at 37 °C overnight. The coated plates were then washed thrice with 100% ethanol, UV sterilised for 20 min and conserved at 4 °C until use.

### 4.7. SCFMs Characterisation

#### 4.7.1. Differential Scanning Calorimetry

DSC was performed using a DSC1 STAR$^e$ System (Mettler-Toledo, Switzerland). About 3 mg dry SCFs were placed in aluminium crucibles and analysed with increasing heat from 0 to 200 °C at a heating rate of 5 °C/min. During the DSC runs, a nitrogen flow at a rate of 20 mL/min was constantly applied.

As a control, 3 mg of a commercial porcine collagen membrane Bio-Gide®(Geistlich Pharma AG, Wolhusen, Switzerland) was dried on a metallic melting pot and analysed on the DSC following the same procedure outlined above.

#### 4.7.2. DMA | DMTA

Dynamic mechanical (DMA) and dynamic mechanical-thermal analysis (DMTA) were carried out on the SCFMs via an MCR 301 rheometer (Anton Paar, GmbH, Graz, Austria) equipped with a universal extensional fixture (UXF) geometry and a CDT-450 chamber. Rectangular specimens (40 mm × 10 mm) were prepared from the samples by using a punch cutter, and each sample thickness was measured via a digital micrometre. A static extensional stress ($\sigma_s$) of 2 MPa was applied for all experiments to ensure the correct sample loading and result reliability.

The linear viscoelastic region (LVER) of the samples was first explored via amplitude sweep tests (AS) at T = 25 ± 1 °C using a frequency ($\nu$) and oscillatory extensional stress ($\sigma$) of 1 Hz and in the range 0.01–10%, respectively. Then, frequency sweep tests (FS) were carried out at T = 25 ± 1 °C with a fixed $\sigma$ = 0.1 MPa, varying the frequency between 0.01 and 10 Hz. Finally, temperature sweep tests (TS) were carried out in the temperature range 25–100 °C with a heating rate of 2 °C/min.

### 4.7.3. In Vitro Degradation Study

To measure the in vitro degradation, each membrane type was weighed (designated as "Wi") and transferred in a test tube containing 10 mL of PBS (pH = 7.4) alone or added with 0.1 mg/mL collagenase from *Clostridium histolyticum* and kept at 37 °C. After 7, 14 and 21 days, the samples were recovered, washed twice with deionised water, dried and weighed again (designated as "Wf"). The percent degradation of the membranes was computed by the following equation:

$$\text{percent degradation (\%)} = (W_i - W_f) / W_i \times 100\%$$

The procedure was carried in triplicate.

To evaluate the release of organic compounds from the SCFMs in saline or collagenase solution withing 21 days, the absorbance at 280 nm was read in the membrane incubation media after 7, 14 and 21 days using PBS or collagenase solution as a blank sample, respectively.

To detect the percentage of collagen material released in saline solution or hydrolysed by collagenase activity from SCFMs during the stability test, 0.4 mL of the incubation media was recovered at 7, 14 and 21 days, hydrolysed in NaOH 2 M at 120 °C at 1 Atm, and finally hydroxyproline content was evaluated as previously described [11].

### 4.7.4. Swelling Test

To evaluate the water binding property of SCFMs, the initial weight of dried membrane (Wi) was measured and then they were soaked in deionised water at 37 °C for 20 h. Finally, the wet weight of the scaffolds (designated as "Ww") was again recorded. A second weighing of the samples after 48 h of incubation without registering a further weight gain ensured that the samples had reached their maximum degree of hydration. Finally, the water content was calculated based on the equation:

$$\text{water content (\%)} = (W_w - W_i) / W_w \times 100\%$$

Experiments were performed in triplicate.

### 4.7.5. DPPH Radical Scavenging Activity

The radical scavenging activity was evaluated on each type of SCFMs as described in [11]. Briefly, 25 × 28 mm membranes were soaked into 500 μL of deionised water, and then embedded into 250 mL of 0.1 mM DPPH in methanol solution (2,2-diphenyl-1-picrylhydrazyl, Calbiochem®, Millipore SpA, Milan, Italy). In the same manner, a negative control sample with deionised water was prepared. The samples were left in incubation for 30 min at room temperature in the dark. Then, the membranes were removed with tweezers, and finally the sample solutions were read at 517 nm using a Beckman spectrophotometer (DU 640). The blank sample was prepared by replacing the DPPH solution with methanol. The antioxidant activity of the samples was evaluated by the inhibition percentage of DPPH radical using the following equation:

$$\text{DPPH radical scavenging activity (\%)} = (A_0 - A)/A_0 \times 100\%$$

where A was sample absorbance rate; A0 was the absorbance of the negative control. The procedure was carried out in triplicate.

## 4.8. SCM Biocompatibility Evaluation

### 4.8.1. Cell Cultures

The L929 mouse fibroblast cell line was obtained by the National Collection of Type Cultures (NCTC), while the human keratinocyte HaCaT cell line (CLS Cell Lines Service, 300493) was obtained by the Cell Lines Service (GmbH, Eppelheim, Germany).

Cells were maintained at 37 °C in a humidified, 5% $CO_2$ atmosphere, in high glucose Dulbecco's modified Eagle's medium (D-MEM) with glutamax (Euroclone, Milan, Italy), which was supplemented with 10% FBS (Euroclone) and with the addition of penicillin/streptomycin as antibiotics.

### 4.8.2. Cell Growth and Cell Adhesion

L929 and HaCaT cell lines were seeded at a density of 50,000 cells/well on 96-well plates that were, or not, pre-coated with each type of SCFs, or rat tail standard collagen as described in Section 4.4 for evaluating cell adhesion. Cells were allowed to adhere for 16 h at 37 °C in complete medium; the medium was subsequently removed, the adhered cells were washed once with PBS to remove the floating unattached ones, and finally MTT (0.5 mg/mL final concentration) test was performed as well to estimate the amount of attached cells when compared to control cells on uncoated wells. Data are means ± S.D. of four independent experiments.

To evaluate cell growth on SCF-coated plates, experiments were performed on 96-well plates. L929 and HaCaT cell lines were both plated at a density of 5000 cells/well on, or not, pre-coated wells. Cells were cultured for 3 days and 6 days at 37 °C in complete medium. At the end of the experiments, the MTT test was once again performed to evaluate cell viability.

For image acquisition, light microscopy cells were seeded at a density of 200,000 cells/well on 12-well plates pre-coated or not, with SCF or rat tail collagen and incubated for 24 h at 37 °C. At the end of the experiment, cells were washed once with PBS, fixed for 30 min at room temperature with 4% paraformaldehyde and then dehydrated in a 70% ethanolic solution. After fixation in buffered 4% paraformaldehyde, cells were rinsed for 5 min three times in PBS (0.1 M, pH 7.4), permeabilised for 10 min in 0.2% Triton-X 100 in PBS and thus rinsed again. Then, they were incubated in a blocking solution with 1% bovine serum albumin and 0.1% Tween 20 in PBS. After rinsing, cells were incubated in a moist dark chamber with Alexa Fluor 488-conjugated Phalloidin (1:40 in PBS, Invitrogen) for 30 min at room temperature. For image acquisition, an inverted optical microscope (IX53 Olympus, Tokyo, Japan) equipped with a CCD camera (U-LH100HG Olympus, Tokyo, Japan) was utilised, and the relative software was used.

### 4.8.3. L929 Fibroblast Gene Expression Analysis

L929 mouse fibroblast cells were seeded at a density of 200,000 cell/well on 12-well plates that were, or not, pre-coated with SCFs, or rat tail standard collagen, and were incubated for 24 h at 37 °C. At the end of the experiment, total RNA was extracted using the RNeasy Mini Kit, (Qiagen, Milan, Italy) according to the manufacturer's instructions.

The cDNA was synthesised by Revert Aid Reverse Transcriptase (Thermo Fisher Scientific, Milan, Italy) using 1 µg of purified total RNA from each sample. Each PCR reaction was performed in 15 µL containing: 1× master mix iQ SYBR®Green (Bio-Rad), 0.2 µM of each primer and 3 µL of a 1:5 diluted reverse transcription reaction buffer. Each sample was analysed in triplicate. The following thermal conditions were used: initial denaturation at 95 °C for 3 min, followed by 45 cycles with denaturation at 95 °C for 15 s and annealing and elongation at 60 °C for 60 s. At the end of each elongation step, fluorescence was measured. Values were normalised to GAPDH (reference gene) mRNA expression. All the PCR primers (Table S1) were designed by means of the Beacon Designer 7.0 software (Premier Biosoft International, Palo Alto, CA, USA) and obtained from TibMolBiol (Genova, Italy). Data analyses were acquired by the DNA Engine Opticon®3 Real-Time Detection System Software program (3.03 version) and, in order to calculate the relative gene expression compared to an untreated (control) calibrator sample, the comparative threshold Ct method was used within the gene expression analysis for iCycler iQ Real Time Detection System Software®(2004 Bio-Rad, Milan, Italy). Data are means ± S.D. of two independent experiments performed in triplicate.

### 4.8.4. L929 Fibroblast Collagen Synthesis Evaluation

Collagen synthesis by L929 fibroblasts was quantified in the cell medium by applying the SIRCOL™ Soluble Collagen Assay (Biocolor Ltd., Carrickfergus, Northern Ireland, UK). Fibroblasts were seeded in tissue culture 12-well plates at a density of 200,000 cells/well that were, or not, pre-coated with each type of SCF and incubated for 48 h at 37 °C.

At the end of the incubation, cell culture media were collected, and the SIRCOL assay was performed according to the manufacturer's instructions. Data are the means ± S.D. of two independent experiments performed in triplicate. Cell culture media alone or pre-incubated for 48 h a 37 °C with the respective coating tested was used as a blank sample for control or for each sample, respectively.

### 4.9. Statistical Analyses

Statistical analyses were performed using one-way ANOVA plus Tukey's post test (GraphPad Software, Inc., San Diego, CA, USA). $p$ values < 0.05 were considered to be significant.

**Supplementary Materials:** The following are available online at https://www.mdpi.com/1660-3397/19/10/563/s1, Figure S1: EDS spectra of *S. foetidus* filaments. Figure S2: *S. foetidus* collagen filament in native tissue. Table S1: S1 primer sequences used in the qPCR analyses.

**Author Contributions:** Conceptualisation, methodology, writing—original draft preparation, M.P.; methodology and software, E.T.; investigation and data curation, A.D., M.C., S.V., S.F., S.A. and D.C.; collection and specie attribution of sponge specimens, M.B.; review, editing and founding acquisition, H.E.; visualisation, I.P.; review and funding acquisition, M.G. All authors have read and agreed to the published version of the manuscript.

**Funding:** This work was supported by University of Genova Funding to M.P. and to DAAD Joint Mobility Program 2017 DAAD-Italy Project "Marine Sponges as Sources for Bioinspired Materials Science". Prog. n. 35474 funding by the Italian Ministry of University and Research (MIUR) to M.G. H.E. was partially supported by MAESTRO 12 project (NCN, Poland) and I.P. by Polish National Agency for Academic Exchange (NAWA) Ulam International Programme PPN/ULM/2020/1/00177.

**Institutional Review Board Statement:** The marine sponge specimens used in this study are not protected species, and were sampled in the protected marine area of Portofino promontory with scientific research authorization n. 4/2012 (prot. No. 409 / 2-1-1).

**Data Availability Statement:** Not applicable.

**Acknowledgments:** The authors are indebted to Laura Negretti for their precious technical support in ESEM analyses; thank Patrizia Arcidiaco, Centro Grandi Strumenti, University of Pavia, Italy, for amino acid analysis; and Francisco Ardini, Department of Chemistry and Industrial Chemistry, for ICP–AES analysis.

**Conflicts of Interest:** The authors declare no conflict of interest.

### References

1. Chevallay, B.; Herbage, D. Collagen-Based Biomaterials as 3D Scaffold for Cell Cultures: Applications for Tissue Engineering and Gene Therapy. *Med. Biol. Eng. Comput.* **2000**, *38*, 211–218. [CrossRef]
2. Jafari, H.; Lista, A.; Siekapen, M.M.; Ghaffari-Bohlouli, P.; Nie, L.; Alimoradi, H.; Shavandi, A. Fish Collagen: Extraction, Characterization, and Applications for Biomaterials Engineering. *Polymers* **2020**, *12*, 2230. [CrossRef]
3. Coppola, D.; Oliviero, M.; Vitale, G.A.; Lauritano, C.; D'Ambra, I.; Iannace, S.; de Pascale, D. Marine Collagen from Alternative and Sustainable Sources: Extraction, Processing and Applications. *Mar. Drugs* **2020**, *18*, 214. [CrossRef] [PubMed]
4. Lim, Y.-S.; Ok, Y.-J.; Hwang, S.-Y.; Kwak, J.-Y.; Yoon, S. Marine Collagen as A Promising Biomaterial for Biomedical Applications. *Mar. Drugs* **2019**, *17*, 467. [CrossRef] [PubMed]
5. Khrunyk, Y.; Lach, S.; Petrenko, I.; Ehrlich, H. Progress in Modern Marine Biomaterials Research. *Mar. Drugs* **2020**, *18*, 589. [CrossRef] [PubMed]
6. Granito, R.N.; Custódio, M.R.; Rennó, A.C.M. Natural Marine Sponges for Bone Tissue Engineering: The State of Art and Future Perspectives. *J Biomed. Mater. Res. Part B Appl. Biomater.* **2017**, *105*, 1717–1727. [CrossRef]

7. Parisi, J.R.; Fernandes, K.R.; Avanzi, I.R.; Dorileo, B.P.; Santana, A.F.; Andrade, A.L.; Gabbai-Armelin, P.R.; Fortulan, C.A.; Trichês, E.S.; Granito, R.N.; et al. Incorporation of Collagen from Marine Sponges (Spongin) into Hydroxyapatite Samples: Characterization and In Vitro Biological Evaluation. *Mar. Biotechnol.* **2019**, *21*, 30–37. [CrossRef] [PubMed]
8. Parisi, J.R.; Fernandes, K.R.; de Almeida Cruz, M.; Avanzi, I.R.; de França Santana, A.; do Vale, G.C.A.; de Andrade, A.L.M.; de Góes, C.P.; Fortulan, C.A.; de Sousa Trichês, E.; et al. Evaluation of the In Vivo Biological Effects of Marine Collagen and Hydroxyapatite Composite in a Tibial Bone Defect Model in Rats. *Mar. Biotechnol.* **2020**, *22*, 357–366. [CrossRef]
9. Fernandes, K.R.; Parisi, J.R.; Magri, A.M.P.; Kido, H.W.; Gabbai-Armelin, P.R.; Fortulan, C.A.; Zanotto, E.D.; Peitl, O.; Granito, R.N.; Renno, A.C.M. Influence of the Incorporation of Marine Spongin into a Biosilicate®: An in Vitro Study. *J. Mater. Sci. Mater. Med.* **2019**, *30*, 64. [CrossRef]
10. Langasco, R.; Cadeddu, B.; Formato, M.; Lepedda, A.J.; Cossu, M.; Giunchedi, P.; Pronzato, R.; Rassu, G.; Manconi, R.; Gavini, E. Natural Collagenic Skeleton of Marine Sponges in Pharmaceutics: Innovative Biomaterial for Topical Drug Delivery. *Mater. Sci. Eng. C* **2017**, *70*, 710–720. [CrossRef]
11. Pozzolini, M.; Scarfi, S.; Gallus, L.; Castellano, M.; Vicini, S.; Cortese, K.; Gagliani, M.C.; Bertolino, M.; Costa, G.; Giovine, M. Production, Characterization and Biocompatibility Evaluation of Collagen Membranes Derived from Marine Sponge Chondrosia Reniformis Nardo, 1847. *Mar. Drugs* **2018**, *16*, 111. [CrossRef]
12. Green, D.; Howard, D.; Yang, X.; Kelly, M.; Oreffo, R.O.C. Natural Marine Sponge Fiber Skeleton: A Biomimetic Scaffold for Human Osteoprogenitor Cell Attachment, Growth, and Differentiation. *Tissue Eng.* **2003**, *9*, 1159–1166. [CrossRef]
13. Pozzolini, M.; Bruzzone, F.; Berilli, V.; Mussino, F.; Cerrano, C.; Benatti, U.; Giovine, M. Molecular Characterization of a Nonfibrillar Collagen from the Marine Sponge Chondrosia Reniformis Nardo 1847 and Positive Effects of Soluble Silicates on Its Expression. *Mar. Biotechnol.* **2012**, *14*, 281–293. [CrossRef]
14. Ehrlich, H.; Wysokowski, M.; Żółtowska-Aksamitowska, S.; Petrenko, I.; Jesionowski, T. Collagens of Poriferan Origin. *Mar. Drugs* **2018**, *16*, 79. [CrossRef] [PubMed]
15. Pozzolini, M.; Scarfi, S.; Mussino, F.; Ferrando, S.; Gallus, L.; Giovine, M. Molecular Cloning, Characterization, and Expression Analysis of a Prolyl 4-Hydroxylase from the Marine Sponge Chondrosia Reniformis. *Mar. Biotechnol.* **2015**, *17*, 393–407. [CrossRef] [PubMed]
16. Pozzolini, M.; Scarfi, S.; Gallus, L.; Ferrando, S.; Cerrano, C.; Giovine, M. Silica-Induced Fibrosis: An Ancient Response from the Early Metazoans. *J. Exp. Biol.* **2017**, *220*, 4007–4015. [CrossRef] [PubMed]
17. Soest, R.W.M.V.; Boury-Esnault, N.; Vacelet, J.; Dohrmann, M.; Erpenbeck, D.; Voogd, N.J.D.; Santodomingo, N.; Vanhoorne, B.; Kelly, M.; Hooper, J.N.A. Global Diversity of Sponges (Porifera). *PLoS ONE* **2012**, *7*, e35105. [CrossRef]
18. Gross, J.; Sokal, Z.; Rougvie, M. Structural and Chemical Studies on the Connective Tissue of Marine Sponges. *J. Histochem. Cytochem.* **1956**, *4*, 227–246. [CrossRef] [PubMed]
19. Jesionowski, T.; Norman, M.; Żółtowska-Aksamitowska, S.; Petrenko, I.; Joseph, Y.; Ehrlich, H. Marine Spongin: Naturally Prefabricated 3D Scaffold-Based Biomaterial. *Mar. Drugs* **2018**, *16*, 88. [CrossRef]
20. Petrenko, I.; Summers, A.P.; Simon, P.; Żółtowska-Aksamitowska, S.; Motylenko, M.; Schimpf, C.; Rafaja, D.; Roth, F.; Kummer, K.; Brendler, E.; et al. Extreme Biomimetics: Preservation of Molecular Detail in Centimeter-Scale Samples of Biological Meshes Laid down by Sponges. *Sci. Adv.* **2019**, *5*, eaax2805. [CrossRef]
21. Garrone, R.; Vacelet, J.; Junqua, S.; Robert, L.; Huca, X. Peculiar Collagen Formation-Filaments of Horny Sponges Ircinia-Ultrastructural, Physicochemical and Biochemical Study. *J. Microsc. -Oxf.* **1973**, *17*, 241–260.
22. Junqua, S.; Robert, L.; Garrone, R.; Ceccatty, M.P.D.; Vacelet, J. Biochemical and Morphological Studies on Collagens of Horny Sponges. Ircinia Filaments Compared to Spongines. *Connect. Tissue Res.* **1974**, *2*, 193–203. [CrossRef] [PubMed]
23. Kölliker, A. *Icones Histiologicae; Oder, Atlas Der Vergleichenden Gewebelehre*, 1st ed.; Wilhel Engelmann: Leipzig, Germany, 1864; pp. 46–59.
24. Towe, K.M.; Rützler, K. Lepidocrocite Iron Mineralization in Keratose Sponge Granules. *Science* **1968**, *162*, 268–269. [CrossRef] [PubMed]
25. Tsurkan, D.; Simon, P.; Schimpf, C.; Motylenko, M.; Rafaja, D.; Roth, F.; Inosov, D.S.; Makarova, A.A.; Stepniak, I.; Petrenko, I.; et al. Extreme Biomimetics: Designing of the First Nanostructured 3D Spongin–Atacamite Composite and Its Application. *Adv. Mater.* **2021**. [CrossRef] [PubMed]
26. Manconi, R.; Pansini, M.; Pronzato, R. *Fauna d'Italia Vol. XLVI - Porifera I - Calcarea, Demospongiae (partim), Hexactinellida, Homoscleromorpha*, 1st ed.; Calderini: Bologna, Italy, 2011; pp. 297–308.
27. Bonfrate, V.; Manno, D.; Serra, A.; Salvatore, L.; Sannino, A.; Buccolieri, A.; Serra, T.; Giancane, G. Enhanced Electrical Conductivity of Collagen Films through Long-Range Aligned Iron Oxide Nanoparticles. *J. Colloid Interface Sci.* **2017**, *501*, 185–191. [CrossRef]
28. Zhuang, J.; Lin, S.; Dong, L.; Cheng, K.; Weng, W. Magnetically Assisted Electrodeposition of Aligned Collagen Coatings. *ACS Biomater. Sci. Eng.* **2018**, *4*, 1528–1535. [CrossRef]
29. Mertens, M.E.; Hermann, A.; Bühren, A.; Olde-Damink, L.; Möckel, D.; Gremse, F.; Ehling, J.; Kiessling, F.; Lammers, T. Iron Oxide-Labeled Collagen Scaffolds for Non-Invasive MR Imaging in Tissue Engineering. *Adv. Funct. Mater.* **2014**, *24*, 754–762. [CrossRef]
30. Burjanadze, T.V.; Veis, A. A Thermodynamic Analysis of the Contribution of Hydroxyproline to the Structural Stability of the Collagen Triple Helix. *Connect. Tissue Res.* **1997**, *36*, 347–365. [CrossRef]

31. Ehrlich, H.; Deutzmann, R.; Brunner, E.; Cappellini, E.; Koon, H.; Solazzo, C.; Yang, Y.; Ashford, D.; Thomas-Oates, J.; Lubeck, M.; et al. Mineralization of the Metre-Long Biosilica Structures of Glass Sponges Is Templated on Hydroxylated Collagen. *Nat. Chem* **2010**, *2*, 1084–1088. [CrossRef]
32. Yamauchi, M.; Sricholpech, M. Lysine Post-Translational Modifications of Collagen. *Essays Biochem.* **2012**, *52*, 113–133. [CrossRef]
33. Garrone, R.; Huc, A.; Junqua, S. Fine Structure and Physicochemical Studies on the Collagen of the Marine Sponge Chondrosia Reniformis Nardo. *J. Ultrastruct. Res.* **1975**, *52*, 261–275. [CrossRef]
34. Swatschek, D.; Schatton, W.; Kellermann, J.; Müller, W.E.G.; Kreuter, J. Marine Sponge Collagen: Isolation, Characterization and Effects on the Skin Parameters Surface-PH, Moisture and Sebum. *Eur. J. Pharm. Biopharm.* **2002**, *53*, 107–113. [CrossRef]
35. Ghosh, A.; Grosvenor, A.J.; Dyer, J.M. Marine Spongia Collagens: Protein Characterization and Evaluation of Hydrogel Films. *J. Appl. Polym. Sci.* **2019**, *136*, 47996. [CrossRef]
36. Carvalho, A.M.; Marques, A.P.; Silva, T.H.; Reis, R.L. Evaluation of the Potential of Collagen from Codfish Skin as a Biomaterial for Biomedical Applications. *Mar. Drugs* **2018**, *16*, 495. [CrossRef] [PubMed]
37. Pozzolini, M.; Millo, E.; Oliveri, C.; Mirata, S.; Salis, A.; Damonte, G.; Arkel, M.; Scarfì, S. Elicited ROS Scavenging Activity, Photoprotective, and Wound-Healing Properties of Collagen-Derived Peptides from the Marine Sponge Chondrosia Reniformis. *Mar. Drugs* **2018**, *16*, 465. [CrossRef]
38. Srivatsan, K.V.; Lakra, R.; Purna Sai, K.; Kiran, M.S. Effect of bimetallic iron:zinc nanoparticles on collagen stabilization. *J. Mater. Chem. B* **2016**, *4*, 1437–1447. [CrossRef]
39. Desimone, M.F.; Hélary, C.; Rietveld, I.B.; Bataille, I.; Mosser, G.; Giraud-Guille, M.-M.; Livage, J.; Coradin, T. Silica–Collagen Bionanocomposites as Three-Dimensional Scaffolds for Fibroblast Immobilization. *Acta Biomater.* **2010**, *6*, 3998–4004. [CrossRef] [PubMed]
40. Jang, D.; Idrobo, J.-C.; Laoui, T.; Karnik, R. Water and Solute Transport Governed by Tunable Pore Size Distributions in Nanoporous Graphene Membranes. *ACS Nano* **2017**, *11*, 10042–10052. [CrossRef]
41. Dodero, A.; Scarfì, S.; Pozzolini, M.; Vicini, S.; Alloisio, M.; Castellano, M. Alginate-Based Electrospun Membranes Containing ZnO Nanoparticles as Potential Wound Healing Patches: Biological, Mechanical, and Physicochemical Characterization. *Acs Appl. Mater. Interfaces* **2020**, *12*, 3371–3381. [CrossRef] [PubMed]
42. Sionkowska, A.; Grabska, S. Preparation and Characterization of 3D Collagen Materials with Magnetic Properties. *Polym. Test.* **2017**, *62*, 382–391. [CrossRef]
43. Schäfer, M.; Werner, S. Oxidative Stress in Normal and Impaired Wound Repair. *Pharmacol. Res.* **2008**, *58*, 165–171. [CrossRef]
44. Merrell, J.G.; McLaughlin, S.W.; Tie, L.; Laurencin, C.T.; Chen, A.F.; Nair, L.S. Curcumin Loaded Poly(ε-Caprolactone) Nanofibers: Diabetic Wound Dressing with Antioxidant and Anti-Inflammatory Properties. *Clin. Exp. Pharm. Physiol.* **2009**, *36*, 1149–1156. [CrossRef]
45. Mehbub, M.F.; Lei, J.; Franco, C.; Zhang, W. Marine Sponge Derived Natural Products between 2001 and 2010: Trends and Opportunities for Discovery of Bioactives. *Mar. Drugs* **2014**, *12*, 4539–4577. [CrossRef]
46. Leal, M.C.; Puga, J.; Serôdio, J.; Gomes, N.C.M.; Calado, R. Trends in the Discovery of New Marine Natural Products from Invertebrates over the Last Two Decades – Where and What Are We Bioprospecting? *PLoS ONE* **2012**, *7*, e30580. [CrossRef]
47. Deshmukh, A.R.; Gupta, A.; Kim, B.S. Ultrasound Assisted Green Synthesis of Silver and Iron Oxide Nanoparticles Using Fenugreek Seed Extract and Their Enhanced Antibacterial and Antioxidant Activities. *BioMed Res. Int.* **2019**, *2019*, 1714358. [CrossRef]
48. Lin, Z.; Solomon, K.L.; Zhang, X.; Pavlos, N.J.; Abel, T.; Willers, C.; Dai, K.; Xu, J.; Zheng, Q.; Zheng, M. In Vitro Evaluation of Natural Marine Sponge Collagen as a Scaffold for Bone Tissue Engineering. *Int. J. Biol. Sci.* **2011**, *7*, 968–977. [CrossRef]
49. Tal, H.; Moses, O.; Kozlovsky, A.; Nemcovsky, C. Bioresorbable Collagen Membranes for Guided Bone Regeneration. In *Bone Regeneration*; Tal, H., Ed.; InTech: Rijeka, Croatia, 2012; pp. 111–134.
50. Rousselle, P.; Montmasson, M.; Garnier, C. Extracellular Matrix Contribution to Skin Wound Re-Epithelialization. *Matrix Biol.* **2019**, *75–76*, 12–26. [CrossRef]
51. Eming, S.A.; Martin, P.; Tomic-Canic, M. Wound Repair and Regeneration: Mechanisms, Signaling, and Translation. *Sci. Transl. Med.* **2014**, *6*, 265sr6. [CrossRef]
52. Brown, R.A.; Prajapati, R.; McGrouther, D.A.; Yannas, I.V.; Eastwood, M. Tensional homeostasis in dermal fibroblasts: Mechanical responses to mechanical loading in three-dimensional substrates. *J Cell Physiol* **1998**, *175*, 323–332. [CrossRef]
53. Pozzolini, M.; Ferrando, S.; Gallus, L.; Gambardella, C.; Ghignone, S.; Giovine, M. Aquaporin in Chondrosia Reniformis Nardo, 1847 and Its Possible Role in the Interaction Between Cells and Engulfed Siliceous Particles. *Biol. Bull.* **2016**, *230*, 220–232. [CrossRef]
54. Tonelli, F.; Cotti, S.; Leoni, L.; Besio, R.; Gioia, R.; Marchese, L.; Giorgetti, S.; Villani, S.; Gistelinck, C.; Wagener, R.; et al. Crtap and P3h1 Knock out Zebrafish Support Defective Collagen Chaperoning as the Cause of Their Osteogenesis Imperfecta Phenotype. *Matrix Biol.* **2020**, *90*, 40–60. [CrossRef]
55. Ardini, F.; Soggia, F.; Abelmoschi, M.L.; Magi, E.; Grotti, M. Ionomic profiling of Nicotiana langsdorffii wild-type and mutant genotypes exposed to abiotic stresses. *Anal. Bioanal. Chem.* **2013**, *405*, 665–677. [CrossRef]
56. Laemmli, U.K. Cleavage of Structural Proteins during the Assembly of the Head of Bacteriophage T4. *Nature* **1970**, *227*, 680–685. [CrossRef]

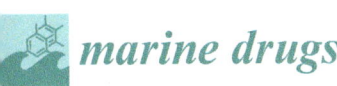 

Article

# Fish Collagen Peptides Protect against Cisplatin-Induced Cytotoxicity and Oxidative Injury by Inhibiting MAPK Signaling Pathways in Mouse Thymic Epithelial Cells

Won Hoon Song [1,2,†], Hye-Yoon Kim [2,3,†], Ye Seon Lim [2,3], Seon Yeong Hwang [2,3], Changyong Lee [2,3], Do Young Lee [2,3], Yuseok Moon [2,4], Yong Jung Song [2,5] and Sik Yoon [2,3,*]

1. Department of Urology, Pusan National University Yangsan Hospital, Yangsan 626-870, Korea; luchen99@hanmail.net
2. Immune Reconstitution Research Center of Medical Research Institute, Pusan National University College of Medicine, Yangsan 626-870, Korea; solarhy77@naver.com (H.-Y.K.); yeseonlim@pusan.ac.kr (Y.S.L.); anatomy2017@pusan.ac.kr (S.Y.H.); qhrrn79@naver.com (C.L.); osldy@naver.com (D.Y.L.); moon@pusan.ac.kr (Y.M.); gynsong@gmail.com (Y.J.S.)
3. Department of Anatomy and Convergence Medical Sciences, Pusan National University College of Medicine, Yangsan 626-870, Korea
4. Department of Convergence Medical Sciences, Pusan National University College of Medicine, Yangsan 626-870, Korea
5. Department of Obstetrics and Gynecology, Pusan National University College of Medicine, Yangsan 626-870, Korea
* Correspondence: sikyoon@pusan.ac.kr; Tel.: +82-51-5108044; Fax: +82-51-5108049
† These authors contributed equally to this work.

**Citation:** Song, W.H.; Kim, H.-Y.; Lim, Y.S.; Hwang, S.Y.; Lee, C.; Lee, D.Y.; Moon, Y.; Song, Y.J.; Yoon, S. Fish Collagen Peptides Protect against Cisplatin-Induced Cytotoxicity and Oxidative Injury by Inhibiting MAPK Signaling Pathways in Mouse Thymic Epithelial Cells. *Mar. Drugs* 2022, 20, 232. https://doi.org/10.3390/md20040232

Academic Editor: Bill J. Baker

Received: 18 February 2022
Accepted: 24 March 2022
Published: 28 March 2022

**Publisher's Note:** MDPI stays neutral with regard to jurisdictional claims in published maps and institutional affiliations.

**Copyright:** © 2022 by the authors. Licensee MDPI, Basel, Switzerland. This article is an open access article distributed under the terms and conditions of the Creative Commons Attribution (CC BY) license (https://creativecommons.org/licenses/by/4.0/).

**Abstract:** Thymic epithelial cells (TECs) account for the most abundant and dominant stromal component of the thymus, where T cells mature. Oxidative- or cytotoxic-stress associated injury in TECs, a significant and common problem in many clinical settings, may cause a compromised thymopoietic capacity of TECs, resulting in clinically significant immune deficiency disorders or impairment in the adaptive immune response in the body. The present study demonstrated that fish collagen peptides (FCP) increase cell viability, reduce intracellular levels of reactive oxygen species (ROS), and impede apoptosis by repressing the expression of Bax and Bad and the release of cytochrome c, and by upregulating the expression of Bcl-2 and Bcl-xL in cisplatin-treated TECs. These inhibitory effects of FCP on TEC damage occur via the suppression of ROS generation and MAPK (p38 MAPK, JNK, and ERK) activity. Taken together, our data suggest that FCP can be used as a promising protective agent against cytotoxic insults- or ROS-mediated TEC injury. Furthermore, our findings provide new insights into a therapeutic approach for the future application of FCP in the prevention and treatment of various types of oxidative- or cytotoxic stress-related cell injury in TECs as well as age-related or acute thymus involution.

**Keywords:** cisplatin; fish collagen peptides; thymic epithelial cells; reactive oxygen species; apoptosis; MAPK (p38 MAPK, JNK, and ERK) pathway

## 1. Introduction

The thymus is the primary lymphoid organ composed of multiple cell types creating a unique microenvironment for producing immunocompetent T cells from bone marrow-derived T cell progenitors/precursors, thereby playing a crucial role in the development of the host adaptive immune system. T cells are not only trained to recognize and eliminate foreign antigens during development in the thymus, but also to tolerate self-antigens through positive and negative selection. This thymic education of T cells is mainly orchestrated by thymic epithelial cells (TECs) that play a pivotal role in the multistep processes, including the homing and clonal expansion, survival, and maturation of the immature T cells [1].

The thymus is a peculiar organ in our body that undergoes progressive involution or atrophy with age. It is called age-related or physiological thymic involution (or atrophy), resulting in a deterioration of its T cell generation ability. In addition, many stimuli including infection, radiation, stress, toxic substances, pregnancy, steroid hormones, malnutrition, immunosuppressive drugs, such as cyclosporine and dexamethasone, chemotherapeutic agents, such as cyclophosphamide, cisplatin, methotrexate, and taxanes, dangerous substances, and harmful biological processes can cause a condition known as acute or accidental thymic involution (or atrophy) [2,3]. Regardless of the type and causative agents of thymic involution, it is usually connected with primary TEC injury [4–6], ultimately leading to a decreased thymus production and outward migration of mature T cells, and increased severity and susceptibility to infections, cancer, and autoimmune diseases [7–9].

Oxidative stress is a disturbance in the balance between reactive oxygen species (ROS) activities and antioxidant defense mechanisms associated with detoxification of the harmful effects of ROS, which affects the induction of thymic involution [10]. Many endogenous and exogenous stimuli trigger ROS production, damaging DNA, cellular proteins/lipids, and cell membrane, and inducing an inflammatory response, leading to apoptotic or necrotic cell death [11].

Chemotherapies with platinum-based anticancer drugs are standard treatments for various cancers, including ovarian cancer, cervical cancer, lung cancer, head and neck cancer, bladder cancer, and lymphoma [12,13]. Cisplatin was the first widely used platinum-based chemotherapy drug and has been the basis agent for treating a broad spectrum of cancers [14]. However, despite its huge potential as a chemotherapy regimen, cisplatin has been linked to several toxic side effects, including nephrotoxicity, lymphosuppression, myelosuppression, ototoxicity, cardiotoxicity, hepatotoxicity, and neurotoxicity, through various mechanisms, such as oxidative stress, apoptosis, inflammation, and autophagy [15,16]. Cisplatin mainly displays its cytotoxic activity by tipping the redox scale favoring oxidative stress, leading to mitochondrial membrane permeabilization and DNA damage [17,18].

Currently, fish collagen peptides (FCP) are gaining increasing attention due to their purported safety [19–21] and diverse biological activities, such as antioxidant activity [22,23], neuroprotective effects [24], anti-aging effects [25], and wound healing effects [26]. Furthermore, oral administration of FCP was reported to diminish the production of pro-inflammatory cytokines, such as tumor necrosis factor-α (TNF-α) and nitric oxide (NO) in rat synoviocytes, and NO and C-reactive protein in diabetic patients with chronic inflammation [27,28]. However, there are still many questions left unanswered about the efficacy of FCP in protecting TEC injury.

Here, the present study shows that FCP protects TECs against cisplatin-induced cytotoxic and oxidative injury by inhibiting MAPK signal transduction pathways.

## 2. Results

*2.1. FCP Promote Cell Proliferation and Inhibit Cisplatin-Induced Cytotoxicity*

A WST-1-based colorimetric cell proliferation assay was used evaluate the ability of FCP to facilitate cell proliferation. Treatment of TECs with FCP for 24 h significantly enhanced cell proliferation at concentrations of 0.01, 0.05, 0.08, 0.1 and 0.15%, by 19.6% ($p < 0.01$), 23.7% ($p < 0.001$), 27.1% ($p < 0.001$), 19.3% ($p < 0.01$), and 11.2% ($p < 0.05$), respectively, compared with the control (Figure 1). At 48 h, the rates of cell proliferation in the FCP-treated group versus the control at concentrations of 0.01%, 0.05%, 0.08%, 0.1%, 0.15%, and 0.2% were greatly increased by 30.9% ($p < 0.001$), 44.8% ($p < 0.001$), 56% ($p < 0.001$), 38.6% ($p < 0.001$), 21.7% ($p < 0.01$), and 12.8% ($p < 0.01$), respectively, compared with the control (Figure 1).

Cellular cytotoxicity and morphology were assessed to examine the level of cisplatin-induced cell injury. Here, the WST-1-based colorimetric cell viability assay after treatment with cisplatin for 24 h at concentrations of 5, 10, and 20 µM revealed a significant decrease in cell number by 26.7% ($p < 0.01$), 36.9% ($p < 0.01$), and 57.9% ($p < 0.001$), respectively, relative to the control (Figure 2). Cisplatin treatment for 48 h at concentrations of 5, 10, and 20 µM strongly reduced cell viability by 61.3% ($p < 0.001$), 87.9% ($p < 0.001$), and 100% ($p < 0.001$), respectively, compared with the control (Figure 2). These cytotoxicity results were also concurrent with the morphological changes observed by phase contrast microscopy (Figure 2), revealing dose- and time-dependent cytotoxic effects of cisplatin in TECs.

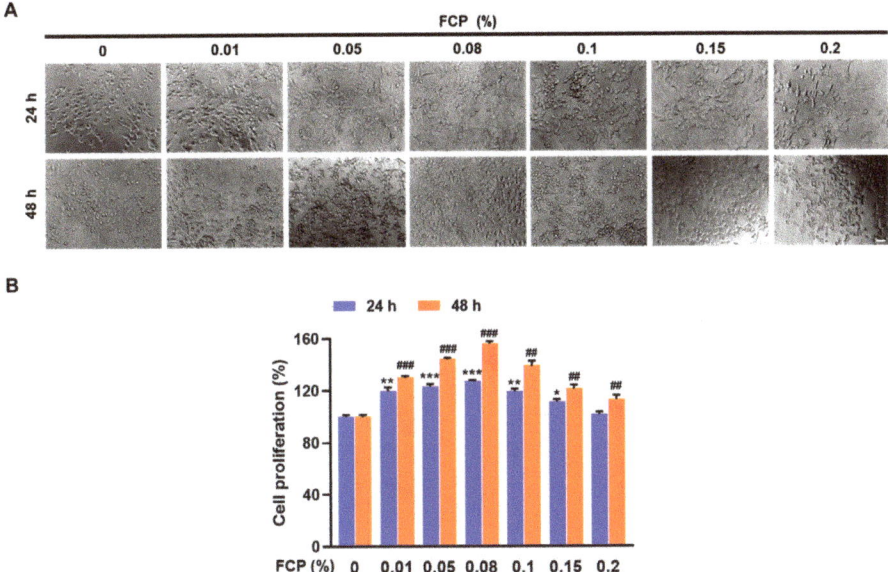

**Figure 1.** Stimulatory effects of FCP on cell proliferation. Proliferation of TECs was measured by phase contrast microscopy (**A**) and cell viability assay (**B**) as described in Materials and Methods. The treatment of TECs with FCP for 24 and 48 h significantly enhanced cell proliferation. Results are presented as the means ± SD of three independent experiments. * $p < 0.05$, ** $p < 0.01$, *** $p < 0.001$ vs. the control at 24 h; ## $p < 0.01$, ### $p < 0.001$ vs. the control at 48 h. Scale bar = 50 µm.

Subsequently, the protective effect of FCP was investigated on cisplatin-induced cytotoxicity in TECs by WST-1 using the phase contrast microscopic assays. As shown in Figure 3, exposure of TECs to cisplatin at concentrations of 5, 7.5, 10 and 15 µM for 24 h led to a reduced cell viability, by 22.5% ($p < 0.01$), 30.3% ($p < 0.001$), 43.1% ($p < 0.001$), and 58.7% ($p < 0.001$), respectively, compared with the control. However, 0.08% FCP pretreatment prior to cisplatin treatment (5, 7.5, 10, and 15 µM for 24 h) resulted in the enhancement of cellular viability, by 41.1% ($p < 0.001$), 42.5% ($p < 0.01$), 36.7% ($p < 0.01$), and 24.04% ($p < 0.001$), respectively, compared with the cisplatin alone treatment group. This result, therefore, indicates the protective role of FCP against cisplatin-induced TEC damage (Figure 3).

Furthermore, molecular mechanisms underlying the protective effect of FCP on TECs injured by cisplatin were explored by analyzing the expression of apoptosis- and cell cycle-related proteins. Cisplatin treatment significantly reduced the expression of anti-apoptotic molecules, Bcl-2 and Bcl-xL, by 24.4% ($p < 0.001$) and 21.2% ($p < 0.001$), respectively, and enhanced the expression of pro-apoptotic molecules, Bax, Bad and cytochrome-c, by 40.1% ($p < 0.001$), 20.8% ($p < 0.001$), and 40.5% ($p < 0.01$), respectively (Figure 4A), whereas it significantly suppressed the expression of the key cell cycle regulatory molecules, cyclin D1 and CDK1 proteins by 52.1% ($p < 0.001$) and 35.5% ($p < 0.001$), respectively, compared with the untreated control (Figure 4B). Notably, all these cisplatin-induced alterations in the expression of apoptosis- and cell cycle-related proteins almost returned to their normal levels after 0.08% FCP pretreatment for 24 h. The cisplatin-induced downregulated expression of Bcl-2, Bcl-xL, cyclin D1, and CDK1 proteins increased due to FCP by 26% ($p < 0.001$),

22.6% ($p < 0.01$), 29.9% ($p < 0.05$), and 42.8% ($p < 0.001$), respectively, (Figure 4A,B), whereas the cisplatin-induced upregulated expression of Bax, Bad and cytochrome-c was reversed following exposure to FCP by 58% ($p < 0.001$), 39.3% ($p < 0.001$), and 29% ($p < 0.001$), respectively, compared with the cisplatin alone treatment group (Figure 4A).

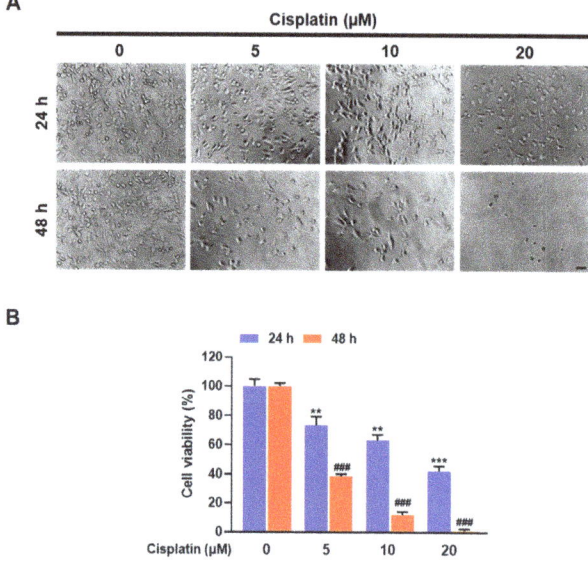

**Figure 2.** Cytotoxic effects of cisplatin on TECs were measured by phase contrast microscopy (**A**) and cell cytotoxicity assay (**B**) as described in Materials and Methods. The treatment of TECs with 5, 10, and 20 µM cisplatin for 24 and 48 h significantly attenuated cell viability. Results are presented as the means ± SD of three independent experiments. ** $p < 0.01$, *** $p < 0.001$ vs. the control at 24 h; ### $p < 0.001$ vs. the control at 48 h. Scale bar = 50 µm.

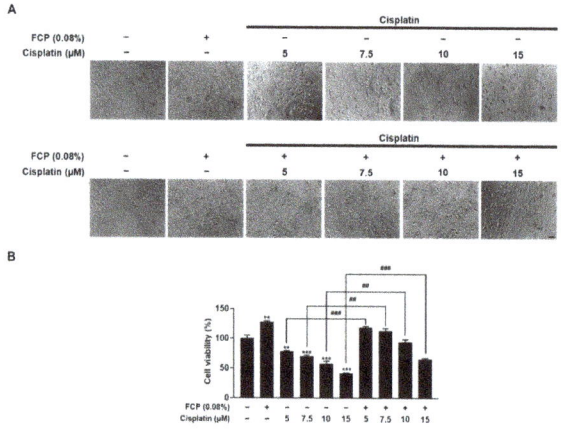

**Figure 3.** Protective effect of FCP on cisplatin-induced cytotoxicity in TECs. Cell viability was measured by phase contrast microscopy (**A**) and WST-1 assay (**B**) in TECs as described in Materials and Methods. The decreased cell number induced by cisplatin treatment (5, 7.5, 10, and 15 µM) was significantly restored by treatment with 0.08% FCP for 24 h. Results are presented as the means ± SD of three independent experiments. ** $p < 0.01$, *** $p < 0.001$ vs. the control. ## $p < 0.01$, ### $p < 0.001$ vs. the cisplatin alone-treated group. Scale bar = 50 µm.

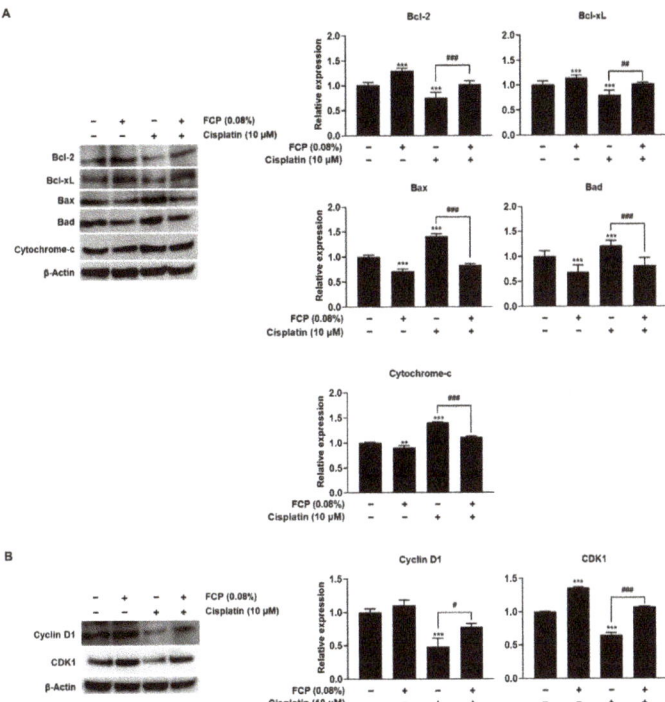

**Figure 4.** Western blot analysis on the inhibitory effects of FCP on cisplatin-induced altered expression of apoptosis- and proliferation-related proteins in TECs. FCP pretreatment in cisplatin alone-treated TECs significantly enhanced the levels of Bcl-2 and Bcl-xL, reduced the levels of Bad, Bax, and cytochrome-c (**A**), and elevated the levels of cyclin D1 and CDK1 compar with the cisplatin alone-treated group (**B**). Results are presented as the means ± SD of three independent experiments. ** $p < 0.01$, *** $p < 0.001$ vs. the control. # $p < 0.05$, ## $p < 0.01$, ### $p < 0.001$ vs. the cisplatin alone-treated group.

### 2.2. FCP Attenuate Cisplatin-Induced ROS Generation

To measure changes in the cellular levels of ROS in response to cisplatin with or without FCP pretreatment, TECs were pretreated with 0.08% FCP for 24 h followed by cisplatin exposure at 10 μM for 24 h (Figure 5A,B). Treatment with cisplatin significantly increased the ROS level as detected by fluorescence microscopy using the oxidant-sensing fluorescent probe 2′,7′-dichlorodihydrofluorescein diacetate (DCFH-DA) by 34.4% ($p < 0.05$) compared with the control (Figure 5A,B).

Pretreatment with FCP showed a significant decrease in the cisplatin-induced ROS release by 72.1% ($p < 0.01$) compared with the cisplatin alone-treated group, indicating its restorative effect on the endogenous antioxidant defense mechanism impaired by cisplatin (Figure 5A,B). Furthermore, treatment with N-acetyl cysteine (NAC), a common ROS scavenger, at a concentration of 5 mM for 2 h, significantly reduced the cisplatin-enhanced ROS level in TECs, by 69.2% ($p < 0.001$) compared with the cisplatin alone-treated group (Figure 5A,B). These findings also indicate that the inhibitory action of FCP on cisplatin-induced cytotoxicity in TECs is attributed to its antioxidant effect.

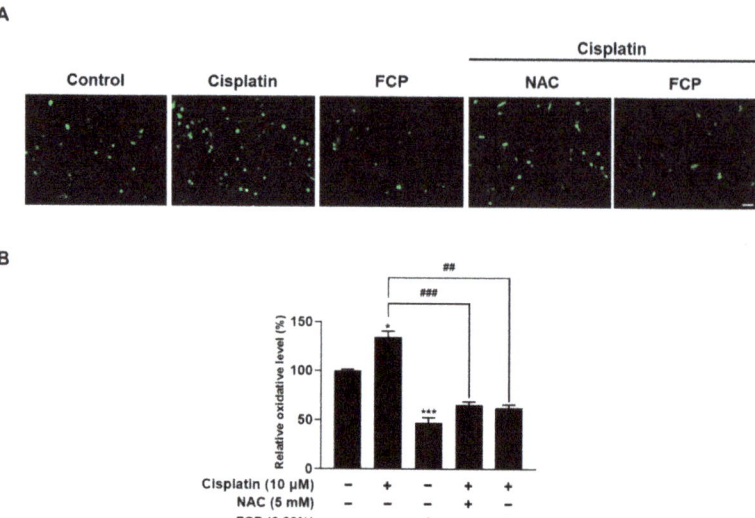

**Figure 5.** Inhibitory effects of FCP and NAC on cisplatin-induced ROS generation in TECs. Intracellular ROS levels were determined via fluorescence microscopy (**A**) and spectroscopy (**B**) using DCFH-DA in TECs. The increased ROS level induced by 10 μM cisplatin treatment was significantly attenuated by pretreatment with 0.08% FCP for 24 h and NAC for 2 h. Quantification of staining intensity was measured by ImageJ software. Results are presented as the means ± SD of three independent experiments. * $p < 0.05$, *** $p < 0.001$ vs. the control. ## $p < 0.01$, ### $p < 0.001$ vs. the cisplatin alone-treated group. Scale bar = 50 μm.

### 2.3. FCP Alleviate Cisplatin-Induced TEC Cytotoxicity through Suppression of MAPK Pathway

MAPK cascades are key signaling pathways that regulate various cellular processes, including stress and inflammatory responses, as well as cell proliferation, differentiation, apoptosis, and motility under both normal and pathological conditions [29,30]. Since cisplatin-induced cell death has been shown to be dependent on the MAPK pathways in several cell types [31], we first tested if cisplatin could activate this pathway in TECs. The results of this study revealed an increase in the expression of p-p38 MAPK, p-JNK, and p-ERK by 57.9% ($p < 0.001$), 16.8% ($p < 0.001$), and 21.8% ($p < 0.001$), in the cisplatin alone-treated group, respectively, than in the control, whereas the expression of total p38 MAPK, JNK, and ERK levels remained unaltered, indicating the activation of p38 MAPK, JNK, and ERK pathways after cisplatin treatment in TECs (Figure 6). However, these elevated levels of p-p38 MAPK, p-JNK and p-ERK were attenuated by the pretreatment with 0.08% FCP for 24 h, by 37.3% ($p < 0.01$), 15.3% ($p < 0.001$), and 58.5% ($p < 0.001$), respectively, compared with the cisplatin alone-treated group (Figure 6).

To further explore the role of MAPK pathways in cisplatin-induced cell cytotoxicity, the cells were treated with a selective p38 MAPK inhibitor (SB203580), JNK inhibitor (SP600125), or ERK inhibitor (U0126). Analysis of the cell viability by WST-1 assay after TECs were treated with 0.08% FCP, 10 μM SB203580, SP600125, and U0126 for 24 h, followed by treatment with or without 10 μM cisplatin for 24 h, showed that FCP pretreatment caused a significant reduction of cisplatin-induced cytotoxicity, similar to all MAPK inhibitor pretreatments, whereas SB203580, SP600125 or U0126 alone did not affect cell viability (Figure 7).

Confirmation of the effect of FCP treatment on the cisplatin-induced expression of MAPK was performed using western blot analysis after TECs were treated with 0.08% FCP and 10 μM SB203580, SP600125, and U0126 for 24 h, followed by treatment with or without 10 μM cisplatin for 24 h. Notably, we observed that FCP pretreatment potently repressed the cisplatin-induced upregulated expression of p-p38 MAPK, p-JNK, and p-ERK, as was the case with MAPK inhibitor pretreatment (Figure 8A–C).

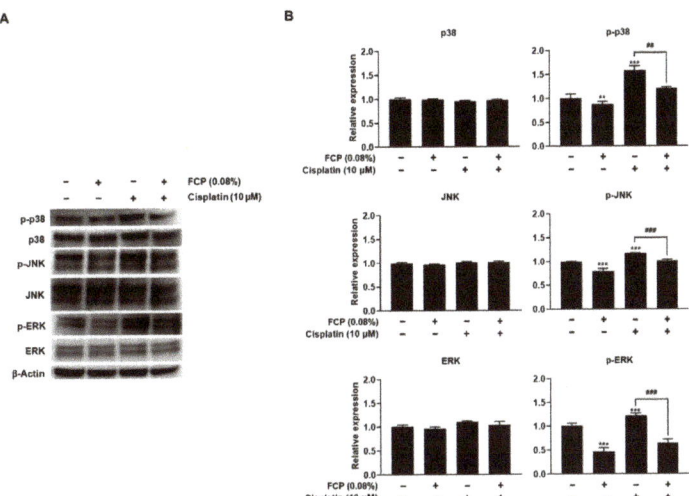

**Figure 6.** Inhibitory effects of FCP on cisplatin-induced activation of p38 MAPK, JNK, and ERK signaling pathway. The expression of p38 MAPK, JNK, and ERK was increased in the cisplatin alone-treated TECs, as assessed by Western blot analysis (**A**). The pretreatment of TECs with FCP blocked the cisplatin-induced phosphorylation of p38 MAPK, JNK, and ERK. Bar graphs depict relative densitometry quantitation of each protein normalized to β-actin (**B**). Results are presented as the means ± SD of three independent experiments. ** $p < 0.01$, *** $p < 0.001$ vs. the control. ## $p < 0.01$, ### $p < 0.001$ vs. the cisplatin alone-treated group.

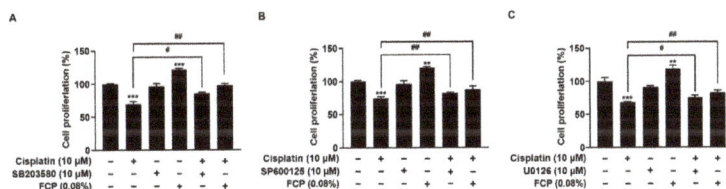

**Figure 7.** FCP promotes TECs proliferation via activation of p38 MAPK (**A**), JNK (**B**), and ERK (**C**) signaling pathways. The treatment of TECs with FCP for 24 h significantly enhanced cell proliferation. The cisplatin-induced cell cytotoxicity was recovered by treatment with FCP, SB203580, SP600125, and U0126 in TECs. Results are presented as the means ± SD of three independent experiments. ** $p < 0.01$, *** $p < 0.001$ vs. the control at 24 h; # $p < 0.05$, ## $p < 0.01$, vs. the control at 48 h.

Together, these results indicate that FCP acts as a potent inhibitor of MAPK pathways, which exerts a protective effect against cisplatin-induced cytotoxicity via suppression of p38 MAPK, JNK, and ERK pathway in TECs.

### 2.4. FCP Prevent Cisplatin-Induced ROS Generation by Inhibition of MAPK Signaling

To investigate whether p38 MAPK, JNK and ERK activation is associated with cisplatin-induced oxidative cell injury in TECs, we examined the effect of p38 MAPK, JNK and ERK inhibition on the cisplatin-induced ROS production. We also assessed the protective effect of FCP on cisplatin-induced ROS release in TECs using the DCFH-DA assay. As shown in Figure 9A–C, the exposure of TECs to 10 µM cisplatin for 24 h caused an increase in ROS level, by 29.5% ($p < 0.01$), 34% ($p < 0.001$) and 33.8% ($p < 0.001$) *versus* the control. However, the enhanced level of ROS induced by cisplatin treatment was significantly declined by the treatment with 10 µM SB203580, 10 µM SP600125 or 10 µM U0126 for 24 h by 25.2% ($p < 0.01$), 46.3% ($p < 0.01$), and 29.6% ($p < 0.05$), respectively, and with 0.08% FCP for 24 h by 37.8% ($p < 0.01$), 79% ($p < 0.001$) and 50.3% ($p < 0.05$), respectively (Figure 9A–C).

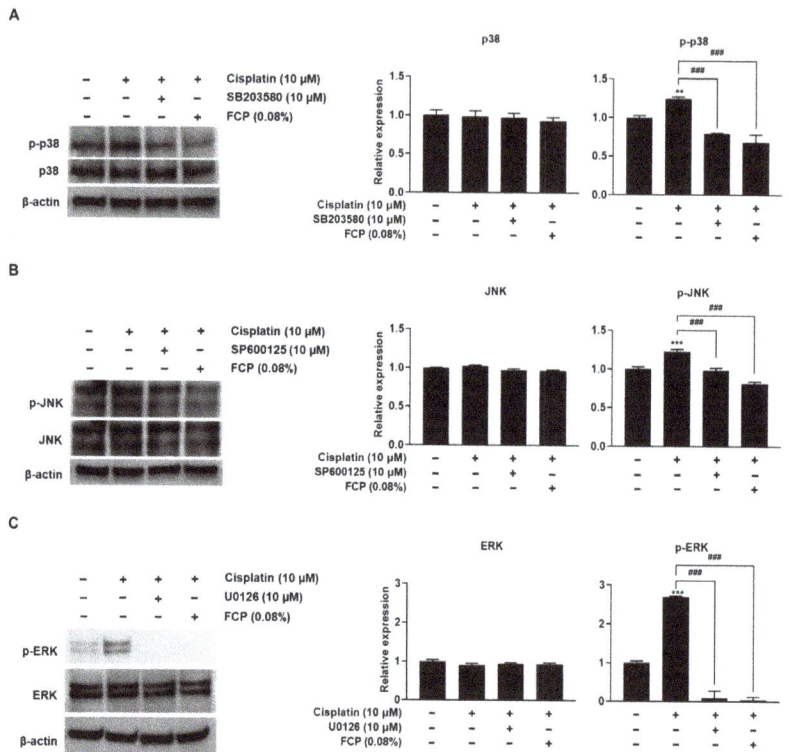

**Figure 8.** Inhibitory effects of FCP, SB203580 (**A**), SP600125 (**B**), and U0126 (**C**) on cisplatin-induced activation of p38 MAPK, JNK, and ERK signaling pathway in TECs. The expression of p-p38 MAPK, p-JNK, and p-ERK was increased in cisplatin-treated TECs. The pretreatment of TECs with FCP, SB203580 (**A**), SP600125 (**B**), and U0126 (**C**) blocked the cisplatin-induced phosphorylation of p38 MAPK, JNK, and ERK. Results are presented as the means ± SD of three independent experiments. ** $p < 0.01$, *** $p < 0.001$ vs. the control. ### $p < 0.001$ vs. the cisplatin alone-treated group.

As shown in Figure 10, the treatment of TECs with 10 µM cisplatin for 24 h resulted in the marked upregulation of p-p38 MAPK, p-JNK, and p-ERK expression compared with the control group by 72.1% ($p < 0.001$), 28.8% ($p < 0.05$), and 56.6% ($p < 0.001$), respectively, while the amount of total p38 MAPK, p-JNK, and p-ERK levels were unaltered. To decipher the role of p38 MAPK, JNK, and ERK in cisplatin-induced oxidative cellular injury in TECs, we investigated the effect of NAC on the cisplatin-induced expression of p-p38 MAPK, p-JNK, and p-ERK in TECs. Pretreatment of cells with FCP for 24 h or NAC for 2 h prior to cisplatin treatment completely abolished the cisplatin-induced phosphorylation of p38 MAPK, JNK, and ERK (Figure 10). These findings indicate that p38 MAPK, JNK and ERK activation is important in cisplatin-induced cellular oxidative stress, and FCP exhibits a strong protective effect against cisplatin-induced oxidative cell injury via the suppression of p38 MAPK, JNK, and ERK pathways in TECs.

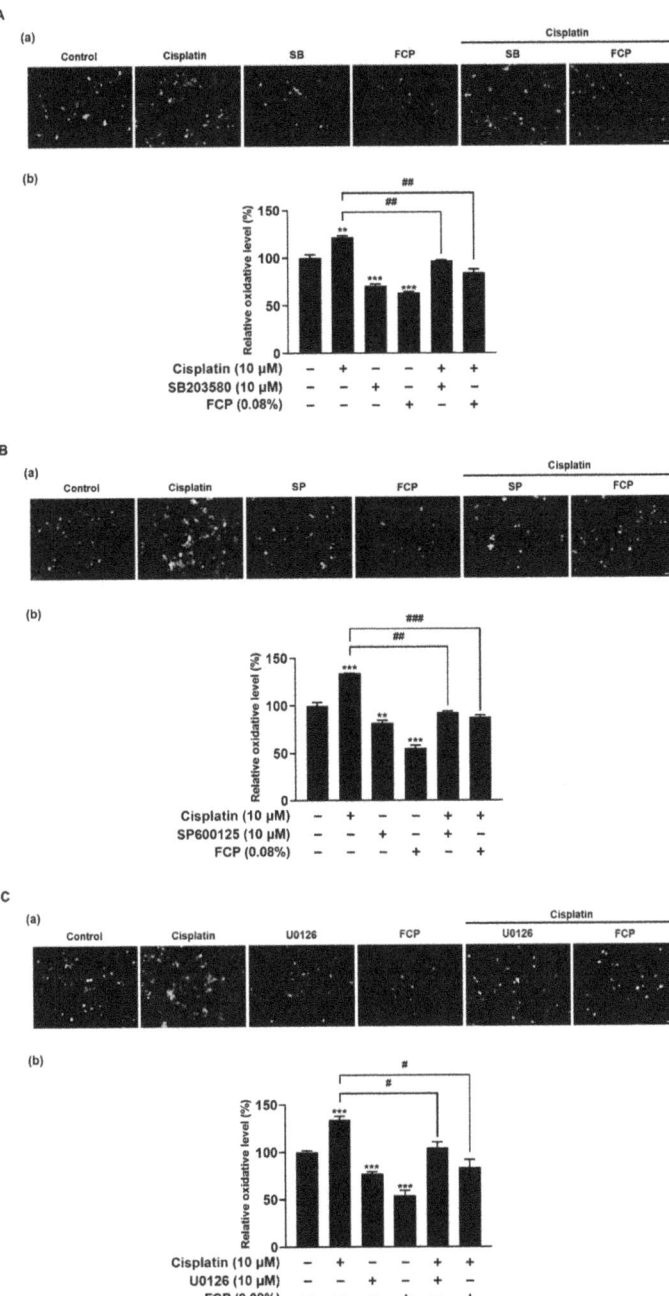

**Figure 9.** Inhibitory effects of FCP on cisplatin-induced ROS generation in TECs via activation of p38 MAPK, JNK and ERK signaling pathway. Intracellular ROS levels were determined via fluorescence microscopy (a) and spectroscopy (b). The increased ROS production induced by cisplatin returned to the control level by treatment with FCP, SB203580 (**A**), SP600125 (**B**) and U0126 (**C**) in TECs. Results are presented as the means ± SD of three independent experiments. ** $p < 0.01$, *** $p < 0.001$ vs. the control. # $p < 0.05$, ## $p < 0.01$, ### $p < 0.001$ vs. the cisplatin alone-treated group. Scale bar = 50 μm.

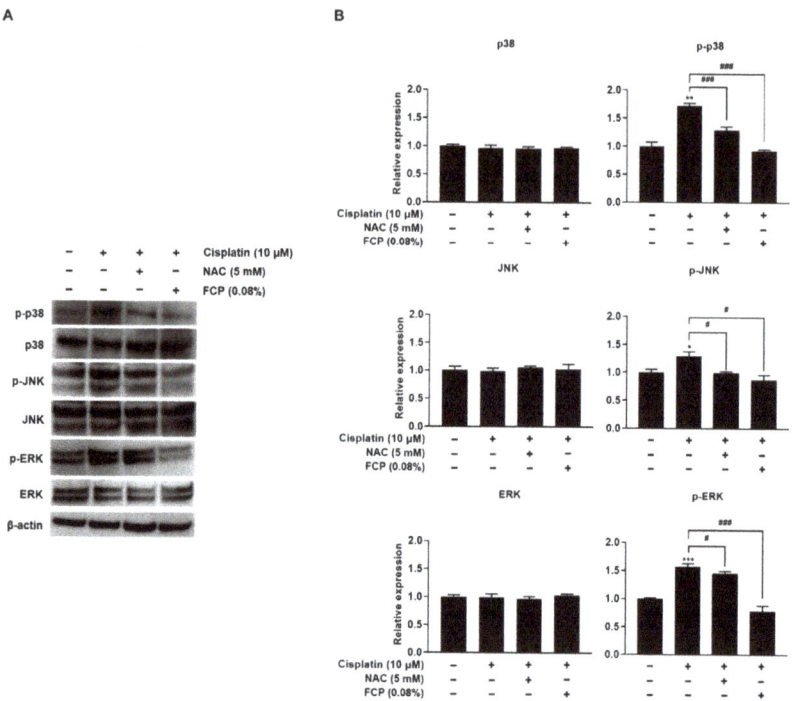

**Figure 10.** Inhibitory effects of FCP and NAC on cisplatin-induced activation of p38 MAPK, JNK, and ERK signaling pathways in TECs. The expression of p38 MAPK, JNK, and ERK was increased in cisplatin-treated TECs, as assessed by Western blot analysis (**A**). The pretreatment of TECs with FCP or NAC blocked the cisplatin-induced phosphorylation of p38 MAPK, JNK, and ERK. Bar graphs depict relative densitometry quantitation of each protein normalized to β-actin (**B**). Results are presented as the means ± SD of three independent experiments. * $p < 0.01$, ** $p < 0.01$, *** $p < 0.001$ vs. the control. # $p < 0.05$, ### $p < 0.001$ vs. the cisplatin alone-treated group.

## 3. Discussion

The results of the present study indicated that FCP derived from tilapia scales exhibited antioxidant and cytoprotective effects on mouse TECs against oxidative stress provoked by cisplatin exposure. In addition, our findings showed increased cellular viability accompanied by FCP-mediated antioxidant activity based on a diminished level of ROS in the cytosol. Furthermore, this study also provides the first molecular evidence for elucidating the function of FCP serving as a cytoprotective agent against TEC damage by cisplatin. Thus, it is proposed that FCP may offer protective effects on TECs against cytotoxic and oxidative stress-induced cellular injury caused by various types of noxious stimuli.

Cisplatin is a highly reactive molecule that exerts its cytotoxic effects mainly through the formation of covalent DNA adducts [32]. In addition, it stimulates the production of intracellular ROS in several types of cells, including hepatocytes [33], pulmonary alveolar cells [34], renal proximal tubule epithelial cells [35], and intestinal epithelial cells [36]. Our findings are consistent with previous studies showing that treatment with antioxidants alleviates the toxic effects of cisplatin, indicating an essential role of oxidative stress in the pathogenesis of cisplatin-induced cell injury in several different types of organs [33,34].

Marine organisms are important sources of bioactive compounds with potential therapeutic applications. In particular, fish collagen-derived peptides are of considerable interest and have drawn great attention recently due to their bioactive functions [37]. Fish collagen has been shown to exhibit microbicidal, anti-inflammatory and anti-skin-aging activities, as well as wound healing and tissue regeneration [37–41]. Despite much having been learnt about the diverse bioactivities of FCP on multiple cell types [42,43]; there is a paucity of information on the biological effects of FCP on TECs. Antioxidant properties of peptides from the diverse sources of fish collagen, such as skin from cod, hoki, and pollock have been demonstrated in many different cell types, such as liver cells [44,45], fibroblasts [46], macrophages [47,48], and keratinocytes [49]. In addition, it was also revealed that FCP enhances the viability of human lung fibroblasts damaged by oxygen radicals [46]. In accordance with these results, the present study showed that FCP from tilapia scales has potent antioxidative and cytoprotective effects on TECs.

Antioxidants, widely used as ingredients in dietary supplements to improve health in sectors of the food and beverage manufacturing industry, have been studied for their potential in the prevention or treatment of several human diseases, such as cardiovascular diseases, diabetes, metabolic syndrome, neurodegenerative disorders, cancer and age-related diseases [50,51]. In addition, they are also used as food preservatives for preventing lipid oxidation. Although synthetic antioxidants, such as butylated hydroxytoluene (BHT) and butylated hydroxyanisole (BHA) have been extensively used due to their high stability, low costs, and wide availability, health risks including carcinogenicity, are of great concern [52]. Thus, there is a growing trend toward replacing synthetic antioxidants with natural antioxidants in the food processing industry [53,54].

It is well documented that ROS generated endogenously or in response to environmental stress have long been implicated in cellular injury, which causes cell death, especially triggered by the dysregulation of the pro- or anti-apoptotic pathways, and tissue damage leading to the development of many diseases [55]. The present study demonstrated that FCP acts as a potent suppressor of TEC apoptosis induced by cisplatin treatment by promoting Bcl-2 and Bcl-xL expression and inhibiting Bad and Bax expression and cytochrome-c release. Taken together, these findings indicate that the amelioration of cisplatin-induced cytotoxicity by FCP in TECs is mediated by their antioxidant and anti-apoptotic properties. The discovery of the protective mechanisms of FCP for repairing cellular injuries induced by oxidative stress and activation of apoptotic cell death pathway in human TECs would advocate the use of FCP for the prevention and treatment of many clinical conditions linked to excessive ROS generation and perturbation in the apoptotic balance in TECs. This is particularly important because oxidative- or cytotoxic stress-mediated injury in TECs can be a significant problem in many clinical settings, and linked to the induction of acute thymic involution, that may cause compromised thymopoietic capacity in TECs, leading to a severe and clinically significant immune deficiency disorder or dysfunction of the adaptive immunity, and causing the body to be unable to generate appropriate immune responses against invading pathogens.

The present study also demonstrated that FCP can promote the proliferation of TECs. In agreement with our study, Liu and Sun [56], also observed the growth-promoting effect of tilapia FCP on rat bone marrow mesenchymal stem cells. In addition, our previous study suggested that nanofibrous scaffolds containing tilapia FCP contribute to the enhancement of mouse TEC proliferation [57]. Furthermore, Liu et al. [58] showed that bovine collagen peptide compounds promote the proliferation and differentiation of MC3T3-E1 preosteoblasts. These investigations, therefore, corroborate that tilapia FCP exhibit significant growth promotion properties in several types of cells.

MAPK signal transduction pathways are involved in the regulation of a wide variety of fundamental cellular processes, such as cell growth, differentiation, survival, apoptosis, migration, inflammation, and environmental stress responses [59]. To determine the role of the p38 MAPK, JNK, and ERK in cisplatin-induced ROS production and the signaling pathway in TECs, the expression levels of p38 MAPK, JNK, and ERK were analyzed by DCFH-DA, cell proliferation, and western blot assays after treatment with NAC, SB203580, SP600125, U0126, and FCP. Consequently, the cisplatin-elicited p38 MAPK, JNK, and ERK activation was abolished by SB203580, SP600125, and U0126 as well as FCP and NAC, suggesting that cisplatin-induced oxidative stress injury in TECs is mediated by p38 MAPK,

JNK and ERK and that FCP, similarly to NAC, notably ameliorates cisplatin-induced oxidative stress in TECs by blocking p38 MAPK, JNK, and ERK activation. In addition, the cisplatin-induced cytotoxic responses were also significantly blocked by SB203580, SP600125, and U0126 as well as FCP. Taken together, these data indicate that FCP plays a critical role in protecting various cytotoxic and oxidative stresses in TECs by repressing the activation of MAPK signal transduction pathways.

## 4. Materials and Methods

### 4.1. Cell Culture and Reagents

Mouse thymic cortical epithelial reticular cells (1308.1) were provided by Dr. Barbara B. Knowles (The Jackson Laboratory, Bar Harbor, ME, USA). The cells were cultured in Dulbecco's modified Eagle's medium (DMEM; Hyclone, GE Healthcare Life Sciences, Logan, UT, USA) supplemented with 10% fetal bovine serum (FBS), 100 IU mL$^{-1}$ penicillin, and 100 mg mL$^{-1}$ streptomycin (all from Gibco, Thermo Fisher Scientific, Waltham, MA, USA) in a humidified atmosphere of 5% $CO_2$ at 37 °C. Subconfluent cells were harvested with trypsin-EDTA and used for further experiments. Media were replaced every second day.

Cisplatin, 2′,7′-dichlorodihydrofluorescein diacetate (DCFH-DA), N-acetyl-L-cysteine (NAC), 4′,6-diamidino-2-phenylindole (DAPI), and bicinchoninic acid (BCA) were obtained from Sigma-Aldrich (St. Louis, MO, USA). Antibodies against ERK, phospho-ERK (p-ERK), JNK, phospho-JNK (p-JNK), p38 MAPK, phospho-p38 MAPK (p-p38 MAPK), cytochrome-c, and cyclin D1 were supplied by Cell Signaling Technology (Cambridge, MA, USA). The antibodies against Bcl-2, Bcl-xL, Bax, Bad, and CDK1 were obtained from Abcam (Cambridge, UK). Additionally, an antibody against β-actin was bought from Santa Cruz Biotechnology (Santa Cruz, CA, USA). The p-p38 MAPK inhibitor (SB203580), p-JNK/MAPK inhibitor (SP600125), and p-ERK/MAPK inhibitor (U0126) were purchased by Tocris Bioscience (Ellisville, MO, USA). FCP extracted from tilapia were provided by Geltech (Busan, Korea), and their physicochemical properties were described in our previous study [49]. All other reagents and compounds used were supplied from Sigma-Aldrich.

### 4.2. Cell Viability Assay

After TECs ($8 \times 10^3$ cells/well) in 96-well flat-bottom culture plates (SPL Life Sciences, Pocheon, Korea) were treated with the indicated doses of FCP for 24 h with or without cisplatin. The cell viability was determined using the colorimetric WST-1 conversion assay (EZ-Cytox assay kit, Daeil Lab Service, Seoul, Korea). A WST-1 reagent (total 10 μL) was added to each well, and cells were incubated for 2 h in a humidified incubator at 37 °C under 5% $CO_2$. The absorbance of the formazan dye, generated by the reaction of dehydrogenase with WST-1 in the metabolically active cells, was measured using a microplate reader (Tecan, Männedorf, Switzerland) at 450 nm according to the manufacturer's instructions, and the percent cell viability was calculated. The experiments were performed in triplicate.

### 4.3. Measurement of ROS

The effect of FCP on the cisplatin-induced generation of ROS in TECs was detected by DCFH-DA, a ROS-sensitive fluorescent probe, under a fluorescent microscope. Cell-permeable DCFH-DA is non-fluorescent, but in the presence of ROS, when this dye is oxidized, it is converted to a highly fluorescent 2′,7′-dichlorofluorescein (DCF) [60]. TECs ($1 \times 10^5$ cells/well) in 6-well culture plates were treated with 0.08% FCP for 24 h before treatment with cisplatin (10 μM) for 24 h. After removing the medium from wells, the cells were washed with phosphate buffered saline and then incubated with 10 μM DCFH-DA in fresh serum-free medium for 30 to 40 min in a humidified incubator at 37 °C with 5% $CO_2$ under dark conditions. The labeled cells were observed with an epi-fluorescence microscope (BX50, Olympus, Tokyo, Japan). Photomicrographs were acquired digitally at $1360 \times 1024$ pixel resolution with an Olympus DP70 digital camera. Furthermore, the DCF fluorescence was measured using a fluorescent microplate reader (SpectraMax M2e, BioTek, Winooski, VT, USA) at 495–529 nm. To minimize the possible photo-oxidation of the probe and or photo-reduction of DCF, the plates were covered with aluminum foil to shield the probe from light.

### 4.4. Western Blot Analysis

To determine protein expression levels, TECs ($8 \times 10^5$ cells/dish), after reaching 70–80% confluency in 60 mm culture dishes (SPL Life sciences), were treated with 0.08% FCP for 24 h before treatment with cisplatin (10 µM) for 24 h. Cells from each set of experiments were harvested and washed twice in cold Tris-buffered saline (TBS, 20 mM Tris-HCl, 150 mM NaCl, pH 7.4). For the western blot analysis, cells were lysed in 100 µL RIPA cell lysis buffer with EDTA (GenDEPOT, Barker, TX, USA) containing a protease inhibitor mixture (Roche, Basel, Switzerland). Samples were kept on ice for 30 min, vortexing briefly (15 s) every 2–3 min. Then, the lysates were centrifuged at 14,000 RPM for 30 min at 4 °C, and the protein concentration was measured using a BCA protein assay (Sigma-Aldrich). Equal amounts of protein samples were heated for 10 min at 70 °C in Bolt LDS sample buffer (Invitrogen, Waltham, MA, USA) and separated by 10% sodium dodecyl sulfate (SDS)-polyacrylamide gel electrophoresis (PAGE, Invitrogen) at 200 V for 25 min, using a Mini-Protean III system (Bio-Rad, Hercules, CA, USA). Proteins were transferred to a polyvinylidene difluoride (PVDF) membrane (GE Healthcare Life science) at 20 V for 1 h. The nonspecific binding was blocked with 3% bovine serum albumin (BSA) in TBS buffer containing 0.1% Tween 20 (TBST buffer), incubated with the indicated primary antibodies at a dilution of 1:500–1:2000 with 5% BSA in TBST overnight at 4 °C with anti-p38 MAPK, anti-p-p38 MAPK, anti-JNK, anti-p-JNK, anti-ERK, anti-p-ERK, anti-Bax, anti-cytochrome-c, anti-Bcl-2, anti-Bcl-xL, anti-Bad, anti-cyclin D1, anti-CDK1, and anti-β-actin (Supplementary Table S1).

On the following day, the membrane was washed with TBST buffer thrice and incubated with secondary antibodies, namely, anti-rabbit IgG HRP conjugate (Cell Signaling Technology) and anti-mouse IgG HRP conjugate (Cell Signaling Technology), at a dilution of 1:10,000 with 3% BSA in TBST for 1 h at room temperature. Subsequently, the membrane was washed thrice with TBST. Immunoreactivity was detected with enhanced chemiluminescence (ECL, Super Signal West Pico Chemiluminescent Substrate kit, Pierce, Rockford, IL, USA) according to the manufacturer's instructions. Images were captured and quantified using a LAS-3000 imaging system (Fujifilm, Tokyo, Japan).

### 4.5. Statistical Analysis

The results of the present study were expressed as the mean ± SD under all conditions. Statistical analysis was performed using a two-tailed Student's $t$-test. Statistically significant differences were considered at $p < 0.05$.

## 5. Conclusions

The findings of the present study demonstrate for the first time that FCP stimulates proliferation, and ameliorates cisplatin-induced cytotoxicity and oxidative stress in TECs. In addition, it was shown that the inhibitory effects of FCP on cytotoxicity are likely associated with suppression of the ROS and MAPK (p38 MAPK, JNK, and ERK) signaling pathways. Therefore, these results suggest that FCP may be a promising protective agent in TEC injury induced by cytotoxicity and oxidative stress elaborated by chemotherapeutic drugs, such as cisplatin and other cytotoxic agents. Furthermore, the data of the current study may provide new insights into the therapeutic approach for the future application of FCP in the prevention and treatment of a variety of the cytotoxic and oxidative stress-mediated injuries in TECs as well as acute or age-related thymic involution.

**Supplementary Materials:** The following supporting information can be downloaded at: https://www.mdpi.com/article/10.3390/md20040232/s1, Table S1: The primary antibodies used for western blotting in the current study.

**Author Contributions:** Conceptualization, W.H.S., H.-Y.K. and S.Y.; methodology, H.-Y.K., C.L., D.Y.L. and Y.S.L.; validation, S.Y.H.; formal analysis, W.H.S., H.-Y.K., Y.S.L. and S.Y.; investigation, S.Y.H. and S.Y.; data curation, W.H.S., H.-Y.K., Y.S.L. and S.Y.; writing—original draft preparation, W.H.S., H.-Y.K. and S.Y.; writing—review and editing; W.H.S., Y.M., Y.J.S. and S.Y.; project administration, S.Y.; funding acquisition, W.H.S. and S.Y. All authors have read and agreed to the published version of the manuscript.

**Funding:** This work was supported by the National Research Foundation of Korea (NRF) funded by the Korean government (MEST) [grant number 2020R1A2C1004529] and [grant number 2021R1F1A1062913].

**Institutional Review Board Statement:** Not applicable.

**Informed Consent Statement:** Not applicable.

**Data Availability Statement:** Not applicable.

**Conflicts of Interest:** The authors declare no conflict of interest.

## References

1. Kadouri, N.; Nevo, S.; Goldfarb, Y.; Abramson, J. Thymic epithelial cell heterogeneity: TEC by TEC. *Nat. Rev. Immunol.* **2020**, *20*, 239–253. [CrossRef] [PubMed]
2. Kinsella, S.; Dudakov, J.A. When the Damage Is Done: Injury and repair in thymus function. *Front. Immunol.* **2020**, *11*, 1745. [CrossRef] [PubMed]
3. Luo, M.; Xu, L.; Qian, Z.; Sun, X. Infection-associated thymic atrophy. *Front. Immunol.* **2021**, *12*, 652538. [CrossRef]
4. Ménétrier-Caux, C.; Ray-Coquard, I.; Blay, J.Y.; Caux, C. Lymphopenia in cancer patients and its effects on response to immunotherapy: An opportunity for combination with cytokines? *J. Immunother. Cancer* **2019**, *7*, 85. [CrossRef] [PubMed]
5. Wang, W.; Thomas, R.; Sizova, O.; Su, D.M. Thymic function associated with cancer development, relapse, and antitumor immunity—A Mini-Review. *Front. Immunol.* **2020**, *11*, 773. [CrossRef] [PubMed]
6. Duah, M.; Li, L.; Shen, J.; Lan, Q.; Pan, B.; Xu, K. Thymus degeneration and regeneration. *Front. Immunol.* **2021**, *12*, 706244. [CrossRef]
7. Lynch, H.E.; Goldberg, G.L.; Chidgey, A.; Van den Brink, M.R.; Boyd, R.; Sempowski, G.D. Thymic involution and immune reconstitution. *Trends Immunol.* **2009**, *30*, 366–373. [CrossRef]
8. Ventevogel, M.S.; Sempowski, G.D. Thymic rejuvenation and aging. *Curr. Opin. Immunol.* **2013**, *25*, 516–522. [CrossRef]
9. Ki, S.; Park, D.; Selden, H.J.; Seita, J.; Chung, H.; Kim, J.; Iyer, V.R.; Ehrlich, L.I.R. Global transcriptional profiling reveals distinct functions of thymic stromal subsets and agerelated changes during thymic involution. *Cell Rep.* **2014**, *9*, 402–415. [CrossRef]
10. Barbouti, A.; Vasileiou, P.V.S.; Evangelou, K.; Vlasis, K.G.; Papoudou-Bai, A.; Gorgoulis, V.G.; Kanavaros, P. Implications of oxidative stress and cellular senescence in age-related thymus involution. *Oxid. Med. Cell. Longev.* **2020**, *2020*, 7986071. [CrossRef]
11. Narendhirakannan, R.T.; Hannah, M.A. Oxidative stress and skin cancer: An overview. *Indian J. Clin. Biochem.* **2013**, *28*, 110–115. [CrossRef] [PubMed]
12. Rose, P.G.; Bundy, B.N.; Watkins, E.B.; Thigpen, J.T.; Deppe, G.; Maiman, M.A.; Clarke-Pearson, D.L.; Insalaco, S. Concurrent cisplatin-based radiotherapy and chemotherapy for locally advanced cervical cancer. *N. Engl. J. Med.* **1999**, *340*, 1144–1153. [CrossRef] [PubMed]
13. Armstrong, D.K.; Bundy, B.; Wenzel, L.; Huang, H.Q.; Baergen, R.; Lele, S.; Copeland, L.J.; Walker, J.L.; Burger, R.A. Intraperitoneal cisplatin and paclitaxel in ovarian cancer. *N. Engl. J. Med.* **2006**, *354*, 34–43. [CrossRef] [PubMed]
14. Zhang, Q.; Lu, Q.B. New combination chemotherapy of cisplatin with an electron-donating compound for treatment of multiple cancers. *Sci. Rep.* **2021**, *11*, 788. [CrossRef] [PubMed]
15. Spanos, W.C.; Nowicki, P.; Lee, D.W.; Hoover, A.; Hostager, B.; Gupta, A.; Anderson, M.E.; Lee, J.H. Immune response during therapy with cisplatin or radiation for human papillomavirus-related head and neck cancer. *Arch. Otolaryngol. Head Neck Surg.* **2009**, *135*, 1137–1146. [CrossRef]
16. Fang, C.Y.; Lou, D.Y.; Zhou, L.Q.; Wang, J.C.; Yang, B.; He, Q.J.; Wang, J.J.; Weng, Q.J. Natural products: Potential treatments for cisplatin-induced nephrotoxicity. *Acta Pharmacol. Sin.* **2021**, *42*, 951–1969. [CrossRef]
17. Rancoule, C.; Guy, J.B.; Vallard, A.; Mrad, M.B.; Rehailia, A.; Magne, N. 50th anniversary of cisplatin. *Bull. Cancer* **2017**, *104*, 167–176. [CrossRef]
18. Rébé, C.; Demontoux, L.; Pilot, T.; Ghiringhelli, F. Platinum derivatives effects on anticancer immune response. *Biomolecules* **2020**, *10*, 13. [CrossRef]
19. Rustad, T. Utilization of marine by-products. *Electron. J. Environ. Agric. Food Technol.* **2003**, *2*, 458–463.
20. Kim, S.; Mendis, E. Bioactive compounds from marine processing byproducts-a review. *Food Res. Int.* **2006**, *39*, 383–393. [CrossRef]
21. Wang, B.; Wang, Y.M.; Chi, C.F.; Luo, H.Y.; Deng, S.G.; Ma, J.Y. Isolation and characterization of collagen and antioxidant collagen peptides from scales of croceine croaker (*Pseudosciaena crocea*). *Mar. Drugs* **2013**, *11*, 4641–4661. [CrossRef] [PubMed]
22. Lai, C.H.; Wu, P.C.; Wu, C.H.; Shiau, C.Y. Studies on antioxidative activities of hydrolysates from fish scales collagen of tilapia. *J. Taiwan Fish. Res.* **2008**, *15*, 99–108.

23. Wang, L.; An, X.; Yang, F.; Xin, Z.; Zhao, L.; Hu, Q. Isolation and characterisation of collagens from the skin, scale and bone of deep-sea redfish (*Sebastes mentella*). *Food Chem.* **2008**, *108*, 616–623. [CrossRef] [PubMed]
24. Cheung, R.C.; Ng, T.B.; Wong, J.H. Marine peptides: Bioactivities and applications. *Mar. Drugs* **2015**, *13*, 4006–4043. [CrossRef]
25. Asserin, J.; Lati, E.; Shioya, T.; Prawitt, J. The effect of oral collagen peptide supplementation on skin moisture and the dermal collagen network: Evidence from an ex vivo model and randomized, placebo-controlled clinical trials. *J. Cosmet. Dermatol.* **2015**, *14*, 291–301. [CrossRef]
26. Ghorpade, V.S.; Yadav, A.V.; Dias, R.J. Citric acid crosslinked cyclodextrin/hydroxypropylmethylcellulose hydrogel films for hydrophobic drug delivery. *Int. J. Biol. Macromol.* **2016**, *93*, 75–86. [CrossRef]
27. Ding, C.H.; Li, Q.; Xiong, Z.Y.; Zhou, A.W.; Jones, G.; Xu, S.Y. Oral administration of type II collagen suppresses pro-inflammatory mediator production by synoviocytes in rats with adjuvant arthritis. *Clin. Exp. Immunol.* **2003**, *132*, 416–423. [CrossRef]
28. Zhu, C.F.; Li, G.Z.; Peng, H.B.; Zhang, F.; Chen, Y.; Li, Y. Treatment with marine collagen peptides modulates glucose and lipid metabolism in Chinese patients with type 2 diabetes mellitus. *Appl. Physiol. Nutr. Metab.* **2010**, *35*, 797–804. [CrossRef]
29. Plotnikov, A.; Zehorai, E.; Procaccia, S.; Seger, R. The MAPK cascades: Signaling components, nuclear roles and mechanisms of nuclear translocation. *Biochim. Biophys. Acta* **2011**, *1813*, 1619–1633. [CrossRef]
30. Kyriakis, J.M.; Avruch, J. Mammalian MAPK signal transduction pathways activated by stress and inflammation: A 10-year update. *Physiol. Rev.* **2012**, *92*, 689–737. [CrossRef]
31. Brozovic, A.; Osmak, M. Activation of mitogen-activated protein kinases by cisplatin and their role in cisplatin-resistance. *Cancer Lett.* **2007**, *251*, 1–16. [CrossRef] [PubMed]
32. Marullo, R.; Werner, E.; Degtyareva, N.; Moore, B.; Altavilla, G.; Ramalingam, S.S.; Doetsch, P.W. Cisplatin induces a mitochondrial-ROS response that contributes to cytotoxicity depending on mitochondrial redox status and bioenergetic functions. *PLoS ONE* **2013**, *8*, e81162.
33. Mansour, H.H.; Hafez, H.F.; Fahmy, N.M. Silymarin modulates cisplatin-induced oxidative stress and hepatotoxicity in rats. *J. Biochem. Mol. Biol.* **2006**, *39*, 656–661. [CrossRef] [PubMed]
34. Afsar, T.; Razak, S.; Almajwal, A.; Khan, M.R. *Acacia hydaspica* R. Parker ameliorates cisplatin induced oxidative stress, DNA damage and morphological alterations in rat pulmonary tissue. *BMC Complement. Altern. Med.* **2018**, *18*, 49. [CrossRef]
35. Soni, H.; Kaminski, D.; Gangaraju, R.; Adebiyi, A. Cisplatin-induced oxidative stress stimulates renal Fas ligand shedding. *Ren. Fail.* **2018**, *40*, 314–322. [CrossRef]
36. Rehman, M.U.; Rather, I.A. Myricetin abrogates cisplatin-induced oxidative stress, inflammatory response, and goblet cell disintegration in colon of wistar rats. *Plants* **2019**, *9*, 28. [CrossRef]
37. Lim, Y.S.; Ok, Y.J.; Hwang, S.Y.; Kwak, J.Y.; Yoon, S. Marine Collagen as A Promising Biomaterial for Biomedical Applications. *Mar. Drugs* **2019**, *17*, 467. [CrossRef]
38. Sivaraman, K.; Shanthi, C. Role of fish collagen hydrolysate in attenuating inflammation—An in vitro study. *J. Food Biochem.* **2021**, *45*, e13876. [CrossRef]
39. Geahchan, S.; Baharlouei, P.; Rahman, A. Marine Collagen: A Promising Biomaterial for Wound Healing, Skin Anti-Aging, and Bone Regeneration. *Mar. Drugs* **2022**, *20*, 61. [CrossRef]
40. Vijayan, D.K.; Sreerekha, P.R.; Dara, P.K.; Ganesan, B.; Mathew, S.; Anandan, R.; Ravisankar, C.N. Antioxidant defense of fish collagen peptides attenuates oxidative stress in gastric mucosa of experimentally ulcer-induced rats. *Cell Stress Chaperones* **2022**, *27*, 45–54. [CrossRef]
41. Yoon, J.; Yoon, D.; Lee, H.; Lee, J.; Jo, S.; Kym, D.; Yim, H.; Hur, J.; Chun, W.; Kim, G.; et al. Wound healing ability of acellular fish skin and bovine collagen grafts for split-thickness donor sites in burn patients: Characterization of acellular grafts and clinical application. *Int. J. Biol. Macromol.* **2022**, *14*, 452–461. [CrossRef] [PubMed]
42. Aleman, A.; Martinez-Alvarez, O. Marine collagen as a source of bioactive molecules. A Review. *Nat. Prod. J.* **2013**, *3*, 105–114. [CrossRef]
43. Silva, T.H.; Moreira-Silva, J.; Marques, A.L.; Domingues, A.; Bayon, Y.; Reis, R.L. Marine origin collagens and its potential applications. *Mar. Drugs* **2014**, *12*, 5881–5901. [CrossRef] [PubMed]
44. Kim, S.K.; Kim, Y.T.; Byun, H.G.; Nam, K.S.; Joo, D.S.; Shahidi, F. Isolation and characterization of antioxidative peptides from gelatin hydrolysate of Alaska pollack skin. *J. Agric. Food Chem.* **2001**, *49*, 1984–1989. [CrossRef] [PubMed]
45. Mendis, E.; Rajapakse, N.; Byun, H.G.; Kim, S.K. Investigation of jumbo squid (*Dosidicus gigas*) skin gelatin peptides for their in vitro antioxidant effects. *Life Sci.* **2005**, *77*, 2166–2178. [CrossRef]
46. Mendis, E.; Rajapakse, N.; Kim, S.K. Antioxidant properties of a radical-scavenging peptide purified from enzymatically prepared fish skin gelatin hydrolysate. *J. Agric. Food Chem.* **2005**, *53*, 581–587. [CrossRef] [PubMed]
47. Ngo, D.H.; Ryu, B.; Vo, T.S.; Himaya, S.W.; Wijesekara, I.; Kim, S.K. Free radical scavenging and angiotensin-I converting enzyme inhibitory peptides from Pacific cod (*Gadus macrocephalus*) skin gelatin. *Int. J. Biol. Macromol.* **2011**, *49*, 1110–1116. [CrossRef]
48. Himaya, S.W.A.; Ngo, D.; Ryu, B.; Kim, S. An active peptide purified from gastrointestinal enzyme hydrolysate of Pacific cod skin gelatin attenuates angiotensin-1 converting enzyme (ACE) activity and cellular oxidative stress. *Food Chem.* **2012**, *132*, 1872–1882. [CrossRef]
49. Subhan, F.; Kang, H.Y.; Lim, Y.; Ikram, M.; Baek, S.Y.; Jin, S.; Jeong, Y.H.; Kwak, J.Y.; Yoon, S. Fish scale collagen peptides protect against $CoCl_2$/TNF-α-induced cytotoxicity and inflammation via inhibition of ROS, MAPK, and NF-κB pathways in HaCaT Cells. *Oxid. Med. Cell. Longev.* **2017**, *2017*, 9703609. [CrossRef]

50. Kebede, M.; Admassu, S. Application of antioxidants in food processing industry: Options to improve the extraction yields and market value of natural products. *Adv. Food Technol. Nutr. Sci. Open J.* **2019**, *5*, 38–49. [CrossRef]
51. Sharifi-Rad, M.; Anil Kumar, N.V.; Zucca, P.; Varoni, E.M.; Dini, L.; Panzarini, E.; Rajkovic, J.; Tsouh Fokou, P.V.; Azzini, E.; Peluso, I.; et al. Lifestyle, oxidative stress, and antioxidants: Back and forth in the pathophysiology of chronic diseases. *Front. Physiol.* **2020**, *11*, 694. [CrossRef] [PubMed]
52. Lourenço, S.C.; Moldão-Martins, M.; Alves, V.D. Antioxidants of natural plant origins: From sources to food industry applications. *Molecules* **2019**, *24*, 4132. [CrossRef] [PubMed]
53. Peschel, W.; Sánchez-Rabaneda, F.; Diekmann, W.; Plescher, A.; Gartzía, I.; Jimenez, D.; Lamuela-Raventos, R.M.; Buxaderas, S.; Codina, C. An industrial approach in the search of natural antioxidants from vegetable and fruit wastes. *Food Chem.* **2006**, *97*, 137–150. [CrossRef]
54. Mira-Sánchez, M.D.; Castillo-Sánchez, J.; Morillas-Ruiz, J.M. Comparative study of rosemary extracts and several synthetic and natural food antioxidants. Relevance of carnosic acid/carnosol ratio. *Food Chem.* **2020**, *309*, 125688. [CrossRef] [PubMed]
55. Ryter, S.W.; Kim, H.P.; Hoetzel, A.; Park, J.W.; Nakahira, K.; Wang, X.; Choi, A.M. Mechanisms of cell death in oxidative stress. *Antioxid. Redox Signal.* **2007**, *9*, 49–89. [CrossRef]
56. Liu, C.; Sun, J. Potential application of hydrolyzed fish collagen for inducing the multidirectional differentiation of rat bone marrow mesenchymal stem cells. *Biomacromolecules* **2014**, *15*, 436–443. [CrossRef]
57. Choi, D.J.; Choi, S.M.; Kang, H.Y.; Min, H.J.; Lee, R.; Ikram, M.; Subhan, F.; Jin, S.W.; Jeong, Y.H.; Kwak, J.Y.; et al. Bioactive fish collagen/polycaprolactone composite nanofibrous scaffolds fabricated by electrospinning for 3D cell culture. *J. Biotechnol.* **2015**, *205*, 47–58. [CrossRef]
58. Liu, C.; Xue, Y.; Sun, J. Hydrolyzed fish collagen inhibits inflammatory cytokines secretion in lipopolysaccharide-induced HUVECs. *Adv. Mater. Res.* **2014**, *1025–1026*, 570–573. [CrossRef]
59. Koul, H.K.; Pal, M.; Koul, S. Role of p38 MAP kinase signal transduction in solid tumors. *Genes Cancer* **2013**, *4*, 342–359. [CrossRef]
60. Marchesi, E.; Rota, C.; Fann, Y.C.; Chignell, C.F.; Mason, R.P. Photoreduction of the fluorescent dye 2′-7′-dichlorofluorescein: A spin trapping and direct electron spin resonance study with implications for oxidative stress measurements. *Free Radic. Biol. Med.* **1999**, *26*, 148–161. [CrossRef]

MDPI
St. Alban-Anlage 66
4052 Basel
Switzerland
Tel. +41 61 683 77 34
Fax +41 61 302 89 18
www.mdpi.com

*Marine Drugs* Editorial Office
E-mail: marinedrugs@mdpi.com
www.mdpi.com/journal/marinedrugs

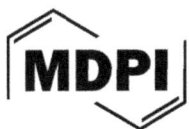

www.ingramcontent.com/pod-product-compliance
Lightning Source LLC
LaVergne TN
LVHW070654100526
838202LV00013B/958